T0264439

Behavioral Emergencies

Editors

NIDAL MOUKADDAM
VERONICA THERESA TUCCI

PSYCHIATRIC CLINICS OF NORTH AMERICA

www.psych.theclinics.com

September 2017 • Volume 40 • Number 3

ELSEVIER

1600 John F. Kennedy Boulevard • Suite 1800 • Philadelphia, Pennsylvania, 19103-2899

http://www.theclinics.com

PSYCHIATRIC CLINICS OF NORTH AMERICA Volume 40, Number 3
September 2017 ISSN 0193-953X, ISBN-13: 978-0-323-54568-6

Editor: Lauren Boyle
Developmental Editor: Kristen Helm

© 2017 Elsevier Inc. All rights reserved.

This periodical and the individual contributions contained in it are protected under copyright by Elsevier, and the following terms and conditions apply to their use:

Photocopying
Single photocopies of single articles may be made for personal use as allowed by national copyright laws. Permission of the Publisher and payment of a fee is required for all other photocopying, including multiple or systematic copying, copying for advertising or promotional purposes, resale, and all forms of document delivery. Special rates are available for educational institutions that wish to make photocopies for non-profit educational classroom use. For information on how to seek permission visit www.elsevier.com/permissions or call: (+44) 1865 843830 (UK)/(+1) 215 239 3804 (USA).

Derivative Works
Subscribers may reproduce tables of contents or prepare lists of articles including abstracts for internal circulation within their institutions. Permission of the Publisher is required for resale or distribution outside the institution. Permission of the Publisher is required for all other derivative works, including compilations and translations (please consult www.elsevier.com/permissions).

Electronic Storage or Usage
Permission of the Publisher is required to store or use electronically any material contained in this periodical, including any article or part of an article (please consult www.elsevier.com/permissions). Except as outlined above, no part of this publication may be reproduced, stored in a retrieval system or transmitted in any form or by any means, electronic, mechanical, photocopying, recording or otherwise, without prior written permission of the Publisher.

Notice
No responsibility is assumed by the Publisher for any injury and/or damage to persons or property as a matter of products liability, negligence or otherwise, or from any use or operation of any methods, products, instructions or ideas contained in the material herein. Because of rapid advances in the medical sciences, in particular, independent verification of diagnoses and drug dosages should be made.

Although all advertising material is expected to conform to ethical (medical) standards, inclusion in this publication does not constitute a guarantee or endorsement of the quality or value of such product or of the claims made of it by its manufacturer.

Psychiatric Clinics of North America (ISSN 0193-953X) is published quarterly by Elsevier Inc., 360 Park Avenue South, New York, NY 10010-1710. Months of issue are March, June, September, and December. Business and Editorial Offices: 1600 John F. Kennedy Blvd., Suite 1800, Philadelphia, PA 19103-2899. Periodicals postage paid at New York, NY and additional mailing offices. Subscription prices are $303.00 per year (US individuals), $628.00 per year (US institutions), $100.00 per year (US students/residents), $369.00 per year (Canadian individuals), $460.00 per year (international individuals), $791.00 per year (Canadian & international institutions), and $220.00 per year (Canadian & international students/residents). Foreign air speed delivery is included in all *Clinics*' subscription prices. All prices are subject to change without notice. **POSTMASTER:** Send address changes to *Psychiatric Clinics of North America*, Elsevier Health Sciences Division, Subscription Customer Service, 3251 Riverport Lane, Maryland Heights, MO 63043. **Customer Service: 1-800-654-2452 (US). From outside the United States, call 1-314-447-8871. Fax: 1-314-447-8029. E-mail: journalscustomerservice-usa@elsevier.com (for print support)** and **journalsonline support-usa@elsevier.com (for online support).**

Reprints. For copies of 100 or more, of articles in this publication, please contact the Commercial Reprints Department, Elsevier Inc., 360 Park Avenue South, New York, New York 10010-1710. Tel.: 212-633-3874, Fax: 212-633-3820, E-mail: reprints@elsevier.com.

Psychiatric Clinics of North America is covered in *MEDLINE/PubMed (Index Medicus)*, *Current Contents/Social and Behavioral Sciences, Social Science Citation Index, Embase/Excerpta Medica,* and PsycINFO.

Contributors

EDITORS

NIDAL MOUKADDAM, MD, PhD
Associate Professor, Menninger Department of Psychiatry and Behavioral Sciences, Baylor College of Medicine, Medical Director, Stabilization, Treatment and Rehabilitation (STAR) Program for Psychosis, Houston, Texas, USA

VERONICA THERESA TUCCI, MD, JD, FAAEM, FACEP
Professor of Emergency Medicine and Research, William Carey University College of Osteopathic Medicine, Academic Chair and Program Director, Merit Health Wesley, Emergency Medicine Residency Program, Hattiesburg, Mississippi, USA

AUTHORS

AWAIS AFTAB, MD
Chief Resident for Education and Research, Department of Psychiatry, University Hospitals Cleveland Medical Center, Case Western Reserve University, Cleveland, Ohio, USA

EVARISTO AKERELE, MD, MPH, DFAPA
Chairman, Department of Psychiatry and Behavioral Health, Interfaith Medical Center, Brooklyn, New York, USA

AL ALAM, MD
Assistant Professor of Psychiatry, Weill Cornell Medical College, NewYork-Presbyterian/Westchester Division, White Plains, New York; Assistant Professor of Internal Medicine, Stony Brook University, Stony Brook, New York, USA

ERIN AUFDERHEIDE, MD
Resident Physician, Department of Emergency Medicine, Baylor College of Medicine, Houston, Texas, USA

SOPHIA BANU, MD
Assistant Professor, Menninger Department of Psychiatry and Behavioral Sciences, Baylor College of Medicine, Houston, Texas, USA

RAKEL C. BEALL, MD, MPH
Assistant Professor, Menninger Department of Psychiatry and Behavioral Sciences, Baylor College of Medicine, Houston, Texas, USA

TERRI BLACKWELL, MD
Assistant Professor of Psychiatry, Carolinas HealthCare System, Charlotte, North Carolina, USA

SHANA COSHAL, MD
Resident Physician, Menninger Department of Psychiatry and Behavioral Sciences, Baylor College of Medicine, Houston, Texas, USA

VISHAL DEMLA, MD
Division of Critical Care Medicine, Critical Care Fellow, Department of Internal Medicine, The University of Texas Health Science Center at Houston, Houston, Texas, USA

SWAPNA DESHPANDE, MD
Rainbolt Family Chair in Child Psychiatry, Clinical Assistant Professor, Training Director, Child/Adolescent Fellowship Program, Department of Psychiatry and Behavioral Sciences, The University of Oklahoma, Oklahoma City, Oklahoma, USA

ARACELI FLORES, PhD
Department of Emergency Medicine, Baylor College of Medicine, Houston, Texas, USA

ANDREW FOOTE, MD
Adult Psychiatrist, Variety Care, Oklahoma City, Oklahoma, USA

LINDSAY FRENCH-ROSAS, MD
Assistant Professor, Menninger Department of Psychiatry and Behavioral Sciences, Baylor College of Medicine, Houston, Texas, USA

RUTH S. GERSON, MD
Director, Bellevue Hospital Children's Comprehensive Psychiatric Emergency Program, Assistant Professor, Department of Child and Adolescent Psychiatry, NYU School of Medicine, New York, New York, USA

SPENCER GREENE, MD, MS, FACEP, FACMT
Director of Medical Toxicology, Assistant Professor, Departments of Emergency Medicine and Pediatrics, Baylor College of Medicine, Houston, Texas, USA

JIN Y. HAN, MD
Assistant Professor, Menninger Departments of Psychiatry and Behavioral Sciences and Family and Community Medicine, Baylor College of Medicine, Houston, Texas, USA

ALI M. HASHMI, MD
Associate Professor of Psychiatry, Mayo Hospital, King Edward Medical University, Lahore, Pakistan

NICHOLAS HAYDEN, BS
Department of Emergency Medicine, Baylor College of Medicine, Houston, Texas, USA

SUNI JANI, MD, MPH
Child and Adolescent Psychiatry Fellow, Massachusetts General Hospital, McLean Hospital, Yawkey Center for Outpatient Care, Boston, Massachusetts, USA

MICHAEL JAUNG, MD
Global Health and International Emergency Medicine Fellow, Department of Emergency Medicine, Baylor College of Medicine, Houston, Texas, USA

CHRISTOPHER KIEFER, MD
Assistant Professor, Department of Emergency Medicine, Health Sciences Center, West Virginia University, Morgantown, West Virginia, USA

JOY M. MACKEY, MD
Assistant Professor, Department of Emergency Medicine, Baylor College of Medicine, Houston, Texas, USA

ANU A. MATORIN, MD
Associate Professor, Menninger Department of Psychiatry and Behavioral Sciences, Baylor College of Medicine, Houston, Texas, USA

LAURA N. MEDFORD-DAVIS, MD, MS
Assistant Professor, Department of Emergency Medicine, Baylor College of Medicine, Houston, Texas, USA

NIDAL MOUKADDAM, MD, PhD
Assistant Professor, Menninger Department of Psychiatry and Behavioral Sciences, Baylor College of Medicine, Medical Director, Stabilization, Treatment and Rehabilitation (STAR) Program for Psychosis, Houston, Texas, USA

ANDREW NEW, MD, MS
Resident Physician, Department of Psychiatry and Behavioral Sciences, Jackson Memorial Hospital, Miami, Florida, USA

TOLU OLUPONA, MD
Director Residency Training and Education, Department of Psychiatry and Behavioral Health, Interfaith Medical Center, Brooklyn, New York, USA

EDORE ONIGU-OTITE, MBBS
Menninger Department of Psychiatry and Behavioral Sciences, Baylor College of Medicine, Houston, Texas, USA

BRITTA OSTERMEYER, MD, MBA
The Paul and Ruth Jonas Chair, Professor and Chairman, Department of Psychiatry and Behavioral Sciences, The University of Oklahoma, Oklahoma City, Oklahoma, USA

JAMES RACHAL, MD
Medical Director of Behavioral Health Charlotte, Vice Chairman and Associate Professor, Department of Psychiatry, Carolinas HealthCare System, Charlotte, North Carolina, USA

JUAN RIOS, MD
Assistant Professor, Department of Clinical Psychiatry, University of Miami Miller School of Medicine, Miami, Florida, USA

GENEVIEVE SANTILLANES, MD, FAAP, FACEP
Associate Professor, Department of Emergency Medicine, Keck School of Medicine of USC, Los Angeles, California, USA

JOHN SAUNDERS, MD, MS
Assistant Professor, Menninger Department of Psychiatry and Behavioral Sciences, Baylor College of Medicine, Houston, Texas, USA

ASIM A. SHAH, MD
Vice Chair for Community Psychiatry, Professor, Menninger Departments of Psychiatry and Behavioral Sciences and Family and Community Medicine, Site Director, Psychiatric Residency Education, Baylor College of Medicine, Director, Community Behavioral Health Program, Executive Director, Psychotherapy Services, Senator, Menninger Department of Psychiatry and Behavioral Sciences, Baylor College of Medicine Faculty Senate, Chief of Psychiatry, Ben Taub Hospital, Harris Health System, Director, Mood Disorder Research Program at Ben Taub, Houston, Texas, USA

ANIM N. SHOAIB, BS
The Honors College, University of Houston, Houston, Texas, USA

WAYNE SPARKS, MD
Assistant Professor of Psychiatry, Medical Director of Telepsychiatry and Regional Behavioral Health, Carolinas HealthCare System, Charlotte, North Carolina, USA

ALLISON TADROS, MD
Associate Professor, Department of Emergency Medicine, Health Sciences Center, West Virginia University, Morgantown, West Virginia, USA

ALEXANDER TOLEDO, MD
Department of Emergency Medicine, Baylor College of Medicine, Houston, Texas, USA

ANH TRUONG, MD
Menninger Department of Psychiatry and Behavioral Sciences, Baylor College of Medicine, Houston, Texas, USA

VERONICA THERESA TUCCI, MD, JD, FAAEM, FACEP
Professor of Emergency Medicine and Research, William Carey University College of Osteopathic Medicine, Academic Chair and Program Director, Merit Health Wesley, Emergency Medicine Residency Program, Hattiesburg, Mississippi, USA

CHRISTINE ZAZZARO, MEd
Assistant Vice President of Behavioral Health Access, Carolinas HealthCare System, Charlotte, North Carolina, USA

Contents

Special Considerations in the Pediatric Psychiatric Population 463

Genevieve Santillanes and Ruth S. Gerson

Youth with psychiatric and behavioral complaints commonly present to emergency departments (EDs), which often lack dedicated mental health staff. This article addresses techniques EDs can use to better care for children in need of psychiatric assessment and medical clearance, specifically addressing the evaluation of youth with suicidal ideation and coexisting medical and psychiatric needs. The evaluation and management of youth with agitation and aggression are also discussed. The article concludes with a discussion of systems changes needed to truly improve emergency care for psychiatrically ill youth.

Addictive Disorders in Adolescents 475

Anh Truong, Nidal Moukaddam, Alexander Toledo, and Edore Onigu-Otite

Addictive disorders in youth represent a dynamic field characterized by shifting patterns of substance use and high rates of experimentation, while retaining the risky behaviors and negative outcomes associated with established drug classes. Youth/adolescents are also at the forefront of use of new technologies, and non–substance-related disorders are pertinent. These disorders present with similar pictures of impairment, and can be diagnosed following the same principles. An underlying mental disorder and the possibility of a dual diagnosis need to be assessed carefully, and optimal treatment includes psychosocial treatments with applicable pharmacologic management, the latter representing an expanding field.

Intensive Care and Its Discontents: Psychiatric Illness in the Critically Ill 487

Ali M. Hashmi, Jin Y. Han, and Vishal Demla

Critically ill patients can develop a host of cognitive and psychiatric complaints during their intensive care unit (ICU) stay, many of which persist for weeks or months following discharge from the ICU and can seriously affect their quality of life, including their ability to return to work. This article describes some common psychiatric problems encountered by clinicians in the ICU, including their assessment and management. A comprehensive approach is needed to decrease patient suffering, improve morbidity and mortality, and ensure that critically ill patients can return to the highest quality of life after an ICU stay.

Drugs of Abuse 501

Evaristo Akerele and Tolu Olupona

Drug abuse and its consequences remain a significant public health issue. An increasing number of individuals are present in the emergency room with life-threatening drug intoxication. It is imperative that emergency room physicians are cognizant of the signs, symptoms, and treatment to improve the chances of early recognition and treatment. As a result, the proportion of lives saved will increase significantly. In this article, we present some of the most prevalent life-threatening drugs that lead to emergency room admission. The signs, symptoms, and treatment modalities are discussed.

Toxicologic Emergencies in Patients with Mental Illness: When Medications Are No Longer Your Friends **519**

Spencer Greene, Erin AufderHeide, and Lindsay French-Rosas

Patients with psychiatric disorders are at risk for toxicologic emergencies. Psychotropic medications have numerous effects on the neurologic, cardiac, and other organ systems and interact with other medications, potentially leading to further side effects. It is important to become familiar with accepted psychiatric practice guidelines, common toxidromes, medical sequelae associated with prescribed medications, and the specific workup and treatment of overdoses of frequently prescribed psychotropics.

The Changing Health Policy Environment and Behavioral Health Services Delivery **533**

Laura N. Medford-Davis and Rakel C. Beall

Deinstitutionalization has left an inadequate supply of inpatient psychiatric beds. Simultaneous cuts to public funding and insurance coverage for outpatient mental health treatment have increased the frequency of acute psychiatric crises. The resulting lack of available options has shifted the burden of treatment to emergency departments and the criminal justice system. Recent legislation has improved insurance access, but rules are not always enforced and there are still few options for care. Discussion of mental health care delivery must acknowledge that many emergent behavioral health crises arise in the context of acute substance intoxication, withdrawal, or dependence.

Legal and Ethical Challenges, Part 1: General Population **541**

Britta Ostermeyer, Anim N. Shoaib, and Swapna Deshpande

Several federal and state laws and regulations, as well as ethical medical principles, govern the emergency clinician's practice of care. Although some common legal-medical and ethical principles are shared with other medical specialties, emergency medicine and emergency psychiatry have unique legal and ethical challenges. This article presents and discusses these challenges, including the physician-patient relationship, malpractice, confidentiality and privilege, duty to report, decision-making capacity and vicarious decision-making, the Emergency Medical Treatment and Labor Act, right to treatment, hospital admissions, involuntary commitment, forced medication administration, and child and elder abuse.

Legal and Ethical Challenges in Emergency Psychiatry, Part 2: Management of Inmates **555**

Andrew Foote and Britta Ostermeyer

Psychiatrists and clinicians encounter unique situations, challenges, and requirements in the treatment of jail and prison inmates in the emergency department. This article reviews the historical legal highlights pertaining to medical and psychiatric care of inpatients, as well as the professional, ethical, and legal aspects that allow clinicians to evaluate, treat, and

properly disposition their inmate patients. In particular, this article discusses the specific suicide risk factors related to inmates and correctional facilities that should be ascertained and managed in a clinician's suicide risk assessment and intervention planning in this special high suicide risk patient population.

International Emergency Psychiatry Challenges: Disaster Medicine, War, Human Trafficking, Displaced Persons **565**

Michael Jaung, Suni Jani, Sophia Banu, and Joy M. Mackey

Mental health disorders are a major cause of morbidity and a growing burden in low-income and middle-income countries; but there is little existing literature on the detailed epidemiology, diagnosis, and treatment in low-resource settings. Special situations with vulnerable populations, such as those created by international humanitarian emergencies, refugees or internally displaced people, and victims of human trafficking, are increasing in prevalence. These victims are often resettled in developed countries and come to the emergency department seeking care. To better care for these populations, knowledge of specialized psychosocial and cultural considerations should inform the comprehensive psychiatric assessment and treatment plan.

Violence in the Emergency Department: A Global Problem **575**

Allison Tadros and Christopher Kiefer

Violence against health care workers is an unfortunately common event. Because of several inherent factors, emergency departments are particularly vulnerable. Once an incident occurs, it often goes unreported and leads to both physical and mental trauma. Health care workers should learn to recognize the cues that patients are escalating toward violence and be familiar with various options for sedating agitated patients. If sedation is not successful, physical restraint may become necessary. There are measures that can be taken that may help minimize the likelihood of violence toward health care workers. These measures include legislation, physical design, and increased security.

Highlight in Telepsychiatry and Behavioral Health Emergencies **585**

James Rachal, Wayne Sparks, Christine Zazzaro, and Terri Blackwell

Carolinas HealthCare System is one of the largest freestanding psychiatric emergency departments in the country. It has grown from a small community mental health center in the 1930s, to one of the largest providers of emergency mental health services in the country. It offers services in person and via telepsychiatry to other emergency departments and primary care clinics. It decreased emergency room wait times and revolutionized where and how patients get their care. This has been the work of several groups from many disciplines. The transition from community mental health center to large-scale mental health emergency department has been a model for the rest of the country.

PSYCHIATRIC CLINICS OF NORTH AMERICA

FORTHCOMING ISSUES

December 2017
Cognitive Behavioral Therapy for Anxiety and Depression
Stefan G. Hofmann and Jasper Smits, *Editors*

March 2018
Geriatric Psychiatry
Daniel German Blazer and Susan Schultz, *Editors*

June 2018
Psychodynamic Psychiatry
Thomas N. Franklin, *Editor*

RECENT ISSUES

June 2017
Women's Mental Health
Susan G. Kornstein and Anita H. Clayton, *Editors*

March 2017
Clinical Issues and Affirmative Treatment with Transgender Clients
Lynne Carroll and Lauren Mizock, *Editors*

December 2016
Violence
James L. Knoll IV, *Editor*

RELATED INTEREST

Emergency Medicine Clinics of North America, November 2015 (Vol. 33, No. 4)
Psychiatric and Behavioral Emergencies
Dick C. Kuo and Veronica Tucci, *Editors*
Available at: http://www.emed.theclinics.com/

THE CLINICS ARE AVAILABLE ONLINE!
Access your subscription at:
www.theclinics.com

Preface

Emergency Psychiatry: Ten Years Later

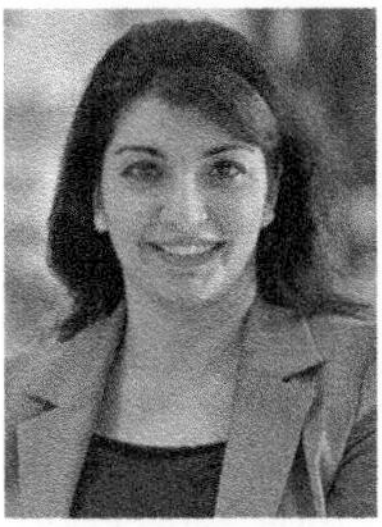

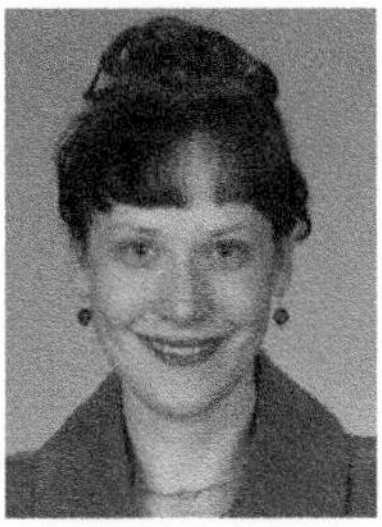

Nidal Moukaddam, MD, PhD
Veronica Theresa Tucci, MD, JD
Editors

The rise of emergency psychiatry as a specialty has been the product of multiple health-care system changes over the past decade: pressures on outpatient care, a decrease in funding of inpatient facilities, and deinstitutionalization have conspired to make emergency departments (ED) the forefront of American mental health care. More often than not, EDs provide longitudinal care as well, by serving the same population again and again when transition to outpatient care fails, and when inpatient care is denied.

Thus, a new face of emergency psychiatry is now conspicuous: we no longer can take comfort in the fact that individuals with mental health problems can safely be tucked away. Rather than be disillusioned, this is a chance to see emergency psychiatry for what it really is: the epitome of multidisciplinary collaboration. Emergency physicians, psychiatrists, social workers, substance use counselors, and nursing staff come together night and day to ensure care of the very vulnerable population of individuals with mental illness who lack the safety net of a regular, dedicated outpatient psychiatrist, and the comfort of an insurance policy that magically makes rehabilitation and psychotherapy services accessible.

True, many issues are still at stake. Emergency psychiatry is a young specialty where unified protocols and guidelines are lacking. Psychiatric and substance use disorder treatments tend to be slow in onset, and for many, this is frustrating. But the biggest hurdle is that many providers in the ED do not know their own abilities, or the possible positive, even life-changing, impact they could have on their patients' lives. This may be related, in part, to lack of knowledge and dedicated research in emergency psychiatry. On the speaker circuit, we often hear surprised, yet happy, comments from the audience about the relief they experience from having their own experiences validated, and from knowing that work is being done to address the issues they face on a daily basis.

Psychiatr Clin N Am 40 (2017) xiii–xiv
http://dx.doi.org/10.1016/j.psc.2017.06.001
0193-953X/17/© 2017 Published by Elsevier Inc.

In this special issue of the *Psychiatric Clinics of North America*, we have strived to gather a collection of articles that highlight the beauty and dedication of emergency psychiatry as well as the specialized knowledge that makes it so challenging, yet so rewarding. Our articles are the product of year-long collaborations between psychiatry and emergency medicine, and we sincerely hope you will enjoy reading them, and find them useful in your practice.

Nidal Moukaddam, MD, PhD
Menninger Department of Psychiatry
Baylor College of Medicine
Stabilization, Treatment & Rehabilitation (STAR)
Program for Psychosis
1504 Taub Loop
Houston, TX 77030, USA

Veronica Theresa Tucci, MD, JD
Baylor College of Medicine
1504 Taub Loop
Houston, TX 77030, USA

E-mail addresses:
nidalm@bcm.edu (N. Moukaddam)
vtuccimd@gmail.com (V.T. Tucci)

Evaluation of Depression and Suicidal Patients in the Emergency Room

Shana Coshal, MD[a], John Saunders, MD, MS[b,*], Anu A. Matorin, MD[b], Asim A. Shah, MD[c]

KEYWORDS

• Depression • Suicide • Emergency room • B-SAFE

KEY POINTS

- Depression is a significant source of disability.
- Suicide is a leading cause of death within the United States.
- It is essential that within the emergency room patients are screened for depression and suicide risk.
- The Basic Suicide Assessment Five-step Evaluation (B-SAFE) model provides a structure for that suicide risk.

DEPRESSION

The World Health Organization, in 2001, recognized depression as a leading cause of disability worldwide and it is identified as the leading cause of disability in their April 2016 review. They also found that fewer than one-half of those affected receive effective treatment for depression. An ultimate potential consequence of untreated depression may be suicide.[1] This further stresses the significance of identification and management of depression in primary care settings. However, depression often goes unrecognized in emergency care settings, further contributing to the increased morbidity and functional decline during these times.[2] Furthermore, emergency department (EDs) serves as a primary care provider for the uninsured and those lacking access to resources.[3,4] Thus, the emergency room provides a critical opportunity for depression identification and intervention.

The authors deny any financial conflicts of interest.

[a] Department of Psychiatry, Baylor College of Medicine, 1502 Taub Loop, Houston, TX 77030, USA; [b] Menninger Department of Psychiatry & Behavioral Sciences, Baylor College of Medicine, One Baylor Plaza - BCM350, Houston, TX 77030, USA; [c] Menninger Department of Psychiatry & Family and Community Medicine, Ben Taub Hospital, Baylor College of Medicine, One Baylor Plaza - BCM350, Houston, TX 77030, USA

* Corresponding author.

E-mail address: John.saunders@bcm.edu

Psychiatr Clin N Am 40 (2017) 363–377
http://dx.doi.org/10.1016/j.psc.2017.05.008
psych.theclinics.com
0193-953X/17/© 2017 Elsevier Inc. All rights reserved.

There remain opportunities to increase the national data in the scientific literature regarding the prevalence of depression in the emergency room setting or the quality of care delivered during those visits.[2,4] Harman and colleagues[4] found annually through 1997 and 2000 that more than 580,000 or 0.6% of all emergency room visits were associated with a primary diagnosis of depression. A cross-sectional study by Kumar and colleagues[2] in 2004 found a 30% yearly prevalence of depression in 4 Boston-area EDs, much higher than the national average of 6.6%. More than one-half of these emergency room visits related to depression resulted in admission, 12% of these admissions involved self-inflicted injury. However, the most common disposition for depressed patients was referral to an outside provider, and certain studies suggest that the adherence to these referrals is poor to fair.[4]

To improve the identification and treatment of depression, the US Preventive Services Task Force recommends screening adults in primary care settings (available from: www.uspreventiveservicestaskforce.org); however, no such recommendations exist for the screening of depression in the emergency room.[2] In light of the general lack of mental health resources and often scarce mental health referral and consultation opportunities, questions about disposition options, can result in frustration and prolonged ED stays.[5]

It has been found that psychotropic medications were prescribed to approximately one-third of discharged patients after evaluating 675 patients discharged from a community-based psychiatric department. Most common prescriptions included antidepressants (64%), benzodiazepines (25%), nonbenzodiazepine sedatives (20%), and mood stabilizers (10%). The decision to prescribe was most significantly associated with a clinical diagnosis of major depressive disorder or bipolar disorder and the established use of psychiatric medicines. Discharged patients with suicidal ideation, substance abuse, or an existing outpatient psychiatrist were most frequently not prescribed psychotropic medication.[6] This practice is in contrast with 61% of discharged patients receiving psychotropic medication who presented to the ED from 1992 to 2001.[7] Follow-up appointments were more likely given to those discharged with a prescription, but this did not increase their compliance in attending the appointment as compared with those discharged without medication. This pattern indicates that initiating medication in the emergency setting may not be a successful method to promote outpatient treatment.[6]

The low rate of antidepressants prescribed from the emergency room may stem from the view that it takes between 2 and 4 weeks to begin to treat the symptoms of depression.[8] Recent evidence has emerged indicating that maximum improvement occurs during the first 2 weeks, with some improvement seen in the first 3 days.[9] In addition, there is some scrutiny related to the time course for when these treatments may be effective.[8,9] Examination of more rapid psychopharmacologic interventions in the ED may be of some benefit. For high-acuity patients requiring admission, a psychiatric medication regimen will be started on the inpatient unit.[4]

There are several types of psychiatric emergencies related to severe depression, the emergencies are relevant given the concern for suicidality in patients struggling with depression. These can include depression leading to self-inflicted injury and suicidality. Approximately 420,000 ED visits occur annually in the United States for attempted suicide and self-inflicted injury, a number that has doubled over the last 20 years. Patients who present to the ED with self-inflicted injuries are more likely to be high users of ED services and have higher suicide mortality rates when compared with the general population.[5] Suicidal emergencies, among other psychiatric emergencies, provide the basis for emergency room visits, and is discussed elsewhere in this article (**Table 1**).[10]

Table 1
Depression screening

Techniques:	Instruments:
History and physical examination	Patient Health Questionnaire-9
Mental status examination	Beck's Depression Inventory
Obtaining collateral information	Geriatric Depression Scale

Data from Sharp LK, Lipsky MS. Screening for depression across the lifespan: a review of measures for use in primary care settings. Am Fam Physician 2002;66(6):1001–8; and Moriarty AS, Gilbody S, McMillan D, et al. Screening and case finding for major depressive disorder using the Patient Health Questionnaire (PHQ-9): a meta-analysis. Gen Hosp Psychiatry 2015;37(6):567–76.

Major Depression with Psychosis

Psychotic features are present in 5% of individuals with depression. Psychotic symptoms increase the severity and distress of the depression and may be associated with increased suicide risk. Electroconvulsive therapy can be considered a potential treatment. Antipsychotics, in addition to antidepressants, are also recommended in most cases and should be monitored closely for akathisia, which itself is a risk factor for violence and suicide.[8]

Catatonia

For the treatment of severe psychomotor retardation and stupor, electroconvulsive therapy can be considered, especially when patients are unable to take oral medication. This type of clinical presentation can occur in the context of various medical and neuropsychiatric disorders, and differential diagnoses including schizophrenia, affective disorders, and organic causes should be reviewed regularly, especially if a history is unavailable.[8] Acute catatonic syndromes have demonstrated response with benzodiazepines and should be administered intramuscularly or intravenously in the emergency setting.[11]

Bipolar Depression

Bipolar or mixed depression is defined as a major depressive episode with cooccurring hypomanic symptoms. Because antidepressants can induce mania in bipolar patients, it is generally recommended in nonemergent situations to avoid antidepressants, especially in high doses. It is also important to note that the prevalence of suicide attempts is very high in those with bipolar depression or during a mixed state (dysphoric mania), with irritability and psychomotor agitation as the strongest predictors of a suicide attempt.[12]

Agitation

Agitated patients are commonly assessed in the ED, and are treated with deescalation, restraint, seclusion, medication, or a combination of these interventions.[13] Behavioral disturbances including the acutely disturbed or violently depressed patient may require the addition of neuroleptics or benzodiazepines as an adjunct to antidepressant therapy.[8] Caution should be exerted with using antipsychotics, particularly with oversedation, QT prolongation, increased agitation, and death in the demented elderly.[13]

It has been suggested that depressed patients who present to the ED may have a distinct sociodemographic and health profile. Some studies have found that depressed patients in the ED were more likely to be female, middle-aged, and of lower socioeconomic status. They found that depressed patients reported more than twice as many health problems, often related to perceived pain, including anxiety, chronic fatigue, back problems, insomnia, headaches, and chronic pain. Depressed patients were also more likely to smoke.[2] This profile could help to identify particularly high-risk groups and target subsequent interventions for depression and suicide, although it is essential to screen all patients for suicidality in this context.

SUICIDE

It is estimated that 1 million people in the world die by suicide each year, a number that is projected to increase to 1.5 million in 2020.[14] In the United States, suicide is the 10th leading cause of death, with more people dying from suicide than traffic accidents and more than double the number who died from homicides.[15,16] In the past 2 decades, the incidence and prevalence of suicide has increased, and continues to increase, whereas rates of heart disease, cancer, and human immunodeficiency virus infection/AIDS are decreasing.[17] Just in 2015, there were 41,149 deaths by suicide in the United States with about 50% from firearms. Suicide rates decreased from 1990 to 2000 from 12.5 suicides per 100,000 to 10.4 per 100,000, but increased again to 13 per 100,000 in 2014. On average there are 117 suicides per day.[15,18] For these reasons, suicide prevention is an urgent public health issue.[19] Furthermore, the ED is an important site for suicide prevention owing to the sheer volume of high-acuity patients at risk for suicide.[20] More than 90% of people who have completed suicide have a major psychiatric disorder, primarily a mood disorder, such as depression; however, suicide risk is also increased in those with neurologic disorders and cancer.[14,17]

Many of those who die by suicide received health care services in the year before their death.[21] Yet, numerous patients deemed high risk for suicide in the period after discharge from EDs and inpatient psychiatric settings do not receive outpatient behavioral treatment in a timely fashion. The Joint Commission of Accreditation of Healthcare Organization's Sentinel Event database records 1089 suicides from 2010 to 2014, among patients within a staffed, supervised setting or within 72 hours of discharge from an inpatient or ED setting. The most common root cause finding among these cases was inadequacies in the assessment, particularly the psychiatric assessment. More than 20% of Joint Commission of Accreditation of Healthcare Organization–accredited behavioral health organizations and one-half of accredited general hospitals were rated noncompliant in 2014 with National Patient Safety Goal 15.01.01 to perform a suicide risk assessment on all patients presenting with psychiatric concerns.[16]

Traditional Risk Assessment

Traditionally, the purpose of the suicide risk assessment is to identify treatable and modifiable risk factors as well as protective factors that inform the patient's treatment and safety management requirements.[22] Acute stressors may include exacerbation of psychiatric illness and psychosocial influences. Chronic, nonmodifiable risk factors may include previous attempts, history of mental illness, and family history of suicide. This process is no different than the risk assessment stratification used to evaluate medical conditions in the ED such as myocardial infarction and the evaluation of current and baseline cardiovascular risk factors.[23] However, psychiatrists do not have specific validated diagnostic tests for evaluating suicidal patients. Instead, the "quintessential" diagnostic instrument available to psychiatrists is systematic suicide risk assessment informed by evidence-based psychiatry, and essentially comes down to reasoned clinical decision making.[22] There is no pathognomonic risk factor or combination of risk factors predictive of suicide (**Table 2**).[22,25]

Table 2
Risk and protective factors of suicide

Acute Risk Factors	Chronic Risk Factors	Protective Factors
Current psychiatric illness	Past psychiatric history	Positive coping and problem-solving skills
Intoxication	Chronic substance use	Sense of family responsibility, that is, children in the home
Recent psychosocial stressors, that is, unemployment, lack of social support	History of trauma	Religious beliefs
Current suicidal thoughts, intent, and plan	Previous history of suicide attempts	Good social supports
Access to lethal means, that is, drugs and weapons	Comorbid physical illness	Positive therapeutic relationship with treatment provider
	Demographics (elderly, Caucasian, male)	Married
	Family history of suicide attempts	

Data from Refs.[14,16,17,23,26]

Safety contracts

Widely used in the past, safety contracts, also known as no-suicide contracts or no-harm contracts, have been out of favor because there is no evidence of their efficacy.[27] The safety or no-suicide contract is not legally binding nor does it protect physicians against negligence in malpractice claims.[23,28] Furthermore, it is erroneous to believe that a document such as the no-suicide contract would actually prevent someone from killing himself or herself, and may leave providers with a false sense of security.[28] Last, they can go against the provider, because judges in case of law suits have argued that if patient needs a safety contract, maybe they need to be safe in a hospital environment.

Traditional discharge criteria

Historically, in some settings to discharge suicidal patients from the emergency room, they must have no prior history of a suicide attempt and no active suicidal ideation. They must be supervised by someone residing with them, who agrees to remove access to lethal means. And, they must be provided with an emergency contact and a follow-up appointment.[13] These criteria were not evidence based. As the evaluation of suicide risk assessment has progressed, so have the criteria for discharge, while remaining focused on patient safety.

Modern Risk Assessment

The modern environment of medicine has brought several challenges to conducting proper suicide risk assessments, mainly time and resources. In addition, the suicide risk assessment has been criticized by some, saying that there is no demonstration of reduced mortality from the implementation of universal screening and evaluation.[22]

Current state of the emergency department

There is time pressure within emergency medicine to see a high volume of patients, including those with high acuity, in the shortest time possible, which has been identified consistently as a predominant barrier in assessing suicide risk.[5] Additionally, the increase in psychiatric visits to the ED further contributes to overcrowding concerns.[13] However, time is required to foster patient rapport and facilitate disclosure of sensitive information.[5] Limited privacy, including ED spatial constraints and presence of family members and visitors, is also repeatedly cited as an obstacle in assessing suicide risk. In addition, the rapid pace of the ED, has led to complaints that ED providers are often "unempathetic" and "unhelpful."[29] Speaking to the patient alone, in a quiet and secure area, using interpersonal skills, such as establishing eye contact and using a nonjudgmental tone and language, help to promote honest communication and patient engagement.[5]

Emergency department–psychiatry relationship

Effective collaboration across multiple disciplines is required to treat psychiatric patients, and is especially critical in emergency settings. However, many ED providers state that they frequently assess suicide risk with insufficient mental health resources both in the ED and in the community.[5] Many EDs use mental health consultations after the determination of a mental health emergency, although not all emergency rooms have access to such consults.[30] Studies have shown discrepancies between emergency physicians' and psychiatrists' decision for admission suggesting an important role for on-site psychiatrists in helping with this decision.[13,30,31] ED providers report "fear," "discomfort," and "lack of confidence" in treating suicidal patients, which is worsened by limited access to psychiatric consultation during evaluation and outpatient resources after discharge. This situation may implicitly deter providers from assessing suicide risk.[5] Negative attitudes toward psychiatric patients in the ED can compromise standard of care and, among psychiatric presentations, suicidal behavior seems to elicit the most negative feelings among staff members. If not acknowledged and addressed, these negative feelings may influence the staff's ability to treat these patients and may even result in adverse patient outcomes, such as premature discharge.[13]

In ED settings where collaboration with psychiatry is possible, there can be disagreement around aspects of treatment, including medical clearance.[32] This tension can delay psychiatric patients from getting timely care. For example, the professional psychiatric and emergency medicine associations recognize the role of laboratory testing in the process of medical clearance, determining if a patient's psychiatric presentation is caused or exacerbated by a medical illness, as a point of contingency. The American College of Emergency Physicians Guidelines state that routine laboratory testing for all patients is of very low yield and that the diagnostic evaluation of patients with primary psychiatric complaints should be guided by the history and physical examination.[33] The American Psychiatric Association Guidelines state that the psychiatrist may have to initiate or request further medical evaluation to address diagnostic concerns that emerge from the psychiatric assessment.[34] Furthermore, the term "medically clear," which used to communicate a psychiatric patient's status, is a misnomer because many patients have ongoing medical needs and it is recommended that a more precise term such as "medically stable" be used to clarify that their medical problems have been addressed.[13]

Acutely intoxicated patients present another dilemma. Patients may make suicidal or homicidal patients when intoxicated, but once sober, may change their minds. This symptomatology change with clinical sobriety needs to be documented in the medical record. A clinical assessment is preferred to laboratory testing when assessing intoxication. The American College of Emergency Physicians guidelines cite normal coordination, reflexes, cognition, and lack of emotional lability as signs of sobriety that indicate when the patient is ready for psychiatric assessment.[13]

Screening

It is necessary to ask every psychiatric patient in the ED about suicidality, and important to never shy away from asking about suicide; some providers have a concern that doing so will cause a patient to think about suicide.[22] The Joint Commission advises screening all patients for suicidal ideation with a brief, standardized, evidence-based screening tool, optimal for the time constraints imposed in the ED. Furthermore, research illustrates that a validated screening tool is more reliable at recognizing those at risk for suicide compared with a clinician's personal judgment or using vague or softened language to interpret suicidal thoughts.[16]

Currently, there is no universally accepted tool or scoring system that predict which patients will eventually complete suicide.[23] However, ED providers have noted that the integration of standardized protocols for suicide screening during initial assessments or intake procedures would increase the likelihood of asking about suicide-related concerns.[5] Screening tools include Patient Health Questionnaire-9 or Patient Health Questionnaire-2 (in past 2 weeks have you experienced depressed mood, anhedonia?), ED-SAFE Patient Safety Screener by Emergency Medicine Network specifically for EDs, and the Suicide Behaviors Questionnaire-Revised. Dallas Parkland Memorial was the first US hospital to implement universal screening for suicide.[16,35] After screening 100,000 patients from the emergency and inpatient units and an additional 50,000 patients from outpatient clinics, they identified 1.8% of patients to be at high risk and 4.5% to be at moderate risk for suicide.[16]

Suicide risk assessment forms with checklists of risk and protective factors, although convenient, lack analysis and synthesis in the process of integrating these variables into an overall comprehensive assessment. These forms, in addition to no-suicide contracts, can create the false sense of security that adequate steps have been taken to treat the patient.[22] Some research suggests that some of these scales including the Patient Health Questionnaire-9, have not been shown to predict psychiatric admissions when used in the emergency room setting.[36] If suicide risk assessment forms are being used, they should be used as an adjunct to clinical decision making and not as the sole treatment decider.[13] Furthermore, they should be modified to include imminent risk factors of suicide, including anxiety and agitation, as well protective factors, which are often overlooked.[22,37]

The Basic Suicide Assessment Five-Step Evaluation

Suicide is a complex, multidimensional event influenced by a host of interacting biological, psychological, environmental, and current situational factors.[10,14] Research into risk factors have shown no definitive results into predicting suicide; therefore, the purpose of the suicide risk assessment has become to develop an informed intervention, uniquely specialized for the patient's needs. A common, simplified, practical approach to suicide risk assessment is the Basic Suicide Assessment Five-step Evaluation (B-SAFE model) proposed by Jacobs and colleagues.[24,25]

Identify risk factors

Identify potential suicidal risk factors using the patient interview, medical records, and collateral information.[25]

Psychopathology Psychopathology, including depression, bipolar disorder, schizophrenia, substance abuse, and personality disorders, is strongly associated with suicide and considered modifiable risk factors that can be diminished with appropriate diagnosis and treatment. Suicidality, in particular, is associated with early depression and bipolar disorder.[25] The period immediately after discharge, up to 3 weeks, from an ED or inpatient psychiatric unit is considered to be a time of heightened risk.[16,25,38] Measures identified that can reduce risk include intensive and early outpatient follow-up.[38]

Self-inflicted injuries and suicide attempts Self-inflicted injuries and suicide attempts presenting to the ED has more than doubled over the past 20 years in all major demographic groups.[39] Self-harm behavior is associated with a 30-fold increased risk in suicide compared with the general population. This suicide risk was higher for females than males, and greatest within the first 6 months after the index self-harm episode.[40] Self-harm behaviors, such as cutting or burning, and impulsive suicide attempts defined as planned for less than 3 hours, performed in the presence of others or where discovery is possible, seem to have less severity and intent to die than those carefully planned and hidden suicide attempts. Hospitalization may be necessary for any patient with self-harm or suicidal behavior who expresses a persistent intent to die.[25]

Psychosocial influences Psychosocial influences have a tremendous impact on people's vulnerability to stress. Specific psychosocial stressors include loss of relationships, identity, status, and employment. Intrapersonal and interpersonal conflict can affect family, social, and occupational functioning. Legal issues can include arrest and possibility of a jail or prison sentence.[17] Other factors include history of trauma and social isolation.[16] Psychosocial variables can also be protective and include patient's support systems and relationships including family, friends, and occupational security.[17]

Physical illness Physical illness is highly prevalent among those who exhibit suicidal behavior.[41] It has been suggested that depression is linked to many other medical conditions, including cardiac disease, stroke, hypertension, diabetes, cancer, and chronic obstructive pulmonary disease.[2] Medical illnesses associated with pain, disfigurement, limited function, or fear of dependence may increase suicide risk.[25] Central nervous system disorders, such as epilepsy, AIDS, Huntington's disease, cerebrovascular accidents, and traumatic brain injury, also carry an increased risk for suicide.[42]

Protective factors

Uncover internal and external protective factors that could help to prevent suicidal thoughts from turning into action. Protective factors, which are significantly valuable, are often overlooked in clinical assessments.[25] Cognitive flexibility, healthy coping strategies, good diet and sleeping patterns, physical exercise, and an active lifestyle, are important protective factors that can be stimulated and strengthened through clinical and community interventions.[14] When counseling patients and conferring these protective effects, it is important to emphasize resilience during past personal crises, family responsibilities, and religious or spiritual beliefs.[25,28] Patients are also encouraged to increase positive cues related to living to make their environment safe, for example, placing pictures of their children or grandchildren on the medicine cabinet. Protective factors shift suicidal ambivalence toward living and reduce the risk of suicide.[17]

Suicidal plans and behavior

Assessment of suicidal thoughts and behaviors are relevant to all physicians.[43] Ask about suicidal plans and behaviors. Probe gently to allow the patient to discuss their feelings and explore options for next appropriate level of care. Those without protective factors, who endorse active and imminent thoughts, with recent behaviors such as writing suicide notes, stocking pills, and buying a weapon, necessitate emergent evaluation for psychiatric admission.[25] For some patients, however, multiple hospitalizations, used solely as a containment strategy, can be counterproductive, indicating that a more effective intervention may be attempting to teach the patient how to cope with their suicidality.[16]

Patients with suicidal thoughts are almost always ambivalent about suicide to some degree, conflicted by simultaneous desires to live and to die. This conflict provides an opportunity for therapeutic intervention by aligning with the part of the patient that wants to live, because some patients may need reasons for living that help to decrease their risk for suicide.[44] Providers must remember that under their suicidal crisis is the result of a pain so intense that it blocks their ability to see any other options to their situation besides death. Edwin Schneidman, founder of modern suicidology, stated that suicide is a permanent solution to a temporary problem.[17] Exacerbation of psychiatric disorders tends to confer acute risk associated with pain, anguish, and a desire to escape. Suicidality related to personality disorders and environmental factors tends to be more chronic in nature with an impulsive quality. Patients with personality disorders may reports feelings of anger, rage, and vengeance associated with their suicidal thoughts.[25]

Intervention

Management of high-risk patients

For patients who screen positive for suicide ideation and decline treatment or minimize risk, it is essential to attempt to gain collateral information. First, request the patient's permission to contact friends, family, or outpatient treatment providers. However, should the patient decline consent and the clinician believes the patient poses a danger to self or others, the Health Insurance Portability and Accountability Act of 1996 (HIPAA) allows the clinician to establish contact without the patient's permission.[16] For further information, please refer to HIPAA Privacy Rule and Sharing Information Related to Mental Health (available from: http://www.hhs.gov/hipaa/for-professionals/special-topics/mental-health/).

Patients who are actively suicidal patients should be kept under one-to-one observation to ensure a safe environment. Patients and their visitors should be checked for items that could be used for self-harm or attempting suicide. Keep patients away from anchor points used for hanging and materials, such as bell cords, bandages, sheets, restraint belts, plastic bags, elastic tubing, and oxygen tubing. These lethal means are easily accessible in hospitals and used in suicides, even in supervised, controlled settings.[16] When it is determined that a patient is at imminent risk for suicide, depending on active plans or severe suicidal ideation, pursue inpatient psychiatric hospitalization.[42]

Management of low-risk patients

Most patients are discharged with some level of risk.[22] For patients who are at lower risk for suicide and safe for outpatient management, a safety plan should be performed. Unlike a no-suicide contract, which states what not to do during a crises, a safety plan provides a written algorithm that can be used during times of distress, which helps to increase the number of options available to navigate an emergency.[45] The Safety Planning Intervention, developed by Stanley and Brown, is used in Veterans Affairs hospitals and is recognized as an evidence-based best practice. The safety plan consists of 6 steps, including warning signs, internal coping strategies, people and social settings that provide distraction, personal contacts, professional contacts, and making the environment safe.[28] The safety plan should be performed collaboratively and implemented in acute care and outpatient settings.[16,28] It should be updated regularly as patients recognize additional warning signs, learn new coping skills, and resources and contacts change, until the suicidal crisis subsides. In addition, patients and family members should be provided with the number to the National Suicide Prevention Lifeline (1-800-273-TALK [8255]) and other information to peer support and local crisis contacts. To increase outpatient compliance, ensure that referrals and appointments to outpatient psychiatric providers for follow-up care have been made within 1 week of assessment, instead of relying on the patient to make their own appointment.[16]

Medications

Because suicidality is often symptomatic of a primary psychiatric disorder, swiftly identifying depression, mania, and psychosis is critical to reducing suicidal thoughts and behaviors. It is important to prescribe appropriate antidepressants, mood stabilizers, and antipsychotics at adequate doses with proper follow-up. Distressing symptoms that may increase imminent suicide risk include anxiety, panic, agitation, insomnia, and pain, and may be rapidly relieved with anxiolytics, sedative-hypnotics, antipsychotics, and analgesics.[25] These agents have rapid onset and resolutions, as opposed to antidepressants, which show maximum improvement in 2 weeks.[9]

Side effects should be monitored carefully for all psychotropic agents. Akathisia, is a common adverse side effect of antipsychotics, and consists of a subjective feeling of inner restlessness and an urge to move accompanied by objective motor component manifesting as rocking, packing, or uncrossing and uncrossing legs. This symptom is very distressing to the patient and itself is associated with an increased risk of suicide. The treatment of akathisia includes discontinuing or holding the antipsychotic in addition to adding either a lipophilic beta-blocker, such as propranolol, or a benzodiazepine. It is imperative to identify accurately; as akathisia is interpreted commonly as worsening agitation, resulting in increased doses of antipsychotics, further worsening the symptoms.[46] Owing to these potential side effects, it is obligatory to arrange outpatient follow-up to ensure clinical monitoring after a prescription is written.[6]

Substance use

Suicide risk assessment must be based on a good qualitative history when the patient is alert, sober, and cooperative.[23] Certain substance use disorders exhibit psychiatric symptoms during times of intoxication and withdrawal, which may include impulsivity. Substance use disorders can be an element of suicidal behavior and identifying prevention strategies is important.[47] The treatment team should aggressively attempt to engage the patient in detoxification and rehabilitation treatments.[25]

Psychosocial

Providers should make every effort to engage in existing support systems, with the patient's permission. Sources of support include family, friends, religious communities, and other health care providers.[45] Therapy referrals for individual, marital, and family counseling can improve interpersonal skills and strengthen coping skills. If social services are available, information about shelter, food, and other community resources should be made available.[25]

Means restriction

Firearms are the most common and lethal method of suicide in the United States.[48] It is imperative that every psychiatric patient in the ED be asked about availability of firearms and intent to obtain firearms.[20] Owing to the politically charged climate surrounding the issue of gun control, Harvard School of Public Health recommends a noncontroversial "lethal means counseling" approach to firearm access.[48] Means restriction is the most effective suicide prevention strategy to date and involves restricting or eliminating access to lethal means in the patient's environment. This may include discarding excess medication, locking up firearms, or limiting access to knives.[28]

Means restriction is crucial, because many suicides occur impulsively during a short-term crisis. Intent is not the only determination of suicide; both intent and means are required for completion.[28,48] The number of guns and method of storage greatly influence suicide risk, with greatest risk occurring with unlocked, loaded handguns.[28] Reaching for a loaded gun takes less time than most other methods of suicide (eg, overdose, hanging, carbon monoxide poisoning).[20] In 2014, one-half of all completed suicides, more than 21,334 people, were committed with a firearm.[49] Tragically, firearms used in youth suicide usually belong to a parent.[48]

If a patient is admitted to a psychiatric unit, gun safety management is transferred to the inpatient team. However, if it the patient is deemed safe for outpatient management, then the ED team should implement and document a gun safety plan. Ideally, if guns are in the home, the patient agrees to have them secured or removed by a responsible, designated person, who then will report back to the physician and confirm that the plan has been carried out. If there is no responsible party available to assist in such process or if there is doubt that the plan can be implemented effectively, then admission is recommended for further evaluation and treatment. It is important to acknowledge that limitations exist on the clinician's ability to ensure compliance with the gun safety management plan.[20]

The "Perfect Depression Care Initiative" of the Michigan's Henry Ford Health System achieved 10 consecutive months without an instance of suicide by focusing on quality improvement measures in the delivery of depression care.[16] A key component to their success was their focus on firearms for those at risk by insisting they provide an inventory of accessible weapons. Through collaboration, lethal means restriction strategies should be discussed and coordinated with patient and family members.[48] Means restrictions has also proven successful in other countries, such as Japan, where suicide rates decreased after carbon monoxide was removed from coal gas.[42]

Malingering

Patients may not be entirely forthcoming and may alter responses to seek admission for secondary gain.[5] Malingering, the intentional production of false or grossly exaggerated symptoms, is motivated by external incentives, such as avoiding arrest or legal charges, or to gain shelter, access to controlled substances, or disability benefits.[50] Use your best judgment when patients endorse suicidal complaints or threats that are believed to be for the purpose of obtaining hospitalization.[25] Providers should be cautious using this term without substantial documentation.

Document Your Assessment

All too often, short of conducting no assessment, providers simply state no suicidal or homicidal ideation; however, the provider must do more.[22] A formal suicide risk assessment highlighting risk and protective factors should be organized and well documented. Modifiable risk factors with their corresponding intervention aimed at addressing that risk factor should be explicitly stated and are enormously helpful in guiding a comprehensive treatment plan. These can include current suicidal thinking and behavior, current psychiatric illness and symptomatology, current personal cries, alcohol or drug use, unemployment, and lack of social support.[26] Last, suicide risk assessment is a process, not a one-time event. Serial assessments and documentation are required at important clinical junctures, because risk and protective factors vary with time and circumstances (**Box 1**).[22,26]

Dynamic formulation

A valuable tool to support the traditional suicide risk assessment is the use of the risk formulation model, an evidence-based practice drawn from prevention research and

Box 1
Documentation

Elements to document
- Summary of the case
- Estimated risk (based on known risk and protective factors)
- Treatment plan (can include medications, tests, consultations, admission, discharge, etc)
- Specific rationale for treatment plan
- Follow-up measures or assessments to be done

Data from Muzina D. Suicide intervention: How to recognize risk, focus on patient safety. Current Psychiatry 2007;6(9):30–46.

violence assessment. This model takes into consideration the dynamic nature of suicide risk, constantly changing owing to level of stressors, access to resources, and compliance with care.[29] This understanding allows for the development of personalized short-term and long-term safety plans for suicidal patients that inform risk management and guide treatment planning.[16]

Education

The best treatment of suicide is prevention.[37] The most efficacious preventive efforts of suicide thus far are restricting access to lethal means and improving education.[19] Education for general practitioners and other health care workers is an evidence-based method for the prevention of suicide that has been shown to decrease rates of suicide significantly.[14] Staff in all patient care settings should be educated on how to properly and sensitively respond to a suicidal patient in a way that is appropriate their role and level of training.[16] Topics that should be covered include the detection and treatment of depression, obtaining help in psychiatric emergencies, and policies for screening, assessing, referring, and treating and suicidal patients.[14,16] This is consistent with the need ED providers identified when surveyed, reporting more confidence in screening for suicide than they did with further assessment, counseling, and referral skills.[51] This increased knowledge improves negative attitudes toward suicidal patients and reduces the stigma associated with suicidal behavior.[14] Regular continuous education should be provided to all health care staff working in acute settings pertaining to psychiatric emergencies to further boost competence and confidence in delivering care.[13] From 1983 to 1984, the Swedish Committee for Prevention and Treatment of Depression demonstrated a reduction in inpatient care and suicide from depression through the delivery of an educational program to all general practitioners.[49]

Collaboration

Although it is ultimately up to the physician to conduct a suicide risk assessment, delegating risk assessment and garnering input from ancillary staff is critical, because they have more contact with the patients.[22] Nurses, particularly, are first line and should be educated on suicide risk; there are clear gaps in knowledge and competencies between mental health and non–mental health nurses, and training should be provided to those working in the ED.[3] Physicians should not carry the burden alone and this multidisciplinary approach is critical to reduce provider burnout and personal distress.[22,29]

Improve access to outpatient care

The Joint Commission urges all health care organizations to integrate comprehensive psychiatric behavioral health, primary care, and community resources, and make these resources accessible to emergency room providers. Continuity and coordination of care require a cohesive health services infrastructure rather than numerous disjointed facilities. Improving the system's ability to expand its community capacity would enable patients to be monitored and treated effectively across services, including mental and general medical health.[49] Asker and Baerum Hospital near Oslo, Norway, achieved a 54% reduction in suicide attempts in a high-risk population with poor history of compliance through the implementation of continuity-of-care strategies, and achieved an 88% success rate for follow-up with aftercare referrals.[16] Considering that the period of discharge from psychiatric hospitals and EDs is a high-risk period for suicidal patients, there is room for improvement patient transitions from inpatient to outpatient psychiatric care.[52]

REFERENCES

1. World Health Organization (WHO). WHO depression fact sheet. 2016. Available at: http://www.who.int/mediacentre/factsheets/fs369/en/. Accessed November 28, 2016.
2. Kumar A, Clark S, Boudreaux ED, et al. A multicenter study of depression among emergency department patients. Acad Emerg Med 2004;11(12):1284–9.
3. Giordano R, Stichler JF. Improving suicide risk assessment in the emergency department. J Emerg Nurs 2009;35(1):22–6.
4. Harman J, Scholle S, Edlund M. Emergency department visits for depression in the United States. Psychiatr Serv 2004;55(55):937–9.
5. Petrik ML, Gutierrez PM, Berlin JS, et al. Barriers and facilitators of suicide risk assessment in emergency departments: a qualitative study of provider perspectives. Gen Hosp Psychiatry 2015;37(6):581–6.
6. Ernst C, Bird S, Goldberg J, et al. The prescription of psychotropic medications for patients discharged from a psychiatric emergency service. J Clin Psychiatry 2006;67(5):720–6.
7. Larkin G, Smith R, Beautrais A. Trends in US emergency department visits for suicide attempts, 1992-2001. Crisis 2008;29(2):73.
8. Porter R, Ferrier N. Emergency treatment of depression. Adv Psychiatr Treat 1999;5:3–10.
9. Mitchell A. Two-week delay in onset of action of antidepressants: new evidence. Br J Psychiatry 2006;108:105–6.
10. Mitchell A, Garand L, Dean D, et al. Suicide assessment in hospital emergency departments: implications for patient satisfaction and compliance. Top Emerg Med 2005;27(4):302–12.
11. Ungvari G, Chiu H, Lok Y, et al. Lorazepam for chronic catatonia: a randomized, double-blind, placebo-controlled cross-over study. Psychopharmacology 1999; 142(4):393–8.
12. Balázs J, Benazzi F, Rihmer Z, et al. The close link between suicide attempts and mixed (bipolar) depression: implications for suicide prevention. J Affect Disord 2006;91(2–3):133–8.
13. Zun LS. Pitfalls in the care of the psychiatric patient in the emergency department. J Emerg Med 2012;43(5):829–35.
14. Wasserman D, Rihmer Z, Rujescu D, et al. The European Psychiatric Association (EPA) guidance on suicide treatment and prevention. Eur Psychiatry 2012;27(2): 129–41.

15. American Foundation for Suicide Prevention (AFSP). Suicide statistics. [webpage]. 2016. Available at: https://afsp.org/about-suicide/suicide-statistics/. Accessed November 29, 2016.
16. Detecting and treating suicide ideation in all settings. Sentinel Event Alert 2016;(56):1–7.
17. Ramirez J. Suicide: across the life span. Nurs Clin North Am 2016;51(2):275–86.
18. Curtin S, Warner, M., Hedegaard, H. Increase in Suicide in the United States, 1999–2014. NCHS Data Brief No. 241, April 2016. 2016. Available at: http://www.cdc.gov/nchs/products/databriefs/db241.htm. Accessed November 29, 2016.
19. Erlich MD, GAP Committee on Psychopathology. Envisioning Zero Suicide. Psychiatr Serv 2016;67(3):255.
20. Simon R. Gun safety management with patients at risk for suicide. Suicide Life Threat Behav 2007;37(5):518–26.
21. Luoma JB, Martin CE, Pearson JL. Contact with mental health and primary care providers before suicide: a review of the evidence. Am J Psychiatry 2002;159(6):909–16.
22. Simon RI. Improving suicide risk assessment: avoiding common pitfals. Psychiatric Times 2011;28(11):16.
23. Ronquillo L, Minassian A, Vilke GM, et al. Literature-based recommendations for suicide assessment in the emergency department: a review. J Emerg Med 2012;43(5):836–42.
24. Jacobs DG, Brewer M, Klein-Benheim M. Suicide assessment: an overview and recommended protocol. San Francisco: Jossey-Bass; 1999.
25. Muzina D. Suicide intervention. Curr Psychiatry 2007;6(9):30–46.
26. Frierson R. The suicidal patient: risk assessment, management, and documentation. Psychiatr Times 2007;24(5):29.
27. Kroll J. Use of no-suicide contract by psychiatrists in Minnesota. Am J Psychiatry 2000;157(10):1684–6.
28. Matarazzo BB, Homaifar BY, Wortzel HS. Therapeutic risk management of the suicidal patient: safety planning. J Psychiatr Pract 2014;20(3):220–4.
29. Deuter K, Galley P, Champion A, et al. Risk assessment and risk management: developing a model of shared learning in clinical practice. Adv Ment Health 2013;11(2):157–62.
30. Douglass AM, Luo J, Baraff LJ. Emergency medicine and psychiatry agreement on diagnosis and disposition of emergency department patients with behavioral emergencies. Acad Emerg Med 2011;18(4):368–73.
31. Garbrick L, Levitt MA, Barrett M, et al. Agreement between emergency physicians and psychiatrists regarding admission decisions. Acad Emerg Med 1996;3(11):1027–30.
32. Williams ER, Shepherd SM. Medical clearance of psychiatric patients. Emerg Med Clin North Am 2000;18(2):185–98, vii.
33. Wiler J, Brown N, Chanmugam A, et al. Care of the psychiatric patient in the emergency department - a review of the literature. American College of Emergency Physicians: Advancing Emergency Care; 2014. Available at: https://www.acep.org/uploadedFiles/ACEP/Clinical_and_Practice_Management/Resources/Mental_Health_and_Substance_Abuse/Psychiatric%20Patient%20Care%20in%20the%20ED%202014.pdf. Accessed December 1, 2016.
34. Vergare MJ, Binder RL, Cook IA, et al. For the work group on psychiatric evaluation. Practice guideline for the psychiatric evaluation of adults. 2nd edition. Washington, DC: American Psychiatric Association; 2006. p. 1–62.

35. Russell B. Parkland pioneers suicide screening program. 2016. Available at: NBCDFW.com. Accessed November 11, 2016.
36. Chang BP, Tan TM. Suicide screening tools and their association with near-term adverse events in the ED. Am J Emerg Med 2015;33(11):1680–3.
37. Hermes B, Deakin K, Lee K, et al. Suicide risk assessment: 6 steps to a better instrument. J Psychosoc Nurs Ment Health Serv 2009;47(6):44–9.
38. Hunt I, Kapur N, Webb R, et al. Suicide in recently discharged psychiatric patients: a case-control study. Psychol Med 2009;39(3):443–9.
39. Ting S, Sullivan A, Edwin D, et al. Trends in US emergency department visits for attempted suicide and self-inflicted injury, 1993-2008. Gen Hosp Psychiatry 2012;34(5):557–65.
40. Cooper J, Kapur N, Webb R, et al. Suicide after deliberate self-harm: a 4-year cohort study. Am J Psychiatry 2005;162(2):297.
41. Tran T, Luo W, Phung D, et al. Risk stratification using data from electronic medical records better predicts suicide risks than clinician assessments. BMC Psychiatry 2014;14(76):1–8.
42. Mann JJ. A current perspective of suicide and attempted suicide. Ann Intern Med 2002;136:302–11.
43. Hirschfeld RM, Russell JM. Assessment and treatment of suicidal patients. N Engl J Med 1997;337(13):910–5.
44. Malone KM, Oquendo MA, Haas GL, et al. Protective factors against suicidal acts in major depression: reasons for living. Am J Psychiatry 2000;157(7):1084–8.
45. Welton R. The management of suicidality: assessment and intervention. Psychiatry 2007;4:24–34.
46. Miller C, Fleischhacker W. Managing antipsychotic-induced acute and chronic akathisia. Drug Saf 2000;22(1):73–81.
47. Vijayakumar L, Kumar MS, Vijayakumar V. Substance use and suicide. Curr Opin Psychiatry 2011;24(3):197–202.
48. Suicide, guns, and public health. Means matter. 2016. Available at: https://www.hsph.harvard.edu/means-matter/means-matter/. Accessed October 1, 2016.
49. Litts D, Berman A, Knesper D. Suicide Attempts and Suicide Deaths Subsequent to Discharge from an Emergency Department or an Inpatient Psychiatry Unit. Suicide Prevention Resource Center; 2011.
50. Resnick P, Knoll J. Faking it: how to detect malingered psychosis. Curr Psychiatry 2005;4(11):12–25.
51. Betz M, Sullivan A, Manton A, et al. Knowledge, attitudes, and practices of emergency department providers in the care of suicidal patients. Depress Anxiety 2013;30(10):1005–12.
52. Olfson M, Marcus SC, Bridge JA. Focusing suicide prevention on periods of high risk. JAMA 2014;311(11):1107–8.

Difficult Patients in the Emergency Department

Personality Disorders and Beyond

Nidal Moukaddam, MD, PhD, Araceli Flores, PhD, Anu Matorin, MD, Nicholas Hayden, BS, Veronica Theresa Tucci, MD, JD*

KEYWORDS

- Difficult patient • High utilizers • Super utilizers • Frequent flyers
- Countertransference • Personality traits/disorders • Borderline

KEY POINTS

- Reasons for difficult physician-patient interactions can be due to patients or the physician, or system factors (wait times, lack of community outreach services, formulary restrictions, and so forth).
- Some difficulty in patient interactions can be due to physicians' counter-transferential feelings.
- The most difficult patients tend to have undiagnosed personality disorders, may be drug seeking, or present repeatedly to the emergency department with recurrent complaints, nonadherence to prescribed treatments, or contingent suicidality.

If the patient says that they want to kill you or your staff, they are psychotic. If the patient makes you and the rest of the staff want to kill them, odds are that you are dealing with a borderline

—*Anonymous*

INTRODUCTION

Part 1: Who are Difficult Patients?

Factors associated with behavioral and psychiatric problems in a medical setting may seem convoluted. Not only will complex medical problems up the ante of an individual's initial presentation to the emergency department (ED) but the addition of a possible psychiatric problem can also muddle up a clear diagnosis and render an ED visit difficult for all health care team members involved as well as for the patients. A full 20% of interactions in the ED can be seen as difficult, though only 0.2% of the US population will have a high frequency of ED service utilization.[1,2] Individuals presenting

Department of Emergency Medicine, Baylor College of Medicine, 1504 Taub Loop, Houston, TX 77030, USA
* Corresponding author.
E-mail address: vtuccimd@gmail.com

Psychiatr Clin N Am 40 (2017) 379–395
http://dx.doi.org/10.1016/j.psc.2017.05.005
psych.theclinics.com
0193-953X/17/© 2017 Elsevier Inc. All rights reserved.

with repeated complaints are typically the most frustrating to health care teams. In the literature, these individuals are referred to as difficult, frequent flyers, superusers, and high and superhigh utilizers.

So who are those difficult patients who seem to consume a disproportionate amount of health care resources? The groups can be roughly divided into presenting with a clear medical complaint versus not: patients with sickle cell disease, for instance, go through periods of heavy ED service utilization but may be managed effectively with thoughtful pain control, thus, reducing ED visits.[3] Similarly, patients with clear medical conditions might be seen often in an ED but are not necessarily considered difficult.

Recent evidence seems to indicate that the difficult population has a higher mental illness burden, higher levels of depression severity, fatigue, sleep difficulties, pain, high alcohol consumption, and anxiety.[4] They have a lower self-perceived quality of health and often have a history of childhood maltreatment.[5,6] Other substance use, obesity, cardiovascular disease, more comorbidity (number and severity), and pain were also noted to increase patients' risk of becoming high utilizers of health care resources.[4] However, others have suggested that the population is not homogeneous and that some more nuanced definitions are needed: according to Pasic and colleagues,[7] using 3 different ways to assess high utilization (2 SD greater than the mean number of visits to an urban psychiatric emergency service, 6 visits in a year, and 4 visits in a quarter), the first high-utilizer group was more likely to be homeless, to have developmental delays, to be enrolled in a mental health plan, to have a history of voluntary and involuntary hospitalizations, to be uncooperative, to have personality disorders, to have unreliable social support, and to have a lifetime history of incarceration and detoxification. However, the second group had more visits, was more likely to have a history of incarceration and psychiatric hospitalization, more likely to be enrolled in mental health plan, and less likely to be homeless. This last group had the highest number of visits by standard deviation (2 greater than the mean; visits were not clustered in a given quarter, suggesting a pattern of use rather than increased use in response to a crisis).

Difficult patients through time-evolving picture and management

Over the course of the past 3 decades, much has changed in the health care system; another layer of complexity was added with the wave of deinstitutionalization that hit the United States in the 70s and 80s. Emphasis moved from humane, professional, and courteous patient management to effectiveness and cost cutting. It is helpful to take a look back to understand how our system arrived at its current state: the aim of the deinstitutionalization movement was better integration of individuals with mental illness into society with expected decrease in care expenditures. Developing countries have seen similar, though less pronounced and less systematic, movements.[8,9]

An unintended consequence of deinstitutionalization is the increase in high utilizers of emergency and urgent care services; though it is not the only reason for the existence of this category of patients, it is certainly a factor. These patients often seem to have intractable social, financial, and medical or mental problems and unfortunately seem to have high rates of nonadherence to treatment recommendations. This group was recognized early, though has had different labels through the years[10]; but no concerted, useful measures have been found for effective management. In addition to the medical complaints that never seem to end, and never seem to get better, it has been suggested that frequent, high utilizers of the ED establish a different relationship dynamic with members of the health care team and almost treat the ED environment, with all its harshness, as a support system and a home: thus, frequent flyers may cause frustration in providers at all levels, seem to have trouble relinquishing control, causing frustration with seemingly unsolvable problems.[11] But frustration is not the only feeling that emerges in the clinician patient relationship in this setting: it is now more understood that there is much ambivalence mired in complexity in these cases, and grounding frequent flyers is better than dismissing or abandoning them.[12] Indeed, the level of difficulty perceived in an interaction depends on the patients' attachment style.[13] And, although emergency providers often think they are doing their best, patients may report they did not feel empathy and a caring emotional response.[14]

System issues and socioeconomic pressures contribute to the woes of interacting with difficult patients (**Figs. 1** and **2**). New hypotheses and new ways of dealing with this population have been slow to emerge,[15] though that population is now recognized as complex, changing, and, simply stated, in need of more care than the ED can offer. Multidisciplinary, individualized care plans may help reduce hospital admissions, readmissions, and costs for complex, high-utilizing patients.[16] Providing a continuous care continuum (in this case a single-payer, citywide system), such as the Camden's model, seems to be efficacious.[17] Focusing on housing helps as well, though most ED providers do not see it a part of their job description.[18] However, in the absence of large system-based solutions, focusing on depression and anxiety, for instance, by using mindfulness-based therapy, provides help for the frequent flyer population and helps reduced unnecessary ED visits.[19] Educating students and residents that care is not limited to one medical problem can also provide a welcome additional positive effect, as evidenced by a proof-of-concept study that allowed students to shadow chaplains during patient care.[20] By learning a new perspective on patient care and expanding the view of patients as human beings, the aforementioned ambivalence and complexity may yield way to more positive feelings.

Meeting patients under urgent or emergency circumstances is challenging and can become increasingly so because of the emotions involved in an acute presentation and the pressure on physicians and other members of the health care team to achieve a good outcome. Family members presenting with patients can cause turmoil as well. As early as 1977, investigators at the Cincinnati Medical Center suggested an

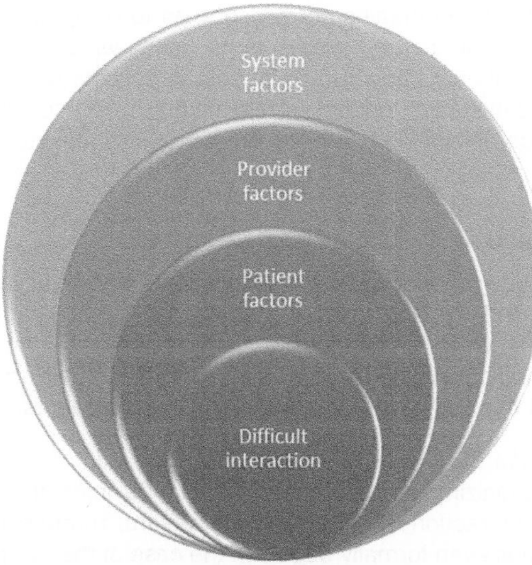

Fig. 1. The interplay between system, patient, and provider factors leading to difficulty in clinical situations.

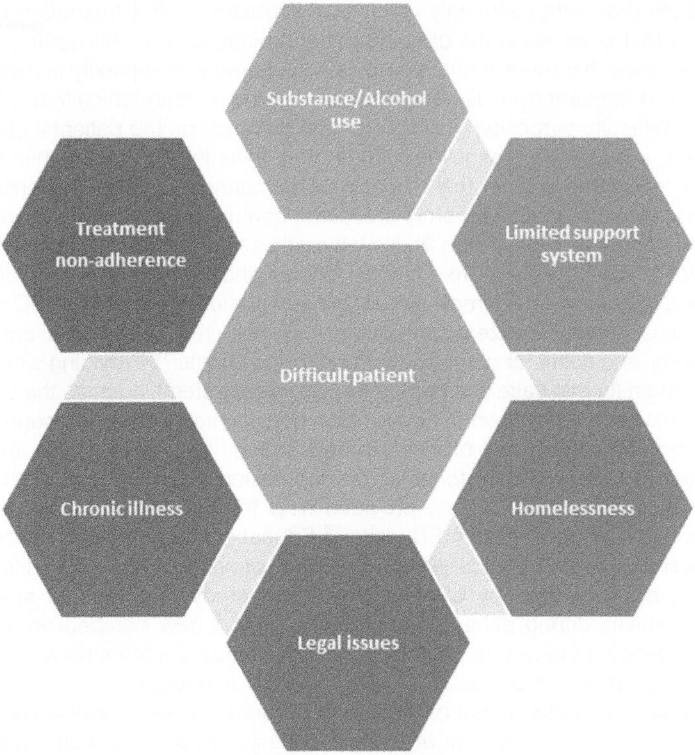

Fig. 2. Factors contributing to difficult patient presentations.

interactional approach to patients, summed in elements, such as remaining calm and empathetic, but also letting family members express themselves and avoid marginalizing them.[21] The literature contains no evidence as to using supportive, cognitive-behavioral, or dialectical therapy elements to management in the ED, though psychosocial treatments are known to be of help in patients who self-harm.[22] More specific recommendations for patients presenting with personality disorders and recurrent somatic complaints have been presented by the authors' group more recently as well.[23]

Part 2: Difficult Patients in the Emergency Department

How would a physician recognize a difficult patient, who may leave them feeling incompetent, frustrated, or, even worse, burned out? The number of visits itself, although a useful marker, is not enough, as some patients present often because of poorly controlled medical issues, as summarized earlier. Next are some behaviors and complaints that may be helpful in identifying difficult patients.

Difficult patients make the health care team uncomfortable

In most settings, recognizing (and reacting to) a patient's name and presenting details is a sign of unusual interaction with the health care team. Treatment starts before the medical encounter has even formally begun: in the case of the ED, physicians should be on the lookout of patients who the ancillary and nursing staff flag ahead of time: *Oh, Mr— is back. I saw one of our patients on my way back from the lunch break. Can you see this patient in triage, she or he is usually making things up.* Although cynicism and negative attitudes should be tolerated in treatment, they are, nevertheless, symptomatic of an intense reaction toward patients. The team might sometimes even request patients be barred access to the clinic or ED.

For the physician, warning signs include dreading an interaction with a patient, delaying calling the patient back until one must absolutely do so, and irritability that does not occur with other patients. Some difficult patients are difficult because of sheer complexity, age (elderly and younger patients requiring collateral will take more time), and unusual presentations; but these categories often do not get labeled as unpleasant.

Difficult patients may affect the team's morale

The demands of patient care sometimes stretch above and beyond what the health care team can offer. Although it is neither the team's nor the patients' fault, such interactions can drain a team's morale unless steps are taken to remedy this situation. Requests perceived as unreasonable are especially challenging: These requests can range from a hot meal when only sandwiches are available to financial help when a health coverage plan fails. One successful program at Metrohealth in Cleveland assigned a one-to-one case manager to such patients for case coordination.[24] But such resources are not readily available outside of dedicated pilot programs; a high frequency of difficult patient interactions may lead to low morale and feelings of helplessness, which may, in turn, increase burnout rate and job turnovers.[25,26] In particular, one aspect of burnout worth mentioning is excessive detachment and dehumanizing patients as a self-protection mechanism, a mechanism that rarely works; instead, a vicious cycle of increased utilization and worsening verbal exchanges may arise when patients are discharged without thinking they have obtained what they sought.

Difficult patients may present with nonadherence

The topic of nonadherence, whether to medications or behavioral modifications, is often a source of frustration for providers. More commonly, in chronic diseases, whether medical or psychiatric, nonadherence represents a quagmire with no answer, requiring lifestyle changes and full patient cooperation to take effect. When in the ED, or the clinic, it is easy for patients to promise adherence. Subsequent visits proving that patients have not followed through with the plan, yet continue to complain, can be difficult, leading the health care team to be less inclined to help patients or less inclined to aggressively plan action beyond immediate stabilization measures. Chronic mental illnesses and drug use are prime examples of this situation, both for conceptual and practical reasons.

Interestingly, from a practical perspective, though both illness groups have some long-acting medication options, these are not used in the ED. In the case of chronic psychosis, patients have a high rate of nonadherence, yet the rates of use of depot antipsychotics, long-acting formulations that can last for 2 to 4 weeks, are practically unheard of in the ED. This reluctance to use long-acting formulations may also be due to the stigmatized image of this medication class and the reluctance of the ED physician/psychiatrist to administer a medication without a clear plan for follow-up for continued care. The same can be said for injectable naltrexone from the ED: Although an attractive option for alcohol cravings with a month-long duration of action, and although most high utilizers (up to half)[27] have alcohol use disorders, this option has not been studied in the ED setting and is not in use. Combined, these 2 examples of underutilization of injectable medications in the ED point out a treatment gap. Additionally, the case of substance use disorders merits particular scrutiny as a conceptual issue, as treatment out of the ED is overwhelmingly psychosocial rather than pharmacologic. Although the addiction medicine field has moved away from the moral model of addiction, the ED-recommended treatments are still inspired by it and shy away from medical or neurobiological conceptualizations of addictive disorders. Therefore, substance users in the ED rarely, if ever, get anticraving medications.

Difficult patients may present with contingent suicidality

It is not uncommon for patients to threaten suicide if something is not going their way. Contingent suicidal ideation (SI) is frequently reported by patients who are homeless or have limited resources but may occur outside these elements. Patients' report of suicidality might be linked to trying to manipulate family members into doing what they want or fulfilling their requests. Contingent SI is not a classified psychiatric problem but mostly explained by character disorder or limited resources. Article – covers the assessment and management of suicidality, whereas the subsequent sections highlight suicidality pertaining to personality disorder. In general, a full safety assessment must be performed regardless of the number of suicidal threats[28]; but thorough team education and learning how to handle contingent SI is essential to avoid acting out.

And lastly, as mentioned earlier, difficult patients may have pathologic personality traits or even disorders, making management difficult. An overview of personality disorders from an ED perspective starts later.

Team strategies for managing difficult patients Management of difficult patients requires a team effort. Most EDs have multidisciplinary teams with various areas of expertise that can comprise physicians, midlevel providers, social workers, psychiatry response teams, or a full psychiatry service and licensed chemical dependency counselors. In academic institutions, residents/trainees and students are also present. A key step to minimize team discomfort and optimize outcomes for patients is to have a multidisciplinary discussion of the case and highlight its difficulty and potential treatments. Time constraints often preclude regular rounding, but communication about patients is essential. Every encounter is a fresh encounter; even the most noncompliant patients may present with delirium, complications, or other serious conditions that need treatment, regardless of how disliked or difficult the patients are. It is also worth reminding teams, especially young trainees, that individuals with chronic mental illness have a shorter life span than those without those illnesses. This subgroup dies of medical causes, not psychiatric causes.[29]

Knowledge of the case at hand is also essential. Long-term staff recall details about patient cases, serving as institutional memory; but care must be taken to not let memories of past treatment failures or nonadherence negatively color the assessment and treatment planning. A more realistic way to reframe repeated ED presentations is to think of patient strengths and weaknesses and suitability for complex discharge plans.

Additionally, an often-overlooked aspect of chronically ill patients is the possibility of cognitive deficits, because of alcohol use,[30] drug use,[31] mental illness, or even head trauma/traumatic brain injuries associated with insecure living situations. Quite often, these deficits are undiagnosed as very few patients get mental status testing in the ED despite guidelines.[32] These deficits essentially render standard explanations of discharge planning insufficient, and it is strongly recommended that simplified language be used. Patients who are seen as high utilizers, although often nonadherent, also have emotional connections to the staff (**Box 1**).

Box 1
Team management strategies for difficult patients

- Set up your team for success:
  - Every encounter is a fresh encounter.
  - Every day is a new day.
- Difficult patients are still patients in need of care. They might be the most complicated of all medically speaking.
- Never forget a thorough safety assessment.
- Difficult patients know they are NOT liked.
- Use the knowledge of experienced staff to promote patient advocacy and find creative solutions for dilemmas at hand.
- Do not assume patients *already know this*. Our patients tend to have cognitive deficits and dysfunctional decision-making.
- No staff member is responsible for system-level limitations, but each kind and professional encounter can change a person's life.

Box 1 summarizes management strategies for team efforts in difficult patient interactions.

Part 3: Personality Traits/Disorders and Instant Countertransference

Mental disorders are one of the 5 most costly conditions in the United States with expenditures at $193.2 billion.[33] Personality psychopathology can be challenging in many ways: it can prevent a clear diagnostic picture and create difficulty in clinical and interpersonal interactions. Personality disorders are persistent patterns of internal and behavioral experiences that differ or deviate from the expected social and cultural norms causing disruption and distress leading to difficulties in daily functioning. (*Diagnostic and Statistical Manual of Mental Disorders, Fifth Edition* [*DSM-5*]) Personality disorder is commonly seen and is noted in 40% to 60% of psychiatric patients. This finding makes individuals with personality disorder the most frequent diagnosis seen by mental health care providers,[34] with misdiagnosis/underdiagnosis not uncommon, as elaborated later.

Why is personality disorder important?

Personality disorders are categorized by symptomatic clusters (A, B, and C) (**Fig. 3**) but are also conceptualized as sharing a spectrum of genetic and environmental risk factors and/or underlying mechanisms.[35] This spectrum makes personality disorders challenging to identify, diagnose, and treat. Comorbidity with other psychiatric disorders is very common, and research suggests a complex picture between clinical and personality disorders.[36] This complicated comorbidity is not lost in ED settings, where patients with personality disorder abound.

Up to 30% of people who require mental services have at least one personality disorder; but because of the very nature of personality disorders, such individuals tend to not seek treatment or quit their treatment about 70% of the time.[34,37] The best treatments for personality disorders consist of a comprehensive, multimodal approach that may include pharmacologic, individual/group/family therapy, high-risk/on-call backup, and long-term follow-up. In the current health care setting, backup call, long-term follow-up, and crisis management often end up being in the ED's realm of experiences. Individuals with personality disorders display enduring, prevalent

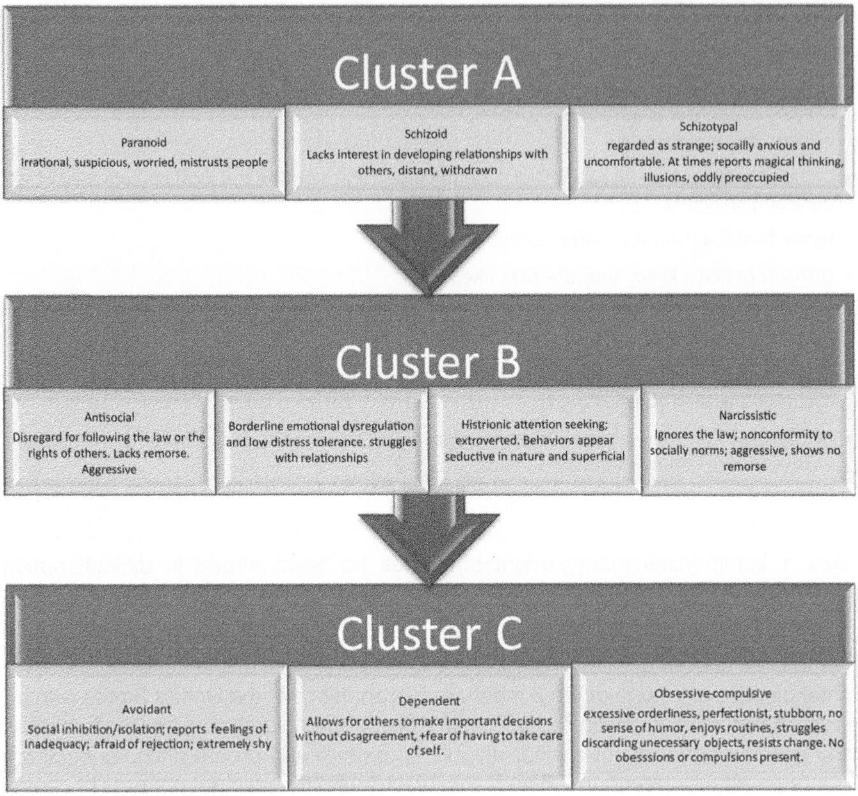

Fig. 3. Personality disorder clusters.

problems getting along with different kinds of people in different contexts. The most researched personality disorder treatment is borderline personality disorder. However, there is not a known definitive permanent treatment of personality disorders.[38]

Further, a common reaction of ED staff is to focus on main clinical diagnoses (previously referred to as Axis I disorders) and not have personality traits properly identified. Specialized treatment strategies for personality traits are not routinely included in staff training.

As the polarity of personality disorders challenges diagnosis, no diagnostic construct is perfect. A cluster model adopts each personality disorder as a distinct category; but the *DSM-5* presents an alternative model, the continuous dimensional model, under consideration with the hopes of addressing current shortcomings in diagnostic procedures. The dimensional model views various personality features along several continuous dimensions (or continuums). In this dimensional approach, personality disorders would be characterized by the level of functioning and pathologic traits in the personality.[33] As the authors expand later, the dimensional model might be more suited for the ED setting.

Cluster versus trait model of personality psychopathology

Personality disorders are connected with thinking and feeling patterns of self and the works that undesirably influence the way individuals function (**Table 1**). In the categorical system currently adopted by the *DSM-5*, there are *10* personality

Table 1
Personality disorders: personality functioning

	Personality Functioning				
	Self		Interpersonal		
	Identity	Self-direction	Empathy	Intimacy	Personality Traits
Antisocial	Egocentrism; self-esteem derived from personal gain, power, or pleasure	Goal setting based on personal gratification; absence of prosocial internal standards, associated with failure to conform to lawful or culturally normative ethical behavior	Lack of concern for feelings, needs, or suffering of others; lack of remorse after hurting or mistreating another	Incapacity for mutually intimate relationships, as exploitation is a primary means of relating to others, including by deceit and coercion; use of dominance or intimidation to control others	Antagonism: manipulative, deceit, callous, hostile Disinhibition: irresponsibility, impulsivity, risk taking
Avoidant	Low self-esteem associated with self-appraisal as socially inept, personally unappealing, or inferior; excessive feelings of	Unrealistic standards for behavior associated with reluctance to pursue goals, take personal risks, or engage in new activities involving interpersonal contact	Preoccupation with, and sensitivity to, criticism or rejection, associated with distorted inference of others' perspectives as negative	Reluctance to get involved with people unless being certain of being liked: diminished mutuality within intimate relationships because of fear of being shamed or ridiculed	Detachment withdrawal, intimacy avoidance, anhedonia Negative affectivity: anxiousness

(*continued on next page*)

Table 1
(*continued*)

	Personality Functioning				
	Self		Interpersonal		
	Identity	**Self-direction**	**Empathy**	**Intimacy**	**Personality Traits**
Borderline	Markedly impoverished, poorly developed, or unstable self-image, often associated with excessive self-criticism; chronic feelings of emptiness; dissociative states under stress	Instability in goals, aspirations, values, or career plans	Compromised ability to recognize the feelings and needs of others associated with interpersonal hypersensitivity (ie, prone to feel slighted or insulted); perceptions of others selectively biased toward negative attributes or vulnerabilities	Intense, unstable, and conflicted close relationships, marked by mistrust, neediness, and anxious preoccupation with real or imagined abandonment; close relationships often viewed in extremes of idealization and devaluation and alternating between overinvolvement and withdrawal	Negative affectivity: emotional lability, anxiousness, separation, hostility, depression Disinhibition: impulsivity, risk taking Antagonism: hostility
Narcissistic	Excessive reference to others for self-definition and self-esteem regulation; exaggerated self-appraisal inflated or deflated or vacillating between	Goal setting based on gaining approval from others; personal standards unreasonably high in order to see oneself as exceptional or too low based on a sense of entitlement; often unaware of own motivations	Impaired ability to recognize or identify with the feelings and needs of others; excessively attuned to reactions of others but only if perceived as relevant to self; overestimate or underestimate of own effect on others	Relationships largely superficial and exist to serve self-esteem regulation; mutuality constrained by little genuine interest in others' experiences and predominance of a need for personal gain	Antagonism: grandiosity, attention seeking

Obsessive-compulsive personality disorder	Sense of self derived predominantly from work or productivity; constricted experience and expression of	Difficulty completing tasks and realizing goals, associated with rigid and unreasonably high and inflexible internal standards of behavior; overly conscientious and moralistic attitudes	Difficulty understanding and appreciating the ideas, feelings, or behaviors of others	Relationships seen as secondary to work and productivity; rigidity and stubbornness negatively affect relationships with others	Compulsivity: rigid perfectionism Negative affectivity: perseveration
Schizotypal personality disorder	Confused boundaries between self and others; distorted self-concept; emotional expression often not congruent with context or internal experience	Unrealistic or incoherent goals; no clear set of internal standards	Pronounced difficulty understanding impact of own behaviors on others; frequent misinterpretations of others' motivations and behaviors	Marked impairments in developing close relationships, associated with mistrust and anxiety	Psychoticism: eccentricity, cognitive and perception dysregulation, unusual beliefs and experience Detachment: restricted affectivity, withdrawal Negative affectivity: suspiciousness

disorders: paranoid personality disorder, schizoid personality disorder, schizotypal personality disorder, antisocial personality disorder, borderline personality disorder, histrionic personality, narcissistic personality disorder, avoidant personality disorder, dependent personality disorder, and obsessive-compulsive personality disorder. Alternatively, the dimensional model for personality suggests assessing and diagnosing by measuring the level of functioning and pathologic traits. This model only sustains *6* personality disorder types: borderline personality disorder, obsessive-compulsive personality disorder, avoidant personality disorder, schizotypal personality disorder, antisocial personality disorder, narcissistic personality disorder and, lastly, personality disorder trait specified.[33]

The dimensional model suggests assessing and diagnosing by measuring the level of functioning and related traits. This model will allow using traits as helpful characteristics of strength in patients even if the person does/does not have a personality disorder. It is expected that some version of this model will eventually replace the current categorical model. There are 2 primary criteria (along with the usual requirement of stability across time, person, and place):

1. Level of functioning: Level of functioning is characterized by a degree of impairment in various areas (identity, self-direction, empathy, intimacy) and a level of impairment ranging from mild to extreme. For a personality disorder to be diagnosed, patients will have to meet the criteria of moderate to extreme impairment.
2. Personality traits: There is one or more personality traits characterized by a combination of maladaptive and adaptive traits in the following areas:
   - Negative affectivity (vs emotional stability)
   - Detachment (vs extraversion)
   - Antagonism (vs agreeableness)
   - Disinhibition (vs conscientiousness)
   - Psychoticism (vs lucidity)

In the ED setting, difficult patients may be prominently affected on one or more dimensions, even if a formal diagnosis of personality disorder is lacking. A common scenario for difficult patient interaction in the ED might be an intoxicated patient yelling at staff, refusing to answer questions, and using profanities, in a manner similar to prior presentations. When intoxication resolves, the patient yells again because he or she was given a sandwich, not a hot tray; the patient asks for an admission and claims no one can help but the inpatient facility. Such a patient would be rated high on negative affectivity, disinhibition, and antagonism, regardless of the actual personality disorder he or she could get diagnosed with. Therapeutic interventions could focus on the maladaptive areas.

Management of personality traits/disorders in the emergency department setting
Overall, the management of individuals with personality traits or disorders requires flexibility on behalf of providers and some modicum of being able to identify one's own emotions. The focus of treatment in nonpsychiatric settings, such as the ED, has a 2-fold goal, the first being avoiding harmful or difficult-to-handle emotional escalations. The second is to avoid personality traits/disorders that interfere with medical treatment. Two major steps facilitate interview and history taking:

1. Obtain a thorough history and provide clear and comprehensive information about treatment; allow patients to be part of the treatment plan: The aim is to have an objective, calm, efficient, and productive interview. Distractions are expected in different forms. In patients with cluster B traits, dramatic comments are often interjected and superfluous and off-topic details can be added. Interviews with these

patients may easily escalate into tears or accusations of the provider not caring, not helping, and so forth, which can greatly slow down the gathering of necessary medical information. Patients with cluster C traits, anxious and worried, may impede the progress of the interview by excessively asking for reassurance and not giving decisive information or answers. On the other end of the spectrum, patients with cluster A traits may underreport symptoms and avoid further interview.

2. Express empathy to patients' fears or concerns: Even the most experienced clinician sometimes forgets that being in an ED is a stressful experience. Expressing empathy and validating the difficulty of the experience usually helps. However, common pitfalls occurring after validation include emotional outpouring, crying, or escalation (cluster B and C as well as drug-seeking patients, high utilizers) or an off-topic, even possibly psychotic or paranoid comment with patients in the cluster A personality group. In some cases, the presence of family may further complicate providing empathy and validation; it is recommended that providers be mindful of those aspects. Asking the family to leave in order to conduct the interview is a useful and sometimes underused tactic. Some patients have neither the medical lingo nor the knowledge to navigate a rushed care visit competently. In those cases, it is very common to witness escalation and misunderstandings in communication with providers. Patients may not ask for clarification of information they do not understand but react to that lack of or misunderstanding in a negative manner. A low-key, casual/modest approach may be helpful in eliciting trust and establishing effective communication. In many cases labeled difficult, patients are asking, requesting, or expecting interventions that are above and beyond the scope of the ED visit. Examples include patients with complicated social situations, such as homelessness; patients with chronic pain; and patients with poor family support. Stating calmly yet kindly that you, the provider, would love to help but cannot fix the aforementioned problem may help significantly in reducing the tension in the interview and allow progress in a more therapeutic direction (**Box 2**).

Countertransference

To improve therapeutic practices, Freud[39] introduced the concept of countertransference, which referred to the emotion or attitude induced in the provider toward patients. This induced emotion should not be considered synonymous or similar to a popular topic, cognitive bias. Cognitive bias refers to the preconceptions that an individual carries, which causes them to deviate from rational thought and and judgement.

Box 2
Summary of management tips for patients with suspected personality traits

- Respect patients' need to feel private.
- Be direct but be respectful of patients' beliefs.
- Set clear limits in interventions.
- Tolerate fluctuations but not full outbursts in patients' mood.
- Show concern for feelings yet focus on objective matters related to treatment.
- Be able to make patients participants in their care. Be factual to reported concerns.
- Exercise patience.
- Provide coping skills to anxiety.
- Provide consistent reassurance.

Bias usually describes the unnoticed actions and logic that can lead to a lack of critical thinking; this causes providers to pursue and treat am inaccurate diagnosis.[40] Countertransference (CT) creates its distinction through describing the mental state that is induced in the provider, whereas cognitive bias refers to the chronic preconceptions individuals possess about others.

The advantage of identifying and managing CT in emergency settings is to enable the physician to collect and analyze more information, which can ultimately lead to an accurate diagnosis and successful treatment. In the 1970s, CT was made relevant to psychiatric practice with a landmark article, "Taking Care of the Hateful Patient,"[41] which did not use the word *countertransference* specifically but espoused its principles. Groves[41] described 4 categories of patients who manipulate their physician into performing various tasks. This manipulation provides key insights into the patients' psyche, and practitioners should not abstain from incorporating this information into their diagnosis.

Groves[41] discusses a relevant stereotypical case that showcases the broad spectrum of situation CT proves useful. In the profile, he describes the "Entitled Demanders" that bully the physician into a role of constant support. These patients can threaten with litigation or with withholding payment to ensure they will not be abandoned by the physician. Without the physician recognizing this behavior, this type of patient can escalate and coerce the physician to practice defensive medicine. Such patients can be very common among high utilizers.

The authors' own data have shown that brief encounters, a few minutes in length, can be riddled with CT feelings that affect medical decision-making (Moukaddam and colleagues, in preparation). Thus, difficult patients in the ED, regardless of cause, can be overlooked or undertreated. The authors have hypothesized that brief interactions characteristic of modern health care encounters carry the same possibility of intense feelings. However, because short encounters do not bring about classic CT, the authors prefer to use the concept of instance CT.[42]

So how does this apply to personality traits and disorders?

Diagnosis of personality disorders often carries, quite intuitively, a judgmental connotation. Evidence suggests that personality disorders might be even more stigmatized than other psychiatric diagnoses. The belief that people with personality disorders should be able to exhibit control over behavior results in symptoms being viewed as manipulations or rejections of help. This can cause patients to be seen as difficult and misbehaving rather than sick. In fact, the public reacts less sympathetically to individuals described as having a personality disorder and is less likely to think these individuals need professional help than those with other psychiatric disorders, despite significant impairments these individuals experience.[43]

CT, as feelings evoked or experienced by providers,[44] can be described as *objective* (induced by patients' attitudes and behaviors) or *subjective* (stemming from provider experiences). The *subjective* feelings that health care providers tend to feel are typically long lasting, whereas objective feelings tend to be more transient and disappear quickly. The concern is that medical decisions are influenced by objective, transitional experiences.[45]

It is imperative that awareness of feelings toward patients is addressed as this might lead to consequences, such as misdiagnosing or preventing treatment. Research suggests that therapists' reactions may vary depending on the type of personality disorder they are treating,[46] though the patients' level of functioning was related to the type of CT experienced by the treating provider as well. Feeling criticized or mistreated was overall a characteristic when treating individuals with cluster A, whereas providers treating individuals with cluster B overall seemed to report feeling overwhelmed, inadequate, helpless, disorganized, and at times overinvolved with their patients. When it came to the feelings reported by providers treating individuals with cluster C, the most common reaction is seeing patients as vulnerable and in need of protection.[45]

In summary, difficult patients are a product of their environment and backgrounds and can sometimes be diagnosed with personality issues. A difficult patient interaction, however, can stem from patients, the provider, or the system in which the two meet. Ultimately, it is wise to focus on the end goal, a healthy encounter that results in a productive resolution of the health problem at hand.

REFERENCES

1. Castillo EM, Brennan JJ, Killeen JP, et al. Identifying frequent users of emergency department resources. J Emerg Med 2014;47(3):343–7.
2. Norman C, Mello M, Choi B. Identifying frequent users of an urban emergency medical service using descriptive statistics and regression analyses. West J Emerg Med 2016;17(1):39–45.
3. Blank FS, Li H, Henneman PL, et al. A descriptive study of heavy emergency department users at an academic emergency department reveals heavy ED users have better access to care than average users. J Emerg Nurs 2005; 31(2):139–44.
4. Robinson RL, Grabner M, Palli SR, et al. Covariates of depression and high utilizers of healthcare: impact on resource use and costs. J Psychosom Res 2016;85:35–43.
5. Barsky AJ, Orav EJ, Bates DW. Somatization increases medical utilization and costs independent of psychiatric and medical comorbidity. Arch Gen Psychiatry 2005;62(8):903–10.
6. Harris LJ, Graetz I, Podila PS, et al. Characteristics of hospital and emergency care super-utilizers with multiple chronic conditions. J Emerg Med 2016;50(4): e203–14.
7. Pasic J, Russo J, Roy-Byrne P. High utilizers of psychiatric emergency services. Psychiatr Serv 2005;56(6):678–84.
8. Murphy JG, Fenichel GS, Jacobson S. Psychiatry in the emergency department: factors associated with treatment and disposition. Am J Emerg Med 1984;2(4): 309–14.
9. Santy PA, Wehmeier PK. Using "problem patient" rounds to help emergency room staff manage difficult patients. Hosp Community Psychiatry 1984;35(5):494–6.
10. Schwartz SR, Goldfinger SM. The new chronic patient: clinical characteristics of an emerging subgroup. Hosp Community Psychiatry 1981;32(7):470–4.
11. Malone RE. Almost 'like family': emergency nurses and 'frequent flyers'. J Emerg Nurs 1996;22(3):176–83.
12. Millard WB. Grounding frequent flyers, not abandoning them: drug seekers in the ED. Ann Emerg Med 2007;49(4):481–6.
13. Maunder RG, Panzer A, Viljoen M, et al. Physicians' difficulty with emergency department patients is related to patients' attachment style. Soc Sci Med 2006; 63(2):552–62.
14. Lin CS, Hsu MY, Chong CF. Differences between emergency patients and their doctors in the perception of physician empathy: implications for medical education. Edu Health (Abingdon) 2008;21(2):144.

15. Mautner DB, Pang H, Brenner JC, et al. Generating hypotheses about care needs of high utilizers: lessons from patient interviews. Popul Health Manag 2013; 16(Suppl 1):S26–33.
16. Mercer T, Bae J, Kipnes J, et al. The highest utilizers of care: individualized care plans to coordinate care, improve healthcare service utilization, and reduce costs at an academic tertiary care center. J Hosp Med 2015;10(7):419–24.
17. Gross K, Brenner JC, Truchil A, et al. Building a citywide, all-payer, hospital claims database to improve health care delivery in a low-income, urban community. Popul Health Manag 2013;16(Suppl 1):S20–5.
18. Mackelprang JL, Collins SE, Clifasefi SL. Housing First is associated with reduced use of emergency medical services. Prehosp Emerg Care 2014;18(4): 476–82.
19. Kurdyak P, Newman A, Segal Z. Impact of mindfulness-based cognitive therapy on health care utilization: a population-based controlled comparison. J Psychosom Res 2014;77(2):85–9.
20. Perechocky A, DeLisser H, Ciampa R, et al. Piloting a medical student observational experience with hospital-based trauma chaplains. J Surg Educ 2014;71(1): 91–5.
21. Levy R, Gale MS. Interactional approach to the difficult emergency department patient. JACEP 1977;6(1):7–9.
22. Hawton K, Witt KG, Taylor Salisbury TL, et al. Psychosocial interventions for self-harm in adults. Cochrane Database Syst Rev 2016;(5):CD012189.
23. Moukaddam N, AufderHeide E, Flores A, et al. Shift, interrupted: strategies for managing difficult patients including those with personality disorders and somatic symptoms in the emergency department. Emerg Med Clin North Am 2015;33(4):797–810.
24. Super-utilizers get red carpet treatment. Hosp Case Manag 2014;22(1):4–5.
25. Bell J, Breslin JM. Healthcare provider moral distress as a leadership challenge. JONAS Healthc Law Ethics Regul 2008;10(4):94–7 [quiz: 98–9].
26. Weberg D. Transformational leadership and staff retention: an evidence review with implications for healthcare systems. Nurs Adm Q 2010;34(3):246–58.
27. Liu SW, Nagurney JT, Chang Y, et al. Frequent ED users: are most visits for mental health, alcohol, and drug-related complaints? Am J Emerg Med 2013;31(10): 1512–5.
28. Hong V. Borderline personality disorder in the emergency department: good psychiatric management. Harv Rev Psychiatry 2016;24(5):357–66.
29. Piatt EE, Munetz MR, Ritter C. An examination of premature mortality among decedents with serious mental illness and those in the general population. Psychiatr Serv 2010;61(7):663–8.
30. Sachdeva A, Chandra M, Choudhary M, et al. Alcohol-related dementia and neurocognitive impairment: a review study. Int J High Risk Behav Addict 2016;5(3): e27976.
31. Verdejo-Garcia A, Chong TT, Stout JC, et al. Stages of dysfunctional decision-making in addiction. Pharmacol Biochem Behav 2017. [Epub ahead of print].
32. Tucci V, Laufman L, Peacock WF, et al. Epic fail! poor neuropsychiatric documentation practices in emergency psychiatric patients. Emerg Med (Los Angel) 2016;6:332.
33. Insel TR. Assessing the economic costs of serious mental illness. Am J Psychiatry 2008;165(6):663–5.
34. Dingfelder SF. Treatment for the 'untreatable'. Monitor on psychology, vol. 35. Washington, DC: American Psychological Association; 2004. p. 46.

35. Diagnostic and statistical manual of mental disorders: DSM-5, fifth edition. Washington, DC: American Psychiatric Publishing; 2013.
36. Links PS, Eynan R. The relationship between personality disorders and axis I psychopathology: deconstructing comorbidity. Annu Rev Clin Psychol 2013;9: 529–54.
37. Saß H. Personality disorders. In: Smelser NJ, Baltes PB, editors. International encyclopedia of social & behavioral sciences. 1st edition. Oxford: Pergamon; 2001. p. 11301–8.
38. Perry JC, Banon E, Ianni F. Effectiveness of psychotherapy for personality disorders. Am J Psychiatry 1999;156(9):1312–21.
39. Freud S. The future prospect of psychoanalytic therapy. Standard edition. London: Hogarth Press; 1910.
40. Elissa Lin Rathe PD. Transference and countertransference from a modern psychoanalytic perspective. Paper presented at the National Association of Clinical Social Workers Convention. Orlando (FL), March 13-14, 2008.
41. Groves JE. Taking care of the hateful patient. N Engl J Med 1978;298(16):883–7.
42. Moukaddam N, Tucci V, Galwankar S, et al. In the blink of an eye: instant countertransference and its application in modern healthcare. J Emerg Trauma Shock 2016;9(3):95–6.
43. Sheehan L, Nieweglowski K, Corrigan P. The stigma of personality disorders. Curr Psychiatry Rep 2016;18(1):11.
44. Handbook of evidence-based psychodynamic psychotherapy: bridging the gap between science and practice. In: Levy RA, Ablon JS, editors. New York: Humana Press; 2009.
45. Colli A, Tanzilli A, Dimaggio G, et al. Patient personality and therapist response: an empirical investigation. Am J Psychiatry 2014;171(1):102–8.
46. Strous RD, Ulman AM, Kotler M. The hateful patient revisited: relevance for 21st century medicine. Eur J Intern Med 2006;17(6):387–93.

A Modern-Day Fight Club? The Stabilization and Management of Acutely Agitated Patients in the Emergency Department

Andrew New, MD, MS[a,*], Veronica Theresa Tucci, MD, JD[b], Juan Rios, MD[c]

KEYWORDS

- Altered mental status • Emergency psychiatry • Treatment • Evaluation
- Management • Agitation • De-escalation

KEY POINTS

- For those who work in an emergency department, agitated patients present a unique challenge of balancing treatment, diagnosis, and patient and staff safety.
- All efforts should be made to maximize patient autonomy while maintaining a safe environment. Medical issues need to be ruled out and triaged appropriately to prevent a delay in diagnosis and/or treatment.
- Verbal de-escalation should be viewed as the gold standard of care, and practitioners should be trained in its implementation and be encouraged to adopt a method that is suitable to their style of practice and their patient population.
- Verbal techniques should include the offering of environmental changes and medications when indicated.

INTRODUCTION

Welcome to Fight Club. The first rule of Fight Club is, you do not talk about Fight Club. The second rule of Fight Club is, you DO NOT talk about Fight Club. The third rule of Fight Club is, someone yells stop, goes limp, taps out, and the fight is over.

It is 3 AM, the devil's hour. All the beds are full and the charts are starting to stack up in the rack. There are more than 20 people and counting in the waiting room when you

---

Disclosures: Nothing to disclose.

[a] Jackson Memorial Hospital System, 1695 Northwest 9th Avenue, Office 3100, Miami, FL 33136, USA; [b] Merit Health Wesley, Department of Emergency Medicine, 5001 Hardy Street, Hattiesburg, MS 39402, USA; [c] University of Miami Miller School of Medicine, 1695 Northwest 9th Avenue, Office 3100, Miami, FL 33136, USA

* Corresponding author.

E-mail address: andrew.new@jhsmiami.org

Psychiatr Clin N Am 40 (2017) 397–410
http://dx.doi.org/10.1016/j.psc.2017.05.002 psych.theclinics.com
0193-953X/17/© 2017 Elsevier Inc. All rights reserved.

hear overhead *code green: security respond to triage stat* followed by unintelligible screaming. You turn the corner and see 3 burly security guards and 2 nurses struggling to put a 30-something man on a gurney in the resuscitation bay. The patient responds with a sea of profanity, and one of the nurses looks at you and asks, "What do you want to do, doctor?"

This scene plays out each and every weekend and weeknight in emergency departments (EDs) across the country. Dealing with acutely agitated patients can make overworked and beleaguered ED staff feel as if they have gone multiple rounds in a street fight and at any moment either they or their patients will go limp or tap out. For emergency personnel, both prospects are equally terrifying as you never know what is coming in the door next and when you have to jump back in the ring.

Altered mental state (AMS) is a common presentation in the ED, perhaps as high as 10% of chief complaints in some locations.[1] The term is still loosely defined, has no standardized definition,[2] and can embody a multitude of medical and psychiatric pathologies.[3] Taking care of patients with AMS is further complicated when patients are acutely agitated. Such agitation increases the risk of harm to both patients and staff.[4] The emergence of agitation can occur in various stages of the evaluation and treatment process. Agitation itself is a symptom of some underlying cause, including medical disorders, psychiatric conditions, chemical ingestion, or even social factors. It is often the patients' response to perceived external stimulus and can indicate a plethora of internal emotions from fear to confusion to anger. The trained clinician will need to be proficient in assessing multiple causative factors while triaging and treating patients on a medical and psychiatric basis. This article specifically focuses on patients who initially present in an agitated state, and it follows the various stages as an encounter would unfold in the ED. **Fig. 1** demonstrates the stages an encounter might take.

PATIENT INTAKE

It is of value to consider how these patients will present in an effort to anticipate what measures should be taken. To present agitated, they were most likely escorted by either ambulance or police and are likely to already be in restraints. When transported by ambulance, patients may be from another hospital, a long-term care facility, or from a 911 call, increasing suspicions of medical comorbidities and requiring possible sources for collateral information. When brought by the police, concerns should be increased for the presence of psychotic disorders, substance abuse, and poor social functioning.[5] Police attempt to attenuate bizarre or inappropriate behaviors that are possibly suggestive of intoxication or psychosis and bring them to an ED or psychiatric facility instead of a police station. Police intervention may exacerbate agitation because of thoughts of arrest, loss of belongings, or forced medical treatment. Regardless of the mode of transportation, one should be cognizant of the level of force that may have been used before arrival.

GATHERING COLLATERAL INFORMATION

When agitated patients present, it is important for one member of the team to gather whatever information is possible while the patient transporter is still present. These individuals may need to immediately return to work after dropping off patients and may be unaware of what specifics would be of most value. Minimal time can be spent to learn valuable information that could greatly enhance management and may be lost at the patient hand-off. Senior staff may also be knowledgeable in the situation if

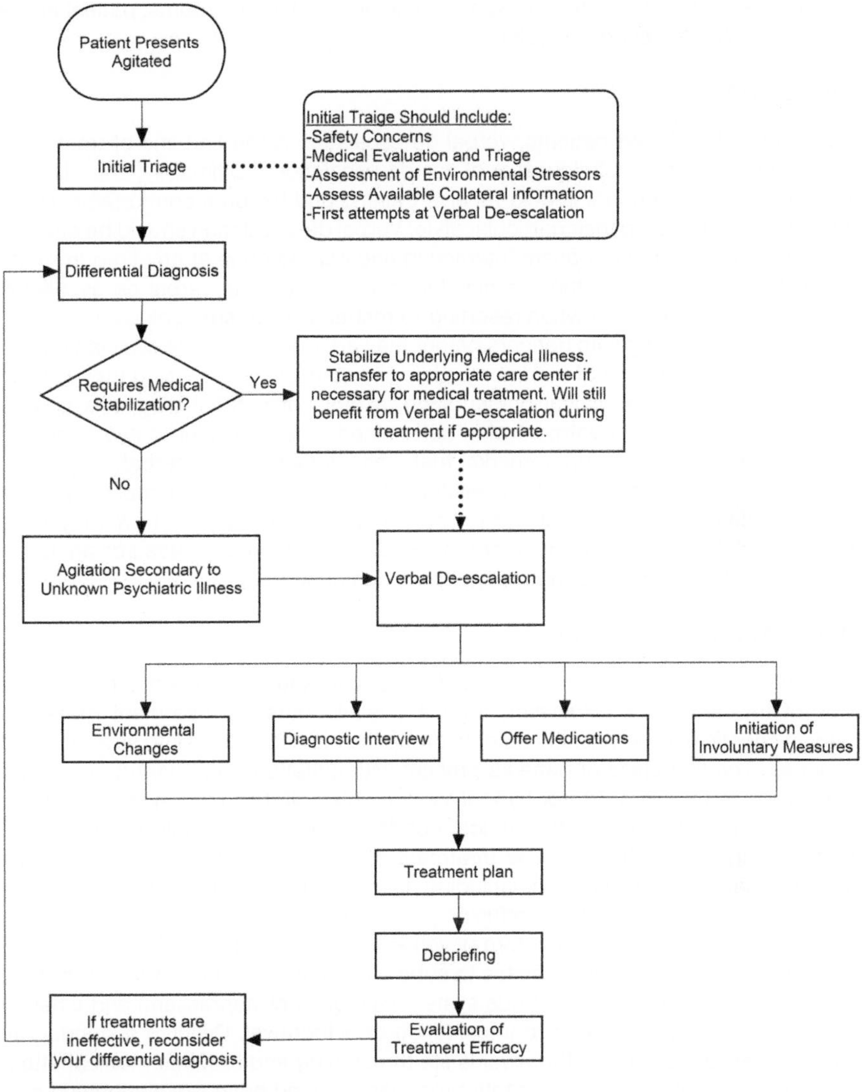

Fig. 1. Patient presents agitated.

patients are known to the unit. Electronic medical records can also provide quick access to previous documented encounters and interventions.

SAFETY CONCERNS

Once it is known agitated patients will be brought into the ED, attention should immediately be given to initial safety concerns. A safe location should be available to gather initial vital signs. This space should be devoid of other patients, medical supplies, and loose objects, which may become weapons in the hands of patients. Ample space can allow for patients to feel less trapped. Elopement is always a concern; precautions should be taken to prevent this, including locked units, seclusion rooms, patient attendants, and, as a last resort, restraints.

INITIAL CONTACT

On contact with agitated patients, verbal de-escalation is the first line of treatment. Various methods and techniques exist for de-escalation.[6] Ultimately, the clinician and ancillary staff members should receive training and become comfortable with a method that is suitable to their particular style. Verbal de-escalation should be attempted in the first moments of patient interaction and can be done at any time from the ambulance to the triage to the examination room. Successful verbal de-escalation usually takes less time than when resorting to restraints or pharmacologic therapies.

By verbally interacting with patients before they are medicated, the clinician can increase the patients' sense of autonomy while simultaneously assessing their level of agitation. Based on the clinical presentation, a rapid differential diagnosis can be formulated and an initial treatment plan determined. It is important to avoid the use of threats or condescending remarks that can worsen or exacerbate agitation. When progressing past verbal de-escalation, it is important to remember a portion of patients can recall details of the encounter and will remember how they were treated. Thus, it is constructive to inform patients why involuntary measures are being used and what behavioral actions they should demonstrate.

INITIAL DIAGNOSTIC CONCERNS

The differential diagnosis for agitation is diverse, and a full discussion is beyond the scope of this article.[3,7–9] However, as it applies to potential treatment measures including chemical anxiolysis, the authors group the causes of AMS into several broad categories. The first class of patients present with agitation secondary to a medical illness, such as thyroid storm or hypoglycemia. This agitation may even result in an agitated delirium. Patients with medical conditions must be rapidly identified and the underlying caused treated. The treatment of such conditions may obviate care in the psychiatric setting. Causes, including fluid and electrolyte disturbances, infections, metabolic disorders, low perfusion states, and medication side effects, may all require medical stabilization before psychiatric treatment (**Table 1**).

The second group of causes relates to substance use. It can be further subdivided into its impact on the central nervous system (stimulant or depressant) and whether the current presentation is due to intoxication or withdrawal. Delirium secondary to alcohol or benzodiazepine withdrawal is life threatening and requires medical attention. Chronic use of these depressants produces reduced brain γ-aminobutyric acid (GABA) levels and increased $GABA_A$-receptor sensitivity resulting in hyperactivity through decreased inhibition. Chronic use also induces increased function of N-methyl-D-aspartate receptors potentiating the seizure-inducing effects of increased glutamate.[10] Screening questionnaires and a rapid breathalyzer can assess the current level of intoxication and likelihood of withdrawal symptoms, including seizures or delirium tremens. Individuals exhibiting clinical symptoms of withdrawal despite an elevated blood alcohol level indicates chronic use and should be closely monitored with appropriate detox measures and pharmaceutical interventions.[11]

The 2 remaining main groups, primary psychiatric disturbance and nonpsychiatric behavioral disturbance, may require less acute medical services but still pose an immediate and potential risk of harm to self or others. These patients ultimately may go on to require a full medical workup, but transfer to a medical service in the acute sense is often unwarranted. The capacity for these patients to cooperate and attenuate to

Table 1
A differential diagnosis of altered mental status

Neurologic	CVA/TIA, ICH/SDH/epidural/SAH, delirium, tumor, dementia
Cardiac	ACS, CHF, CMO, arrhythmia, pericarditis, myocarditis, endocarditis
Vascular	Aortic dissection, AAA, mesenteric ischemia, carotid stenosis, VBI
Pulmonary	PNA, PE, pleural effusion; low suspicion for pneumothorax, hemothorax, rib fracture
GI	GIB, gastritis, PUD, Boerhaave /Mallory-Weiss tear, pneumoperitoneum, colitis, diverticulitis, appendicitis.
GU	UTI, pyelonephritis, infected stone
Toxicology/medication	Medication side effect, intentional vs accidental overdose, poisoning
Endocrine	Thyroid storm, myxedema, Addisonian crisis, myasthenia crisis
Electrolyte	Hyponatremia/hypernatremia, Hypocalcemia/hypercalcemia, and so forth
Infectious	Sepsis secondary to UTI/PNA/ulcer; any infectious process
Environmental	Heat vs cold emergencies, dehydration, sun exposure
Psychiatric	Primary psychiatric illness, psychosis, substance use/withdrawal, personality disorder, secondary gain

Abbreviations: AAA, abdominal aortic aneurysm; ACS, acute coronary syndromes; CHF, congestive heart failure; CMO, cardiomyopathy; CVA, cerebrovascular accident; GI, gastrointestinal; GIB, gastrointestinal bleed; GU, genitourinary; ICH, intracerebral hemorrhage; PE, pulmonary embolism; PNA, pneumonia; PUD, peptic ulcer disease; SAH, subarachnoid hemorrhage; SDH, subdural hemorrhage; TIA, transient ischemic attack; UTI, urinary tract infection; VBI, vertebrobasilar ischemia.

the interview will influence the degree to which verbal de-escalation can be implemented.

Various clinical instruments have been developed to assess for delirium, including the Delirium Rating Scale,[12] Confusion Assessment Method (CAM),[13,14] Memorial Delirium Assessment Scale,[15,16] Delirium Symptom Interview,[17,18] and Confusional State Evaluation Scale.[19] These scales can take 1 to 10 minutes on average and in some instances, such as with the CAM, can be 94% to 100% sensitive and 90% to 95% specific in identifying delirium as the most probable diagnosis.[20] Individuals with delirium often display decreased attention and cognition with visual hallucinations that fluctuate in severity making verbally interventions less efficacious.

EVALUATING AGITATION

Agitation can be viewed as an extreme state of arousal that leads to excessive verbal and motor activity. It can be grossly divided into aggressive and nonaggressive varieties. Examples of aggressive behaviors include screaming, fighting, destruction of property, and self-harm. Nonaggressive behaviors can include pacing, impulsivity, rocking, restlessness, wandering, repetitive behaviors, hyperverbal speech, and the recurrent need for redirection. Multiple scales have been developed to assess for the level of agitation depending on the skill of the practitioner and the location of the evaluation (**Box 1**). The common elements to these scales include an emphasis on observation of behaviors, ability for patients to respond to simple commands, level of consciousness, and ability to attenuate the interview. Severe agitation requires rapid treatment and may necessitate the use of involuntary measures. If patients are

Box 1
Scales for evaluating agitation

Agitation Behavior Mapping Instrument[21]

Behavioral Activity Rating Scale[22]

Cohen-Mansfield Agitation Inventory[23]

Overt Agitation Severity Scale[24]

Pittsburgh Agitation Scale[25]

Richmond Agitation-Sedation Scale[26]

Riker Sedation-Agitation Scale[27]

able to cooperate with an interview, a thorough history should be gathered as in a standard psychiatric evaluation.

OFFERING ENVIRONMENTAL CHANGES

If patients are communicable but still agitated, it is advantageous to offer a suitable location for the encounter. Depending on the layout of your facility, other patients might be present during the encounter and witness how it develops. Their perception of the event can be impactful to a therapeutic alliance, especially if coercion or involuntary measures are used. Attempts at verbal de-escalation can demonstrate the staff's dedication to patient autonomy and improve the perceptions of the medical team. Lastly, those patients with secondary gain may witness the encounter and mimic specific behaviors with the aim of receiving medication or gaining admittance.

If patients are presenting agitated, they can be triaged and evaluated in a suitable seclusion room. However, if patients become agitated while in a waiting area, offering a location change at the onset can prevent incidental harm to staff and other patients. It is also important to evaluate if the encounter zone has enough space for additional staff should the situation call for it.

Beyond location, environmental changes can include a variety of elements. Decreasing the amount of ambient noise, dimming the lights, offering oral hydration, or adjusting the temperature can all be beneficial.[28] Some patients displaying paranoia may prefer additional light or prefer specific positioning within a room. In areas with low socioeconomic status and high rates of homelessness, providing sustenance can often be beneficial. The ability of patients to entertain these options indicates how cooperative they can be and may suggest the agitation is behavioral or situational in nature.

OFFERING MEDICATIONS

Once medications are indicated, it is important to involve patients in the process. As their personal bias toward medications is unknown, initial probing questions are of benefit. Secondary to their presentation, a full triage may not have been completed and a medication allergy review is warranted. Then various persuasive strategies can be used with an aim of maximizing patient autonomy. Educating patients on the potential rate of onset may lead them to choose an injection over an oral medication. Providing additional information as to what effects (sedation, anxiolysis, antipsychotic) and average onset may also help comfort patients. Coercion should be used as a last resort as it begins to infringe on the rights of the individual.

It is important to consider the environmental factors that might impact the initiation of pharmacotherapy. Fatigued staff may push for additional sedation, resulting in less management issues. Previous encounters with the same patient may also lead staff to experience anecdotal fears and preconceptions of anticipated patient behavior. Conversely, a previous history of violence is an important risk factor and predictor of future violence and should be incorporated into risk assessments. Pharmacotherapy resulting in excess sedation may also lengthen the total amount of time patients spend in the ED.

MEDICATIONS TO CONSIDER

When determining which medications to offer, multiple elements need to be considered, including but not limited to patient factors (age, past medical/psychiatric history, pregnancy, allergies, current medications, medication tolerance), environmental factors (rate of onset, route of administration, availability of medications), and medication profile (method of action, level of sedation, adverse side effects). A wide variety of medications have been demonstrated as efficacious in various situations (**Table 2**). These medications can be used to target underlying causes of agitation in some specific instances, though may attenuate agitation regardless of cause secondary to common pathways.[29] In agitation, abnormal neurotransmitter levels and dysfunctional neuronal activity can occur in dopamine, glutamate, serotonin, and GABA signaling,[30] creating multiple theorized targets for treatment. Recommendations for treatment based on diagnostic assessment are demonstrated in **Fig. 2**.

Various routes of administration have been developed, each with their own pros and cons. Almost all of the medications are available in an oral formulation. It has equal efficacy in the treatment of agitation and minimal time disadvantage compared with intramuscular preparations.[31] Oral medications can be susceptible to diversionary tactics. If this is a concern, dissolvable preparations can be considered. Intravenous options, common in medical-surgical patients, can be used for rapid effect but demonstrate no benefit after 3 hours[32] and come with the risk of leaving a line in agitated patients. Intramuscular agents should be considered second line.[30] They have beneficial properties, including increased bioavailability and rapid absorption. However, these medications are costlier than their oral counterparts and may be viewed as a greater incursion on patient autonomy.[33] Recently, inhaled oral formulations have been developed for use, and recent studies have begun to evaluate safety and efficacy.[34]

First-generation antipsychotics (FGAs) have an established history of use in the treatment of agitation. Haloperidol (Haldol) has been demonstrated in numerous studies and is widely used. Recent studies have suggested use of second-generation antipsychotics (SGAs) based on equal efficacy and reduced rates of extrapyramidal symptoms. In patients with alcohol withdrawal, GABAergic medications, such as benzodiazepines, can be used to reduce aberrant autonomic instability.

Combinations of haloperidol, lorazepam, and diphenhydramine are widely used for agitation,[35,36] though they may lead to excess sedation.[37] Minimizing extrapyramidal symptoms, by use of an SGA or combining an FGA with diphenhydramine or benzodiazepines, may also contribute to increased medication compliance and motivation to continue treatment. Recent studies have begun to study the efficacy of ketamine for treatment of agitation, as it has regular use in the ED for procedural sedation.[38,39] Ketamine has been associated with an increased risk of intubation compared with Haldol[40] but has been effective in treating agitation.[41,42] Ketamine may also require

Table 2
Specific medications for treatment of agitation by class

Medication Class	Medication	Routes of Administration: Oral (mg)	IM (mg)	IV (mg)	Inhaled (mg)	Maximum (mg/d)	Adverse Effects
First-generation antipsychotic	Haloperidol	5–10	2.5–5.0	2.5–5.0	—	100	EPS, dystonia, tardive dyskinesia
	Thiothixene	5–10	10–20	—	—	60	EPS, hypotension, irregular menses
	Droperidol	—	2.5–5.0	—	—	5	QT prolongation
	Loxapine	25	10–15	—	10	100	Seizures, agranulocytosis, hypotension
	Chlorpromazine	100	50	—	—	1000	Agranulocytosis, hypotension
Second-generation antipsychotic	Olanzapine	2.5–5.0	2.5–10.0	—	—	30	Orthostatic hypotension, metabolic dysfunction
	Aripiprazole	9.75	10–30	—	—	30	Weight gain, headache, insomnia, nausea
	Risperidone	2–3	—	—	—	16	Similar to typical antipsychotics
	Ziprasidone	40–160	10–20	—	—	40	Similar to typical antipsychotics
Benzodiazepines	Lorazepam	1–2	0.5–1.0	—	—	10	Respiratory depression
	Diazepam	5–10	—	—	—	40	Respiratory depression
Antihistamines	Diphenhydramine	25–50	25–50	—	—	300	Anticholinergic, sedation

Abbreviations: EPS, extrapyramidal symptoms; IM, intramuscular; IV, intravenous.

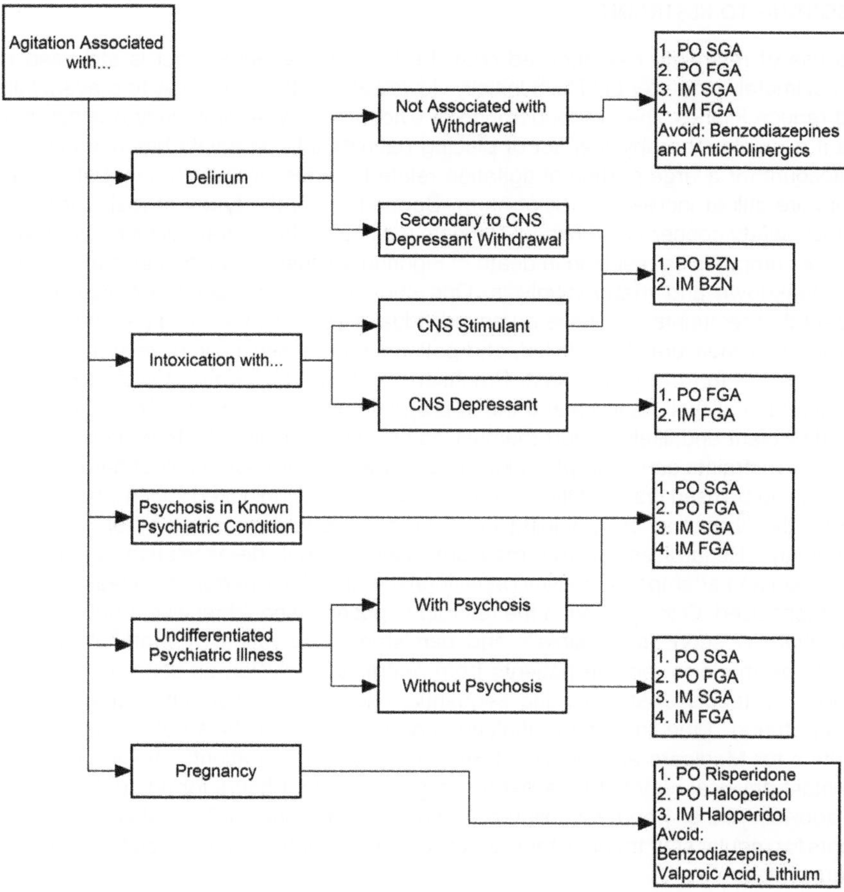

Fig. 2. Indications and protocol for pharmacotherapy of agitation. BZN, Benzodiazepine; CNS, central nervous system; FGA, first generation antipsychotic; IM, intramuscular; PO, oral; SGA, second generation antipsychotic. (*Data from* Roffman JL, Stern TA. Alcohol withdrawal in the setting of elevated blood alcohol levels. Primary Care Companion to The Journal of Clinical Psychiatry 2006;8(3):170–3.)

additional treatment in a large portion of patients.[41] Ketamine can exacerbate schizophrenia and should be avoided in patients with this condition.[43]

The minimal effective dose should be used when treating special populations, including elderly, pregnant, and pediatric patients, as no medication has been found to be truly safe. In the elderly, no more than half of the normal starting dose should be used. Olanzapine is often used in the elderly, as it is the SGA with the lowest risk of hypotension and lacks the common side effects of FGA. In pregnant patients, Haldol is commonly used as first-line treatment despite associations with cleft palates, micromelia, and malformations of skeletal muscle and the central nervous system.[44–49] Risperdal has been shown to have no known teratogenic effects[50,51]; it is a suitable oral option, especially in the first trimester. Medications such as valproic acid,[52–54] lithium,[55–58] and carbamazepine[59,60] should be avoided in pregnant patients secondary to known teratogenic effects, especially in the first trimester.

RESORTING TO RESTRAINTS

The use of restraints has declined over the last few decades[61] but is still used in approximately a quarter of EDs.[62] Initially viewed as an efficacious way to prevent falls and reduce injuries, the preponderance of evidence now recommends against their use if possible. The physical act of placing patients into restraints has been shown to account for a large portion of agitation-related injuries. While in the restraints, patients are still at increased risk of harm. Depending on the types of restraint used, various safety concerns are raised. Patients may suffer from strangulation, asphyxiation, or compression resulting in death.[63] Fighting against restraints can lead to muscle breakdown and rhabdomyolysis. One should also consider the psychological impact that restraints may have on an individual and the surrounding patients.[64]

If all other measures have failed, and patients require seclusion or restraint, determining which form to use is next. Practitioners should be aware of what measures are available at their facilities and the appropriate use of those measures. If patients remain violent and likely to hurt themselves or others despite all other interventions, physical restraints can be applied. However, if patients are not at risk of harm, seclusion should be used first.[65] Patients may be in a locked or unlocked seclusion depending on the likelihood of remaining in seclusion and willingness to enter seclusion voluntarily. Regardless of the measure used, verbal de-escalation should be continued and attempts to convey behavioral modifications warranting release should be emphasized. Once placed in the restraints, patients should receive a physical examination as soon as possible[66] and persistent observation by staff.[67,68] Efforts should be made to remove patients from restraints/seclusion as soon as possible. Various protocols exist regarding sequential release from restraints depending on the institution. Time limits and regulations on use of restraints is determined by the Centers for Medicare and Medicaid Services. They state patients should remain in constant physical restraint for a period no greater than 4 hours for an adult, 2 hours for adolescents, or 1 hour for children younger than 9 years old. They also list requirements for regular staff training, reporting of adverse events, and the need for adequate documentation.

DEBRIEFING

After treatment has been initiated, it is important to debrief all parties involved. This debriefing can encompass staff, the treated patient, and those patients who witnessed the event. Staff debriefing is important for continual efforts to improve care. This debrief can be short or extensive, time permitting, but should include a discussion of the case presentation, differential diagnosis, treatment plan, disposition, areas for improvement, appropriate documentation, and possible emotional impacts the event may have had. Discussions with patients can help direct future behaviors, establish appropriate expectations, and foster an environment of safety. This discussion is especially important when patient or environmental factors led to the most extreme limitations on patient autonomy, including physical restraints and forced chemical anxiolysis.

SUMMARY

For those who work in an ED, agitated patients present a unique challenge of balancing treatment, diagnosis, and patient and staff safety. All efforts should be made to maximize patient autonomy while maintaining a safe environment. Medical issues need to be ruled out and triaged appropriately to prevent a delay in diagnosis and/or treatment. Verbal de-escalation should be viewed as the gold standard of care, and practitioners should be trained in its implementation and be encouraged to adopt a method that is suitable to their style of practice and their patient population. Verbal techniques should include the offering of environmental changes and medications when indicated. Patients should be informed of the treatment plan and what behavioral modifications should take place to prevent future behaviors. Involuntary restraints should be viewed as a last resort, and their use should be closely monitored. The management of agitated patients and the treatment outcome is subject to a litany of factors; only through close observation, reflection, study, and further education can we continue to improve.

REFERENCES

1. Xiao H. Evaluation and treatment of altered mental status patients in the emergency department: life in the fast lane. World J Emerg Med 2012;3(4):270.
2. Morandi A, Pandharipande P, Trabucchi M, et al. Understanding international differences in terminology for delirium and other types of acute brain dysfunction in critically ill patients. Intensive Care Med 2008;34(10):1907–15.
3. Kanich W, Brady W, Huff J, et al. Altered mental status: evaluation and etiology in the ED. Am J Emerg Med 2002;20(7):613–7.
4. Gacki-Smith J, Juarez A, Boyett L, et al. Violence against nurses working in us emergency departments. J Nurs Adm 2009;39(7–8):340–9.
5. Dhossche D, Ghani S. Who brings patients to the psychiatric emergency room? Gen Hosp Psychiatry 1998;20(4):235–40.
6. Richmond J, Berlin J, Fishkind A, et al. Verbal de-escalation of the agitated patient: consensus statement of the American Association for Emergency Psychiatry Project BETA de-escalation workgroup. West J Emerg Med 2012;13(1):17–25.
7. Han JH, Wilber ST. Altered mental status in older patients in the emergency department. Clin Geriatr Med 2013;29(1):101–36.
8. Wilber ST, Ondrejka JE. Altered mental status and delirium. Emerg Med Clin North Am 2016;34(3):649–65.
9. Joseph J, Kennedy M, Mattu A, et al. Altered mental status in the elderly. Geriatric emergencies: a discussion-based review. Hoboken (NJ): John Wiley & Sons; 2016.
10. Trevisan LA, Boutros N, Petrakis IL, et al. Complications of alcohol withdrawal: pathophysiological insights. Alcohol Health Res World 1998;22(1):61–6.
11. Roffman JL, Stern TA. Alcohol withdrawal in the setting of elevated blood alcohol levels. Prim Care Companion J Clin Psychiatry 2006;8(3):170–3.
12. Trzepacz PT. Validation of the delirium rating scale-revised-98: comparison with the delirium rating scale and the cognitive test for delirium. J Neuropsychiatry 2001;13(2):229–42.
13. Ely EW, Margolin R, Francis J, et al. Evaluation of delirium in critically ill patients: validation of the Confusion Assessment Method for the Intensive Care Unit (CAM-ICU). Crit Care Med 2001;29(7):1370–9.
14. Inouye SK, Van Dyck CH, Alessi CA, et al. Clarifying confusion: the confusion assessment method: a new method for detection of delirium. Ann Intern Med 1990;113(12):941–8.
15. Breitbart W, Rosenfeld B, Roth A, et al. The memorial delirium assessment scale. J Pain Symptom Manage 1997;13(3):128–37.

16. Lawlor PG, Nekolaichuk C, Gagnon B, et al. Clinical utility, factor analysis, and further validation of the Memorial Delirium Assessment Scale in patients with advanced cancer. Cancer 2000;88(12):2859–67.
17. Albert MS, Levkoff SE, Reilly C, et al. The delirium symptom interview: an interview for the detection of delirium symptoms in hospitalized patients. J Geriatr Psychiatry Neurol 1992;5(1):14–21.
18. Trzepacz PT, Mittal D, Torres R, et al. Validation of the Delirium Rating Scale-revised-98: comparison with the delirium rating scale and the cognitive test for delirium. J Neuropsychiatry Clin Neurosci 2001;13(2):229–42.
19. Grover S. Assessment scales for delirium: a review. World J Psychiatry 2012;2(4): 58.
20. Wei LA, Fearing MA, Sternberg EJ, et al. The confusion assessment method: a systematic review of current usage. J Am Geriatr Soc 2008;56(5):823–30.
21. Choy CNP, Lam LCW, Chan WC, et al. Agitation in Chinese elderly: validation of the Chinese version of the Cohen-Mansfield Agitation Inventory. Int Psychogeriatr 2001;13(03):325–35.
22. Swift RH, Harrigan EP, Cappelleri JC, et al. Validation of the behavioural activity rating scale (BARS)™: a novel measure of activity in agitated patients. J Psychiatr Res 2002;36(2):87–95.
23. Finkel SI, Lyons JS, Anderson RL. Reliability and validity of the Cohen–Mansfield agitation inventory in institutionalized elderly. Int J Geriatr Psychiatry 1992;7(7): 487–90.
24. Kunik M. The Overt Agitation Severity Scale for the objective rating of agitation. Neuroscience 1997;9:541–8.
25. Rosen J, Burgio L, Kollar M, et al. The Pittsburgh agitation scale: a user-friendly instrument for rating agitation in dementia patients. Am J Geriatr Psychiatry 1995; 2(1):52–9.
26. Sessler CN, Gosnell MS, Grap MJ, et al. The Richmond Agitation–Sedation Scale: validity and reliability in adult intensive care unit patients. Am J Respir Crit Care Med 2002;166(10):1338–44.
27. Khan BA, Guzman O, Campbell NL, et al. Comparison and agreement between the Richmond Agitation-Sedation Scale and the Riker Sedation-Agitation Scale in evaluating patients' eligibility for delirium assessment in the ICU. Chest J 2012; 142(1):48–54.
28. Freudenreich O. Emergency management of acute psychosis. In: Freudenreich O, editor. Psychotic disorders: a practical guide. New York: Wolter Kluwer/Lippincott Williams & Wilkins; 2008. p. 72–8.
29. Lindenmayer JP. The pathophysiology of agitation. J Clin Psychiatry 2000; 61(Suppl 14):5–10.
30. Wilson MP, Pepper D, Currier GW, et al. The psychopharmacology of agitation: consensus statement of the American Association for Emergency Psychiatry Project BETA Psychopharmacology Workgroup. West J Emerg Med 2012;13(1): 26–34.
31. Dubin WR, Waxman HM, Weiss KJ, et al. Rapid tranquilization: the efficacy of oral concentrate. J Clin Psychiatry 1985;46(11):475–8.
32. Müller-Oerlinghausen B, Berghöfer A, Ahrens B. The antisuicidal and mortality-reducing effect of lithium prophylaxis: consequences for guidelines in clinical psychiatry. Can J Psychiatry 2003;48(7):433–9.
33. Fitzgerald P. Long-acting antipsychotic medication, restraint and treatment in the management of acute psychosis. Aust N Z J Psychiatry 1999;33(5):660–6.

34. Currier G, Walsh P. Safety and efficacy review of inhaled loxapine for treatment of agitation. Clin Schizophr Relat Psychoses 2013;7(1):25–32.
35. MacDonald K, Wilson MP, Minassian A, et al. A retrospective analysis of intramuscular haloperidol and olanzapine in the treatment of agitation in drug- and alcohol-using patients. Gen Hosp Psychiatry 2010;32:443–5.
36. Battaglia J, Moss S, Rush J, et al. Haloperidol, lorazepam, or both for psychotic agitation? A multicenter, prospective, double-blind, emergency department study. Am J Emerg Med 1997;15(4):335–40.
37. Allen MH. Managing the agitated psychotic patient: a reappraisal of the evidence. J Clin Psychiatry 2000;61(14 Suppl):S11–20.
38. Green SM, Roback MG, Kennedy RM, et al. Clinical practice guideline for emergency department ketamine dissociative sedation: 2011 update. Ann Emerg Med 2011;57(5):449–61.
39. Green SM, Rothrock SG, Lynch EL, et al. Intramuscular ketamine for pediatric sedation in the emergency department: safety profile in 1,022 cases. Ann Emerg Med 1998;31(6):688–97.
40. Cole JB, Moore JC, Nystrom PC, et al. A prospective study of ketamine versus haloperidol for severe prehospital agitation. Clin Toxicol 2016;54(7):556–62.
41. Hopper AB, vilke GM, Castillo EM, et al. Ketamine use for acute agitation in the emergency department. J Emerg Med 2015;48(6):712–9.
42. Vrana B. Use of intranasal ketamine for the severely agitated or violent ED patient. J Emerg Nurs 2016;42(3):198–9.
43. Lahti A. Subanesthetic doses of ketamine stimulate psychosis in schizophrenia. Neuropsychopharmacology 1995;13(1):9–19.
44. Abdel-Hamid HA, Abdel-Rahman MS, Abdel-Rahman SA. Teratogenic effect of diphenylhydantoin and/or fluphenazine in mice. J Appl Toxicol 1996;16(3):221–5.
45. Wertelecki W, Purvis-Smith SG, Blackburn WR. Amitryptyline/perphenazine maternal overdose and birth defects (abstract). Teratology 1980;21:74A.
46. McGarry JM. A double-blind comparison of the anti-emetic effect during labour of metoclopramide and perphenazine. Br J Anaesth 1971;43(6):613–5.
47. Vorhees CV, Brunner RL, Butcher RE. Psychotropic drugs as behavioral teratogens. Science 1979;205(4412):1220–5.
48. Kopelman AE, McCullar FW, Heggeness L. Limb malformations following maternal use of haloperidol. JAMA 1975;231(1):62–4.
49. Briggs GD, Freeman RK, Yaffe SJ. Drugs in pregnancy and lactation. 5th edition. Baltimore: Williams & Wilkins; 1998. Haloperidol.
50. Ratnayake T, Libretto SE. No complications with risperidone treatment before and throughout pregnancy and during the nursing period. Am J Psychiatry 2002; 63(1):76–7.
51. Mackay FJ, Wilton LV, Pearce GL. The safety of risperidone: a post-marketing study on 7684 patients. Hum Psychopharmacol 1998;13(6):413–8.
52. Wyszynski DF, Nambisan M, Surve T, et al. Increased rate of major malformations in offspring exposed to valproate during pregnancy. Neurology 2005;64(6): 961–5.
53. Hernandez-Diaz S, Smith CR, Shen A, et al. Comparative safety of antiepileptic drugs during pregnancy. Neurology 2012;78(21):1692–9.
54. Jentink J, Loane MA, Dolk H, et al. Valproic acid monotherapy in pregnancy and major congenital malformations. N Engl J Med 2010;362(23):2185–93.
55. ACOG practice bulletin: clinical management guidelines for obstetrician-gynecologists number 92, April 2008 (replaces practice bulletin number 87,

November 2007). Use of psychiatric medications during pregnancy and lactation. Obstet Gynecol 2008;111(4):1001–20.
56. Cohen LS, Friedman JM, Jefferson JW, et al. A reevaluation of risk of in utero exposure to lithium. JAMA 1994;271(2):146–50.
57. Correa-Villasenor A, Ferencz C, Neill CA, et al. Ebstein's malformation of the tricuspid valve: genetic and environmental factors. The Baltimore-Washington Infant Study Group. Teratology 1994;50(2):137–47.
58. Cohen LS. Treatment of bipolar disorder during pregnancy. J Clin Psychiatry 2007;68(Suppl 9):4–9.
59. Savarese DMF, Zans JM. Carbamazepine: drug information. Waltham (MA): UpToDate; 2014.
60. Rosa FW. Spina bifida in infants of women treated with carbamazepine during pregnancy. N Engl J Med 1991;324(10):674–7.
61. Cleary KK, Prescott K. The use of physical restraints in acute and long-term care. J Acute Care Phys Ther 2015;6(1):8–15.
62. Zun LS, Downey L. The use of seclusion in emergency medicine. Gen Hosp Psychiatry 2005;27:365–71.
63. Berzlanovich AM, Schöpfer J, Keil W. Deaths due to physical restraint. Dtsch Arztebl Int 2012;109(3):27–32.
64. Frueh BC, Knapp RG, Cusack KJ, et al. Patients' reports of traumatic or harmful experiences within the psychiatric setting. Psychiatr Serv 2005;56:1123–33.
65. Knox D, Holloman G. Use and avoidance of seclusion and restraint: consensus statement of the American Association for Emergency Psychiatry Project BETA Seclusion and Restraint Workgroup. West J Emerg Med 2012;13(1):35–40.
66. Rose A, Slack P. Physical examination of patients postrestraint on psychiatric inpatient units. J Psychiatr Intensive Care 2016;12(1):45–9.
67. Glezer A, Brendel RW. Beyond emergencies: the use of physical restraints in medical and psychiatric settings. Harv Rev Psychiatry 2010;18(6):353–8.
68. Brown HE, Stoklosa J, Freudenreich O. How to stabilize an acutely psychotic patient. Curr Psychiatry 2012;11(12):10–6.

Emergency Department Medical Clearance of Patients with Psychiatric or Behavioral Emergencies, Part 1

Veronica Theresa Tucci, MD, JD[a,*], Nidal Moukaddam, MD, PhD[b], Al Alam, MD[c,d], James Rachal, MD[e]

KEYWORDS

- Medical clearance • Medical screening • Medical stability
- Psychiatric and behavioral emergencies

KEY POINTS

- Up to 7% of all adult emergency department (ED) patients now present with a primary psychiatric complaint.
- Emergency physicians must stabilize and medically clear patients with behavioral and psychiatric emergencies before these patients are accepted for inpatient hospitalization.
- Emergency physicians, emergency psychiatrists, and inpatient psychiatry teams often disagree on the extent of ancillary testing necessary to medically clear patients for inpatient admission.
- In fact, at the time of this publication, there are still no interdisciplinary algorithms regarding the medical clearance and stability process.
- Moreover, the guidelines from the American College of Emergency Physicians and the American Psychiatric Association directly conflict, adding layers of frustration to an already overburdened system.

INTRODUCTION

I feel the need, the need for speed.

—*Maverick, Top Gun*

Disclosure Statement: The authors have nothing to disclose.
[a] Merit Health Wesley, Department of Emergency Medicine, 5001 Hardy Street, Hattiesburg, MS 39402, USA; [b] Menninger Department of Psychiatry and Behavioral Sciences, Baylor College of Medicine, 1502 Taub Loop, NPC Building 2nd Floor, Houston, TX 77030, USA; [c] Weill Cornell Medical College, NewYork-Presbyterian/Westchester, 21 Bloomingdale Road, White Plains, NY 10605, USA; [d] Stony Brook University, Stony Brook, NY, USA; [e] Carolinas Health Care System, Behavioral Health, 501 Billingsley Road, Charlotte, NC 28211, USA
* Corresponding author.
E-mail address: vtuccimd@gmail.com

Psychiatr Clin N Am 40 (2017) 411–423
http://dx.doi.org/10.1016/j.psc.2017.04.001
psych.theclinics.com
0193-953X/17/© 2017 Elsevier Inc. All rights reserved.

Emergency physicians (EPs) are usually painted as the medical mavericks, the so-called cowboys whose egos write checks that their "bodies can't cash." In the same vein, inpatient psychiatrists are often cast in the role of Ice Man. Slow and deliberate, inpatient psychiatry is replete with men and women who look askance at their emergency colleagues, remarking "You're everyone's problem. That's because every time you go up in the air, you're unsafe. I don't like you because you're dangerous." Indeed, to the inpatient psychiatrist, the EP is often seen as rushing through the examination and assessment of the psychiatric patient with the sole goal of getting the patient out of their emergency department (ED). Little do they realize that the EP is protecting her and his wingman's flank, waiting for the next proverbial patient land mine to go off. Plagued by visions of the inferior wall myocardial infarction sitting in the waiting room, the EP watches her or his charts stack up while staring at the boarded psychiatric patient taking up yet another bed. Despite their frequent misgivings, the inpatient team still relies on these mavericks to diagnose, stabilize, and manage their patients. Perhaps straddling the line between these players are the emergency psychiatrists who embody the wisdom and spirit of Viper, and "rules of engagement are written for your safety and for that of your team. They are not flexible, nor am I. Either obey them or you are history." The 3 sides to the medical clearance triangle are emergency medicine, emergency psychiatry, and inpatient psychiatry. When they work in harmony, hard-fought battles are won and the patient's needs are served. On the other hand, when the sides fight among themselves, the war is lost before it begins and the patient is the one who loses the most, left to linger in the ED, an environment ill-suited to address their needs. Is it any wonder that their problems steadily worsen and even reach a tipping point, at which they may become a danger to ED staff or themselves? This article explores the more challenging aspects of the medical clearance process and offers strategies for interdisciplinary collaboration and addresses the unique challenges of special populations.

Primary psychiatric chief complaints currently account for roughly 6% of all adult ED visits and 7% of all pediatric ED visits.[1,2] In 2006, 4.7 million visits involved a primary psychiatric diagnosis, a rate of 20 visits per 100 adults.[3] According to the National Hospital Ambulatory Medical Care Survey (NHAMC), by 2012, 5.25 million visits were for a primary psychiatric diagnosis. Perhaps even more important, those 5.25 million visits did not account for patients who presented with issues such as self-inflicted traumas or poisonings. Indeed, known self-inflicted wounds accounts for another 419,000 visits.[4] Moreover, the NHAMC Survey does not take into account the occult suicidality of the ED patient population or those for whom mental illness was a secondary diagnosis that, nonetheless, still needed to be managed. Indeed, even in 2005, more than 8% of ED patients who presented to the ED with a medical complaint also had active suicidal ideation when asked.[5]

The data are clear: patients with psychiatric and behavioral issues are increasingly presenting to the ED to manage both their acute crises and chronic conditions. Despite being chronically overworked and understaffed, the ED functions as the safety net for society. EPs must begin the diagnostic and treatment process for this patient population. As previously noted, the ED setting is not therapeutic for most patients suffering the ravages of mental illness. Before these patients can be admitted to an inpatient ward, the EP must medically clear of these patients.

MEDICAL CLEARANCE DEFINITION AND BACKGROUND

Before a patient may be transferred to an inpatient psychiatric facility from an ED for treatment of their psychiatric or behavioral condition, the inpatient team generally requires emergency providers to perform a medical assessment of the patient and identify and stabilize any medical conditions that may be contributing to the patient's psychiatric symptoms. The process is commonly referred to as medical clearance.

Although the intent of medical clearance may seem apparent, there is an ambiguity inherent in the process itself that leads to misdiagnoses, clinical delays, and provider frustration.[6–9] So why the ambiguity?

To some physicians, the term medical clearance entails a medical blessing wherein the patient is free from all medical problems or comorbid conditions. To others, it is acceptable to clear a patient if the patient's medical problems are not causing their psychiatric symptoms (eg, bronchitis in an otherwise healthy young adult). Finally, other providers would permit patients to be medically cleared even when a medical illness may have caused or contributed to the patients' symptoms but in which treatment is no longer needed (eg, history of hypertensive encephalopathy in a patient who is now normotensive).

These approaches are not specific to a specialty but rather are specific to the provider and institution. They are not evidence-based and often the result of anecdote and traditional practices. Consequently, some emergency psychiatrists willingly embrace the broadest categorization of clearance. Likewise, some EPs apply the narrowest definition and admit those patients in the gray area to the medical services for treatment before inpatient psychiatric evaluation. This provider variability, coupled with the lack of an interdisciplinary gold-standard definition of medical clearance, results in vastly different approaches to process, even within the same geographic region.[10]

Despite the ambiguity in defining medical clearance, the process itself is an essential step in the evaluation and treatment of patients with psychiatric and behavioral emergencies. Multiple studies reported that 34% to 50% of patients who present with psychiatric emergencies have coexisting medical diseases that can be causing or exacerbating their psychiatric illness.[11–15]

Individuals with new onset psychiatric symptoms should be assumed to have an underlying medical disorder causing the presentation unless proved otherwise. First, staff should exhaust all resources to determine whether the patient has had similar events in the past. The presence or absence of a past psychiatric history is among most important determinants of psychiatric versus medical illness. Most alert adult patients with new psychiatric symptoms who present to the ED have an organic cause.[16] Those patients will require an extensive medical work up to identify any medical emergencies that are causing the patient's psychotic picture before the patient is admitted to a psychiatric facility.

Medical illness is highly prevalent in patients with severe mental illness (SMI), such as schizophrenia, bipolar disorder, and schizoaffective disorder, with 50% to 90% of patients having at least 1 chronic medical condition.[17] Several reviews and studies have shown that people with SMI have an excess mortality, being 2 or 3 times as high as that in the general population.[18–21] This mortality gap, translates to a shortened life expectancy of 8 to 30 years and about 60% of this excess mortality is due to physical illness.[22]

This decrease in life expectancy is likely due to both patient (eg, poor insight, noncompliance) and provider (eg, countertransference and bias) factors.[23] Moreover, psychiatric patients have a higher incidence of medical conditions,[24–26] as well as a greater risk of injury.[27,28]

As part of the medical assessment, providers should identify any conditions that require ongoing or scheduled treatment or further attention (eg, hypertension, obstructive sleep apnea requiring continuous positive airway pressure, hemodialysis), medication choice (eg, true allergies, pregnancy), or which may affect placement at a given inpatient facility or medication decisions (eg, the presence of indwelling catheters). Receiving facilities vary greatly in their staffing and ability to manage complex medical issues and often have separate requirements outside the medical clearance process, known as exclusionary criteria.[29,30] A discussion of exclusionary criteria is beyond the scope of this article.

CLINICAL EVALUATION

Approach to the Patient with Psychiatric Complaints

Overall, the approach to patient presenting with behavioral complaints should be the same as the approach to those with general medical conditions. The patient's clinical findings should guide further diagnostic testing, including laboratory tests, imaging, consultations, and interventions. The approach to the psychiatric patient in the ER begins with the ABCs, and addressing any life-threatening concerns. As previously discussed, mentally ill patients are at increased risk for traumatic injury and morbidity from underlying and untreated medical conditions. The authors recommend that EPs treat all psychiatric patients as occult trauma patients and perform an assessment similar to advanced trauma life support.

First, the primary survey should be completed. All threats to airway, breathing, and circulation (ie, threats to life or limb) should be addressed. Next, the EP should establish a baseline mental status and neurologic function looking at disability. The EP should then expose the patient (if he or she is not already in a gown) and search for evidence of illness and injury and attend to the patient's environment, both from a medical and therapeutic perspective. After the ABCDE of the primary survey has been completed, the EP should obtain the history, review system, and perform a secondary survey with a head-to-toe physical examination looking for any conditions that might have been missed at first glance. A systematic approach ensures that the patient will receive a thorough evaluation.

History

Willie Sutton, among most famous bank robbers in American history was asked why he robbed banks. He answered because that's where the money is. The history is arguably the most important part of the medical clearance evaluation. Indeed, a study showed a sensitivity of 94% for picking up the medical conditions found to be present.[31] That is where the so-called money is.

Despite the importance of obtaining an adequate history, a study found that 80% of the patients who were medically clear had a medical disease that should have been identified.[11] In 1978, Hall and colleagues found that in 658 consecutive psychiatric outpatients, 9.1% of the patients had a medical disorder (eg, delirium, thyroid disease, diabetic complications) masquerading as a psychiatric condition.[32] Three years later, a Canadian study virtually replicated Hall and colleagues' findings and noted that 7% of the patient population had symptoms attributable to their medical problems (most commonly, alcoholism and chronic organic brain conditions).[12,33]

To prevent improper psychiatric diagnoses, EPs must elicit a detailed description of the patient's symptoms, including timing, provoking, and palliative features (ie, triggers), any previous episodes, and establish how the patient's current behavior has changed from baseline. Unfortunately, obtaining a psychiatric history can be difficult because, although many patients are forthcoming with the details, others are unable or unwilling to give history. Often, the physician must obtain additional history from collateral sources such as family, friends, police, or emergency medical services.

Acute changes or rapid deterioration in mental status suggests an underlying organic cause.[34]

MEDICAL PROBLEMS PRESENTING AS PSYCHIATRIC COMPLAINTS

There are a myriad of medical conditions that may present with psychiatric complaints or exacerbate symptoms of previously diagnosed psychiatric problems. A broad differential diagnosis must be entertained, particularly when confronted with new-onset psychosis and altered mental status (AMS). A prospective study found that 63% of 100 consecutive patients, ages 16 to 65 years, with new psychiatric symptoms, had an organic cause for their symptoms. The medical history was telling in 42% of the patients with medical causes of their symptoms. Likewise, this study showed that 11% of the patients had relevant physical examination findings.[16] Another report found 34% to 46% of inpatients on a psychiatric ward have medical disorders causing or exacerbating psychiatric illness.[14,15]

The patient's history and examination should guide the diagnostic evaluation and ordering of tests. All red flags, including symptoms of infection, thought disturbances, and fluctuations of consciousness, must be evaluated and delirium ruled out. Failure to properly diagnose delirium leads to high morbidity and mortality.[35]

Similarly, EPs should obtain the patient's medication history, including any recent medication changes and document compliance or adherence with their treatment regimen.

Medical comorbidities and medical complaints should also be evaluated thoroughly because these can both cause and/or exacerbate psychiatric symptoms. There may also be treatment implications for both acute and chronic medical disorders if the patient is admitted to an inpatient psychiatric facility. All acute medical conditions should be addressed and stabilized before patient transfer to an inpatient psychiatric facility. EPs should also schedule all chronic medications when possible (eg, antihypertensive regimen) and make recommendations for treating any other acute medical problems (eg, a course of clindamycin for purulent cellulitis).

Review of Systems

The review of systems is another way to uncover medical conditions, given the limited insight of some psychiatric patients. Risk factors should also be probed, including drug and alcohol use and sexual behaviors, as well as any recent trauma. As with the history of present illness, positive pertinent findings should guide ancillary testing.

Physical Examination

An appropriate physical examination should unearth medical pathologic conditions responsible for causing or worsening the patient's psychiatric presentation and guide the care the patient needs during inpatient hospitalization. When EPs have limited history or are confronted with an altered patient, she or he should conduct a thorough physical examination and assess the patient for evidence of infection, trauma, or other pathologic conditions, including toxidromes.[36] For patients with known psychiatric illnesses who are alert and cooperative with the EP, the examination should be focused and guided by the history and review of systems. Physical findings suggestive of organic disease are delineated in **Table 1**.

Differentiating primary psychosis from secondary organic psychosis (eg, medical or toxic causes) can be difficult. What could make it more complicated is that a positive finding on an examination or a positive laboratory test result alone (eg, a urine drug test

Table 1
Physical examination findings suggestive of organic conditions

Vital Sign abnormalities	Infection, toxidrome or withdrawal, Central nervous system (CNS) disease, hypertensive encephalopathy, endocrine abnormalities, autoimmune dysfunction
Oculomotor dysfunction	CNS disease, toxidromes or withdrawal
Cranial nerve abnormalities	Encephalitis, mass, stroke
Gait abnormality	Wernicke, syphilis, B12 deficiency
Lymphadenopathy	Human immunodeficiency virus, lymphoma, infection
Enlarged or nodular thyroid	Graves disease, thyroid storm
Rash	Meningitis
Battle sign or raccoon eyes	Intracranial hemorrhage
Stiff neck, Brudzinski and Kernig signs	Meningitis
Ascites	Hepatic dysfunction or encephalopathy
Jaundice	Hepatic dysfunction
Uremic frost	Kidney failure

positive for cannabis) does not establish causality. The MADFOCS scale is a useful mnemonic that can be used for differentiating organic from primary psychoses.[37,38]

At times, an observation period with attention to the psychotic symptoms and repeated cognitive testing might still be necessary to make an accurate diagnosis. The American College of Emergency Physicians (ACEP) suggests that clinicians consider using a period of observation to determine if psychiatric symptoms resolve as the episode of intoxication resolves (level C recommendation).

Providers should perform a mental status examination to help differentiate functional from organic pathologic conditions.[39] A detailed extensive mental status examination is not necessary in every patient with AMS. Indeed, this examination should be systematic, focused, brief, and practical in the ED setting. At a minimum, the 3 key elements of orientation, memory, and judgment should be addressed.[40]

The authors recommend that EPs adopt the Quick Confusion Scale (QCS) because it is as reliable as a full Mini-Mental Status Examination and much quicker to use.[40]

Deficiencies in the Initial Assessment

Unfortunately, multiple studies demonstrate that EPs do not obtain adequate histories or perform sufficient examinations. Not only does this lead to missed diagnoses, patient safety issues and inappropriate dispositions, it also results in an increased dependence on ancillary testing or imaging.

In 1981, the Journal of the American Medical Association published a paper on diagnostic errors in the evaluation of behavior disorders. They found that in 215 patients referred to a specialized medical-psychiatric inpatient unit, thorough neuropsychiatric evaluation resulted in a therapeutically important alteration of the referring diagnosis in 41%. Of patients referred for a tentative diagnosis of dementia, 63% were found to have treatable conditions. They found that these erroneous diagnoses were provided roughly equally by psychiatric and medical practitioners; they suggested that evaluation would ideally be done by neurologists or psychiatrists with specialty expertise in neuropsychiatric evaluation.[15]

In a study performed by Tintinalli and colleagues[8] more than a decade later, the investigators found multiple deficiencies in the physical examination of the emergency psychiatric patient. Once again, physicians failed to perform a mental status in more than 50% of patients.

In 2000, another study by Reeves and colleagues[7] performed a root cause analysis to determine why medical emergencies went unrecognized and patients were admitted to psychiatric units instead of the appropriate medical floor. Approximately one-third of missed cases involved severe alcohol or drug intoxication. One-eighth of the cases involved withdrawal or delirium tremens. Similarly, one-eighth of the incorrectly diagnosed patients involved prescription drug overdoses. According to the investigators, more than 40% of the patients had inadequate examinations and physicians failed to obtain an adequate history in more than one-third of the cases. Physicians also failed to address abnormal vital signs in almost 8% of patients.

A 2008 study by Szpakowicz and Herd[41] revealed that physicians were still performing inadequate physical examinations. Specifically, providers failed to record a complete set of vital signs in almost half of the cases.

In 2015, Tucci and colleagues[42] performed a retrospective chart review of 50 consecutive psychiatric patients that focused on the neurologic and psychiatric examinations of the emergency psychiatric patient. Despite working at a county hospital that sees more than 9500 psychiatric patients each year (representing almost 10% of the census), providers still performed (or at least documented) abysmally lacking examinations. Mood and affect were documented in less than 50% of cases. Suicidality was documented in less than one-third of the patients who presented with a chief complaint of suicidal ideation. Only 1 out of the 50 patients had any kind of mental status examination documented. Sixteen percent of patients did not have their orientation status documented (even when AMS and behavioral conditions are commonly included for psychiatric referral). More than half did not have a cranial nerve examination. Less than 25% had their gait or reflexes tested. Twenty eight percent of patients had their strength tested and 12% had a sensory examination performed.

The authors cannot find a single study that supports the contention that EPs perform adequate histories and physical examinations on patients who present with psychiatric or behavioral emergencies.

LABORATORY AND ANCILLARY TESTING

Importance and Utility

Many studies demonstrate that broad ordering of tests is low yield and that the appropriate standard is to tailor such testing to the patient's history and physical examination findings.

In a retrospective study by Korn and colleagues,[43] the investigators concluded that EPs could skip ancillary testing in patients with primary psychiatric complaints who denied current medical problems, had a documented psychiatric history, stable vital signs, and normal physical examinations and refer immediately to psychiatry.

Another observational analysis of 345 psychiatric patients noted that almost all medical problems and substance abuse in ED psychiatric patients could be identified by vital signs, and history and physical examination and did not require confirmatory testing.

In 2004, Gregory and colleagues[44] found that routine laboratory studies were generally low yield except in higher risk categories: the elderly, substance users, patients with no prior psychiatric history, and patients with preexisting medical disorders or concurrent medical complaints.

So then, why are there still inpatient facilities requiring extensive workups for patients with known psychiatric history who present with a primary psychiatric problem?

This dilemma is memorialized in the conflicting guidelines issued by the ACEP and the American Psychiatric Association (APA). In 2006, ACEP published a clinical policy on the medical clearance of the psychiatric patient. This policy declares that routine laboratory testing of all patients is unnecessary and that the history and physical examination findings should guide the ordering of ancillary testing. Moreover, ACEP noted that urine drug screen tests do not affect patient management, are not required, and if they are performed, should not delay transfer to inpatient psychiatric facilities. Similarly, EPs were counseled that the patient's cognitive ability or clinical sobriety that should determine when an appropriate psychiatric interview may be conducted and not the patient's blood alcohol level. ACEP did allow for a reasonable observation period to determine if the patient's mood disorder and psychiatric symptoms were secondary to intoxication.[45]

The APA guidelines include a much broader list of requirements for medical clearance and include assessments of comorbid drug and alcohol use.[46]

Psychiatrists cannot diagnose patients with a new psychiatric condition while the patient is acutely intoxicated or under the influence of mind-altering substances. Additionally, intoxication and withdrawal syndromes can mimic mental illness even in patients with primary psychiatric diagnoses who have otherwise been well-controlled in an outpatient setting (eg, suicidal ideation only present during acute intoxication in a patient with a documented history of major depressive disorder). Concomitant drug and alcohol may also affect the patient's placement in a facility equipped to handle rehabilitation and withdrawal. Consequently, the APA places more importance on drug and alcohol testing.

As can be seen from the previous summaries, ACEP and the APA have issued guidelines that directly conflict with each other in the setting of patients with known psychiatric history who present with a primary psychiatric complaint.

In general, there tends to be less disagreement between specialties when faced with new onset AMS or psychosis for which an extensive work up is required. A thorough evaluation and laboratory tests are necessary for (1) broad screening, (2) exclusion of specific diseases informed by treatability and epidemiology, and (3) medical baseline measures to allow monitor for iatrogenic morbidity such as obesity and metabolic disorders.[47] **Box 1** shows recommended workup for individuals with first-episode psychosis. All of the recommended tests may be started but do not need to be completed in the ED. The authors recommend that such patients be admitted to the general medical floor with a presumptive diagnosis of delirium or altered mental state.

At the time of this publication, the breadth of laboratory testing for the purpose of medical clearance still remains controversial. Unfortunately, however, there is no interdisciplinary consensus regarding the number and types of ancillary testing required for medical clearance.

The authors hail from emergency medicine and psychiatry, and recognize that the controversy of ancillary testing is rooted in that, although individual physicians may perform proper histories and physical examinations, currently, the specialty of emergency medicine as a whole is not. Psychiatrists believe they need to rely on more objective measures to ascertain whether the patient has a medical problem causing his or her psychiatric symptoms. Borrowing from the trauma literature, the authors recommend EPs adopt a more regimented or check-list approach to the history and physical examination of the emergency psychiatric patient. Once regimented histories and physical examinations become the norm instead of the exception, the authors expect our psychiatric colleagues will be more sanguine in accepting tailored testing

Box 1
Recommended work up for first episode of psychosis

Medical work-up in first-episode psychosis

Complete blood count

Full chemistry, liver function test

Syphilis serology venereal disease research laboratory (the rapid plasma regain)

Human immunodeficiency virus test

Vitamin B12

Electrocardiogram (if cardiac risk)

Urine drug screen

Ethanol level

Drug levels if indicated

Considered if indicated by clinical picture

Brain imaging with computed tomography or MRI

Electroencephalogram

Chest radiograph

Lumbar puncture

to address specific patient complaints or elements in their medical histories, instead of the current, seemingly required, shot-gun approach.

Common Pitfalls in the Medical Clearance Process

The failure to properly diagnose medical pathologic conditions as the root cause of (or exacerbating feature of) psychiatric illness leads to increased morbidity and mortality. As previously discussed, a thorough history and physical, including mental status examination, is extremely important to identify these causes and guide further testing. However, studies show that many providers skip these crucial steps. Moreover, as

Box 2
Common errors in the medical clearance process

Poor history taking

Failure to obtain collateral information from family, emergency medical services, police, and so forth.

Failure to perform a thorough physical examination

Failure to address vital sign abnormalities (eg, sustained tachycardia, hypoxemia)

Failure to develop a differential diagnosis based on the totality of the patient's history and physical examination

Anchoring early on a primary psychiatric diagnosis

Inadequate laboratory and radiographic testing

Shotgun laboratory and radiographic testing

discussed in our separate article on Moreover, as discussed in this issue of Al Alam and colleagues' article, "Emergency department medical clearance of patients with psychiatric or behavioral emergencies: part 2: special psychiatric populations and considerations," special populations, a higher portion of geriatric, pediatric, and pregnant patients may have symptoms caused by medical conditions and providers should entertain a broad differential when approaching these patients. special populations, a higher portion of geriatric, pediatric, and pregnant patients may have symptoms caused by medical conditions and providers should entertain a broad differential when approaching these patients.

Common pitfalls are summarized in **Box 2**.

SUMMARY

EPs must diligently investigate whether a patient's psychiatric symptoms are caused or worsened by an organic condition. Moreover, if a condition is identified, the EP must stabilize it before the patient can be transferred to an inpatient facility for longer term treatment and management. To rule out medical causes, the EP must perform a thorough physical examination and take an adequate history and/or obtain collateral information. Laboratory and ancillary testing should be guided by what is indicated based on clinical assessment.

The sheer complexity of the medical stability, clearance, and admission process sometimes lead EPs to ask, like Maverick, "So you think I should quit?" Viper, "I didn't say that....Now I'm not gonna sit here and blow sunshine up your ass, Lieutenant. A good pilot is compelled to evaluate what's happened, so he can apply what he's learned. Up there, we gotta push it. That's our job. It's your option Lieutenant. All yours." Like fighter pilots in high-stress situations, it is time to apply what has been learned and advocate for a uniform, interdisciplinary standard of medical clearance from the professional societies ACEP, APA, and AAEP (The American Association for Emergency Psychiatry).

REFERENCES

1. Larkin GL, Claassen CA, Emond JA, et al. Trends in U.S. emergency department visits for mental health conditions, 1992 to 2001. Psychiatr Serv 2005;56(6):671–7.
2. Simon AE, Schoendorf KC. Emergency department visits for mental health conditions among US children, 2001-2011. Clin Pediatr 2014;53(14):1359–66.
3. Zun LS, Downey L. Pediatric health screening and referral in the ED. Am J Emerg Med 2005;23(6):737–41.
4. National Hospital Ambulatory Medical Care Survey: 2012 Emergency Department Summary Tables. 2012. Available at: https://www.cdc.gov/nchs/data/nhamcs_emergency/2012_ed_web_tables.pdf. Accessed May 26, 2017.
5. Claassen CA, Larkin GL. Occult suicidality in an emergency department population. Br J Psychiatry 2005;186:352–3.
6. Zun LS, Hernandez R, Thompson R, et al. Comparison of EPs' and psychiatrists' laboratory assessment of psychiatric patients. Am J Emerg Med 2004;22(3):175–80.
7. Reeves RR, Perry CL, Burke RS. What does "medical clearance" for psychiatry really mean? J Psychosoc Nurs Ment Health Serv 2010;48(8):2–4.
8. Tintinalli JE, Peacock FWt, Wright MA. Emergency medical evaluation of psychiatric patients. Ann Emerg Med 1994;23(4):859–62.

9. Tucci V, Siever K, Matorin A, et al. Down the rabbit hole: emergency department medical clearance of patients with psychiatric or behavioral emergencies. Emerg Med Clin North Am 2015;33(4):721–37.
10. Weissberg MP. Emergency room medical clearance: an educational problem. Am J Psychiatry 1979;136(6):787–90.
11. Hall RC, Gardner ER, Stickney SK, et al. Physical illness manifesting as psychiatric disease. II. Analysis of a state hospital inpatient population. Arch Gen Psychiatry 1980;37(9):989–95.
12. Carlson RJ, Nayar N, Suh M. Physical disorders among emergency psychiatric patients. Can J Psychiatry 1981;26(1):65–7.
13. Schumacher Group. Emergency department challenges and trends: 2010 survey of hospital emergency department administrators. Available at: asa.pdf@newsroom.acep.org. Accessed May 26, 2017.
14. Hall RC, Gardner ER, Popkin MK, et al. Unrecognized physical illness prompting psychiatric admission: a prospective study. Am J Psychiatry 1981;138(5):629–35.
15. Hoffman RS. Diagnostic errors in the evaluation of behavioral disorders. JAMA 1982;248(8):964–7.
16. Henneman PL, Mendoza R, Lewis RJ. Prospective evaluation of emergency department medical clearance. Ann Emerg Med 1994;24(4):672–7.
17. Gold KJ, Kilbourne AM, Valenstein M. Primary care of patients with serious mental illness: your chance to make a difference. J Fam Pract 2008;57(8):515–25.
18. Lack D, Holt RI, Baldwin DS. Poor monitoring of physical health in patients referred to a mood disorders service. Ther Adv Psychopharmacol 2015;5(1):22–5.
19. Rossler W, Salize HJ, van Os J, et al. Size of burden of schizophrenia and psychotic disorders. Eur Neuropsychopharmacol 2005;15(4):399–409.
20. Roshanaei-Moghaddam B, Katon W. Premature mortality from general medical illnesses among persons with bipolar disorder: a review. Psychiatr Serv 2009;60(2):147–56.
21. Ross LE, Vigod S, Wishart J, et al. Barriers and facilitators to primary care for people with mental health and/or substance use issues: a qualitative study. BMC Fam Pract 2015;16:135.
22. Druss BG, von Esenwein SA, Compton MT, et al. Budget impact and sustainability of medical care management for persons with serious mental illnesses. Am J Psychiatry 2011;168(11):1171–8.
23. Moukaddam N, Tucci V, Galwankar S, et al. In the blink of an eye: instant countertransference and its application in modern healthcare. J Emerg Trauma Shock 2016;9(3):95–6.
24. Warren MB, Campbell RL, Nestler DM, et al. Prolonged length of stay in ED psychiatric patients: a multivariable predictive model. Am J Emerg Med 2016;34(2):133–9.
25. Keenan TE, Yu A, Cooper LA, et al. Racial patterns of cardiovascular disease risk factors in serious mental illness and the overall U.S. population. Schizophr Res 2013;150(1):211–6.
26. Daumit GL, Dickerson FB, Appel LJ. Weight loss in persons with serious mental illness. N Engl J Med 2013;369(5):486–7.
27. Baughman KR, Bonfine N, Dugan SE, et al. Disease burden among individuals with severe mental illness in a community setting. Community Ment Health J 2016;52(4):424–32.

28. Piatt EE, Munetz MR, Ritter C. An examination of premature mortality among decedents with serious mental illness and those in the general population. Psychiatr Serv (Washington, DC) 2010;61(7):663–8.
29. Tucci V, Moukaddam N, Matorin A, et al. Inpatient psychiatric facility exclusionary criteria and the emergency pediatric psychiatric patient. Int J Acad Med 2017;3: 44–52.
30. Tucci V, Liu J, Matorin A, et al. Like the eye of the tiger: inpatient psychiatric facility exclusionary criteria and its "knock out" of the emergency psychiatric patient. J Emerg Trauma Shock, in press.
31. Olshaker JS, Browne B, Jerrard DA, et al. Medical clearance and screening of psychiatric patients in the emergency department. Acad Emerg Med 1997; 4(2):124–8.
32. Hall RC, Popkin MK, Devaul RA, et al. Physical illness presenting as psychiatric disease. Arch Gen Psychiatry 1978;35:1315–20.
33. Summers WK, Munoz RA, Read MR, et al. The psychiatric physical examination - Part II: findings in 75 unselected psychiatric patients. J Clin Psychiatry 1981; 42(3):99–102.
34. Tintinalli JE, Stapczynski JS, John Ma O, et al. Tintinalli's Emergency medicine: a comprehensive study guide. 7th edition. New York: McGraw Hill; 2011.
35. Evans DL. Bipolar disorder: diagnostic challenges and treatment considerations. J Clin Psychiatry 2000;61(Supp 13):26–31.
36. Baren JM, Mace SE, Hendry PL, et al. Children's mental health emergencies–part 2: emergency department evaluation and treatment of children with mental health disorders. Pediatr Emerg Care 2008;24(7):485–98.
37. Frame DS, Kercher EE. Acute psychosis. Functional versus organic. Emerg Med Clin North Am 1991;9(1):123–36.
38. McGee DL. Clinical pearls for the evaluation of the psychotic patient. Scientific Assembly of the American College of Emergency Physicians. San Diego (CA), October 1998.
39. Irons MJ, Farace E, Brady WJ, et al. Mental status screening of emergency department patients: normative study of the quick confusion scale. Acad Emerg Med 2002;9(10):989–94.
40. Bauer J, Roberts MR, Reisdorff EJ. Evaluation of behavioral and cognitive changes: the mental status examination. Emerg Med Clin North Am 1991;9(1): 1–12.
41. Szpakowicz M, Herd A. "Medically cleared": how well are patients with psychiatric presentations examined by emergency physicians? J Emerg Med 2008;35(4): 369–72.
42. Tucci V, Laufman L, Peacock WF, et al. Epic Fail! Poor neuropsychiatric documentation practices in emergency psychiatric patients. Emerg Med (Los Angel) 2016;6:332.
43. Korn CS, Currier GW, Henderson SO. "Medical clearance" of psychiatric patients without medical complaints in the emergency department. J Emerg Med 2000; 18(2):173–6.
44. Gregory RJ, Nihalani ND, Rodriguez E. Medical screening in the emergency department for psychiatric admissions: a procedural analysis. Gen Hosp Psychiatry 2004;26(5):405–10.
45. Lukens TW, Wolf SJ, Edlow JA, et al. Clinical policy: critical issues in the diagnosis and management of the adult psychiatric patient in the emergency department. Ann Emerg Med 2006;47(1):79–99.

46. Association AP. American Psychiatric Association practice guidelines for the treatment of psychiatric disorders: compendium 2006. Arlington (VA), 2006.
47. Freudenreich O, Schulz SC, Goff DC. Initial medical work-up of first-episode pyschosis: a conceptual review. Early Interv Psychiatry 2009;3(1):10–8.

Emergency Department Medical Clearance of Patients with Psychiatric or Behavioral Emergencies, Part 2

Special Psychiatric Populations and Considerations

Al Alam, MD[a,b,*], James Rachal, MD[c],
Veronica Theresa Tucci, MD, JD[d], Nidal Moukaddam, MD, PhD[e]

KEYWORDS

- Pediatric medical clearance • Geriatric medical screening • Medical stability
- Psychiatric and behavioral emergencies

KEY POINTS

- Psychiatric patients are high-risk medical patients who are seen more frequently in the emergency department.
- More than 5% of all pediatric emergency patients involve a primary psychiatric complaint.
- Emergency physicians must stabilize and medically clear patients with behavioral and psychiatric emergencies before these patients are accepted for inpatient hospitalization.
- Emergency physicians, emergency psychiatrists, and inpatient psychiatry teams often disagree on the extent of ancillary testing necessary to medically clear patients for inpatient admission.
- Elderly patients presenting with psychiatric complaints likely have underlying medical conditions that warrant a comprehensive evaluation and routine laboratory testing before being admitted to a psychiatric facility.

Disclosure: The authors have nothing to disclose.
[a] Weill Cornell Medical College, NewYork-Presbyterian/Westchester, 21 Bloomingdale Road, White Plains, NY 10605, USA; [b] Stony Brook University, Stony Brook, NY, USA; [c] Carolinas Health Care System, Behavioral Health, 501 Billingsley Road, Charlotte, NC 28211, USA; [d] Section of Emergency Medicine, Baylor College of Medicine, 1504 Taub Loop, Houston, TX 77030, USA; [e] Menninger Department of Psychiatry and Behavioral Sciences, Baylor College of Medicine, 1502 Taub Loop, NPC Building 2nd Floor, Houston, TX 77030, USA
* Corresponding author. NewYork-Presbyterian/Westchester, 21 Bloomingdale Road, White Plains, NY 10605.
E-mail address: aba9030@med.cornell.edu

Psychiatr Clin N Am 40 (2017) 425–433
http://dx.doi.org/10.1016/j.psc.2017.05.001
psych.theclinics.com
0193-953X/17/© 2017 Elsevier Inc. All rights reserved.

INTRODUCTION

Patients with psychiatric disorders have a higher incidence of chronic medical conditions as well as injury, including serious head injury, than the general population. These patients deserve a thorough evaluation just as any other patient who presents to the emergency department (ED). The medical clearance is often the first step of the evaluation and treatment of those psychiatric patients before they are admitted to a psychiatric hospital. This medical clearance of patients with known psychiatric disorders follows the same principle of first screening whether the patient has a medical condition that is causing or exacerbating the psychiatric presentation. Second, the emergency physician must identify any other medical conditions that may require treatment or further attention.

Emergency physicians need to be aware that many psychiatrists view the patient's initial presentation in the ED and the medical clearance as the only opportunity to diagnose an underlying organic illness. Therefore, this process should be able to identify any and all acute medical emergencies before a patient is admitted to a psychiatric care unit, where resources for diagnosis and medical treatment modalities may not be readily available. Furthermore, discovery of major medical abnormalities can alert psychiatrists to the possibility that complaints appearing psychiatric in origin might be the manifestations of underlying medical conditions.[1]

Although the evaluation of psychiatric patients is not as daunting as might be thought, emergency physicians frequently have negative attitudes toward psychiatric patients. Stefan[2] noted that emergency care providers regard psychiatric patients as problems or nuisances. Considerable evidence indicates that mentally ill patients often do not receive adequate recognition, monitoring, or care for their medical illnesses.[3] There are several contributing factors to these findings, including societal attitudes and personal biases, inadequate educational preparation, organizational climate, safety concerns, crowding, caregiver lack of confidence, and lack or guidelines.[2] This approach, if not acknowledged and properly handled, may lead to poor outcomes as significant medical disorders otherwise go undetected and potentially lead to morbidity or even mortality.

This article focuses on the medical clearance process for specific psychiatric disorders, including patients with eating disorders and special populations including pediatric, obstetric, and geriatric psychiatric patients.

PATIENTS WITH EATING DISORDERS

Eating disorders are increasingly recognized as an important cause of morbidity and mortality in young individuals. Anorexia nervosa is a serious psychiatric illness characterized by an inability to maintain an adequate, healthy body weight. These patients often require admission to the hospital and are seen frequently in the ED. However, many opportunities to intervene are lost and, unless the patient endorses suicidal ideation, the emergency physician may simply discharge the patient or attend to the stated medical problem.

Admission criteria for both medical and psychiatric units vary but a thorough emergency evaluation is critical. Medical work-up and screening are essential because these patients often have multiple physiologic abnormalities and can decompensate quickly. A thorough history is an important first step, because it can indicate risk factors and help predict morbidity and mortality. Duration of eating disorder as well as chronicity of comorbidities such as hypokalemia can indicate risk of sudden death; the greater the period of illness, the greater the risk.[4] In patients who purge, understanding the methods of purging is critical because each form of purging has unique risks.[5] History of abdominal pain is important and could lead to concerns about pancreatitis, and questions about muscle weakness and tea-colored urine could lead to an evaluation for rhabdomyolysis.[5] History of suicidal thoughts should be thoroughly assessed because patients with anorexia nervosa have a 20% risk of completed suicide.[6]

On initial evaluation, a weight should be obtained and the ideal body weight (body mass index [BMI]) should be calculated. Admission criteria vary from BMI less than 80% to less than 70%. Significant loss of body weight over a 3-month time frame or little to no nutritional intake in last 10 days also should be considered for admission.[7] Vital signs with orthostatic blood pressures and electrocardiogram should be obtained. Hypotension is common in anorexia nervosa and needs to be treated. Patients can be hypothermic and temperature less than 35.6°C (96°F) also can indicate admission to a medical unit.[8] Sinus bradycardia caused by increased vagal tone is common. Although there is no supporting clinical evidence, many experts recommend hospitalizing when bradycardia reaches less than 40 beats/min (bpm) in adults and less than 50 bpm in adolescents, and patients with severe bradycardia (30–40 bpm) should be admitted to a telemetry unit.[6,7] Prolonged corrected QT (QTc) may also be an indication for telemetry monitoring, especially while refeeding. In addition, patients presenting with syncope or other symptoms concerning for cardiac arrhythmia require hospitalization with telemetry monitoring.[6]

Laboratory tests should include a basic metabolic panel with the addition of calcium, magnesium, and phosphorus.[6,9] Magnesium and phosphorus are rarely ordered by emergency physicians for medical clearance of adult psychiatric patients and so must be processed separately. Calcium or ionized calcium is frequently included in the metabolic panel. Hypokalemia is commonly seen in anorexia nervosa because of purging via vomiting, laxatives, or using diuretics.[10] Hypokalemia is known to progressively increase the risk of serious cardiac arrhythmias, including ventricular arrhythmia. K+ level less than 3.3 mEq/L must be actively corrected orally and less than 2.8 mEq/L should be corrected intravenously in an inpatient setting.[11] Hyponatremia tends to be caused by loss of fluid during purging behaviors, or may indicate diuretic use or be caused by volume depletion.[11] Complete blood counts (CBCs) can show anemia, leukopenia, or thrombocytopenia.[6,8] Liver function tests, such as aspartate transaminase/alanine transaminase as well as bilirubin levels, can be increased, especially in patients with prolonged starvation.[12] An human chorionic gonadotropin pregnancy test is recommended in every childbearing female patient and a urine drug screen if drug use is suspected.

Patients with eating disorders seen in the ED require special attention. A low BMI, a greater severity of social and psychological problems, self-induced vomiting, and purgative abuse have been identified as predictors of poor outcome in this disorder.[13]

THE PEDIATRIC PATIENT

Over the past decade there has been a significant increase in pediatric ED visits for mental health reasons.[14] Between 1995 and 2001, 5% of all ED visits were mental health related. Admission rates of psychiatric patients are double those of patients without significant mental health complaints.[15] Mean length of stay for pediatric psychiatric patients was 61 to 722 minutes longer than for patients without psychiatric complaints. Prolonged ED lengths of stay contribute to ED overcrowding, are costly, and delay the disposition of potentially aggressive or suicidal patients.[15]

Medical clearance for pediatric psychiatric admissions has long lacked an interdisciplinary consensus. A study by Santillanes and colleagues[16] suggested that, if a pediatric patient presents for an isolated psychiatric issue meets basic criteria (no altered mental status, no history of ingestion, no history of hanging, no traumatic injury, no unrelated medical complaint or sexual assault), then the patient could be directly transferred to psychiatric hold and perhaps even admitted as an inpatient without a medical screen.

Emergency physicians must elicit whether the patient's psychiatric symptoms are primary psychiatric or secondary to a medical issue. Features from history that could indicate an organic cause include new-onset illness, onset before the age of 12 years, sudden onset of symptoms, visual or tactile hallucinations, seizure, and no family history of mental illness[17,18] (**Table 1**). Concerning physical examination findings include abnormal vital signs (these could indicate infection, toxidrome, or cardiac or endocrine abnormality); fluctuating mental status examination (could indicate delirium); focal neurologic finding (could indicate trauma or stroke); evidence of physical trauma, especially to the head or neck area; and abnormal skin examination (this could indicate autoimmune disorder, hepatic disorders, nutritional disorders, and some genetic disorders).[18]One study indicated that younger patients had a much higher chance of a missed medical diagnosis.[19]

Ancillary testing of patients with no abnormal findings on history or examination has been an increasingly controversial topic as well. According to Donofrio and colleagues,[20] an 18-month study started in 2009 showed that 871 of a total 1082 patients received ancillary testing at an average cost of $1235, and that 94.3% of the patients had examinations that were not concerning and had test results that were clinically insignificant. In another study, by Janiak and Atteberry,[21] 19% had abnormal laboratory tests that changed the disposition of the patient. The study also discussed testing of asymptomatic patients, which has been shown to cause harm to the patient (through further invasive testing that would not otherwise have been performed) and waste to the health care system.[21,22] According to Janiak and Atteberry,[21] many of the tests were repeated once the patient arrived on the inpatient unit.[21] Routine thyroid-stimulating hormone (TSH) and a rapid plasma reagin (RPR) were particularly unhelpful. Shihabuddin and colleagues[23] and Fortu and colleagues[24] also state that routine urine drug screen testing provides little additional help in treating patients. In one study, urine drug screen results did not change the management of any of the children with positive results.[23,24]

Table 1
Historical features distinguishing organic causes of psychiatric complaints from functional disorders

Organic	Functional
Age <13 y	Previous psychiatric diagnosis, age >13 y (peak onset, 15–30 y)
Rapid onset of initial symptoms	Insidious development of symptoms
Rapid progression of symptoms	Insidious progression of symptoms
Visual or tactile hallucinations	Auditory hallucinations
Substance abuse history	No history of illicit drugs, alcohol, or prescription drug abuse
New medications or dose change	No new medications or changes in dose
Seizures	No seizures
Absent family history of psychiatric disorders	Family history of psychiatric disorder

The controversy regarding medical clearance is likely to continue until histories and examinations are standardized and psychiatrists become more comfortable relying on these examinations. Until such time, many inpatient facilities will continue to require more extensive testing through their exclusionary criteria.[25] The authors recommend checking urine drug screens, urine pregnancy tests, and alcohol levels (if there is any concern for intoxication).

Irrespective of inpatient facility testing requirements, placement of pediatric psychiatric patients also presents unique challenges, in part because of comorbid conditions as noted in **Box 1**, so emergency teams must be aware of the individual psychiatric facility exclusionary requirements. Exclusionary criteria are a separate part of the admission process that addresses the psychiatric facility's capability of taking care of a certain kind of patient and generally includes both the challenges that a facility faces (eg, feeding tubes) and the concerns that they want addressed (eg, drug and alcohol abuse).

PREGNANT PATIENTS

Psychiatric illnesses can worsen or appear for the first time during pregnancy and may necessitate admission to an inpatient psychiatric hospital unit. These admissions can be challenging for the psychiatric team because the patient is going through physiologic changes that could be complicating the psychiatric presentation.[26] In those patients, the medical clearance is an important step not only for the safety of the patient and the fetus but also to elicit any possible medical illnesses that may be causing or contributing to the psychiatric presentation.

Psychiatric medications might be needed and consideration should be given to possible teratogenic effects depending on the gestational age of the fetus. If possible, the results of the patient's dating ultrasonography scan should be obtained; if not, last menstrual period can estimate gestational age but this is considered much less accurate.[27]

It is important to ask about vaginal bleeding, leakage of fluid, and fetal movement.[28] If patients are not reliable or disorganized, it is important to examine the patients for any signs of vaginal bleeding. Vital signs, especially blood pressure, are very important. If the physician has any concern about the possibility of preeclampsia, an immediate obstetric consult should be obtained, because this can be life threatening.[29]

An acute change in mental status in a pregnant patient requires a thorough neurologic evaluation, because pregnancy is a hypercoagulable state and the patient is at higher risk for stroke.[30] Both hypothyroidism and hyperthyroidism mimic or might complicate psychiatric disorders such as depression and bipolar disorder. Patients with new-onset psychiatric symptoms such as depression, anxiety, or mood lability might benefit from getting a TSH test to screen for any thyroid abnormalities.[31]

Box 1
Comorbid and confounding conditions in the pediatric population

- Autism spectrum disorders
- Intellectual and neurodevelopmental disabilities (eg, mental retardation)
- Speech and language disability
- Substance use or abuse
- Trauma and stressor-related disorders

Also, in patients with a history of hypothyroidism, pregnancy may require an increased dose of thyroid replacement therapy.[31]

Anemia is common in pregnancy and can share some symptoms with depression. In pregnant patients with new-onset or worsening depression, a CBC may be appropriate to assess for possible anemia.[27] Patients with severe anemia require more attention and immediate obstetric consult because it can compromise the fetus.[32]

Psychiatric disorders in women of childbearing years are common and might require psychiatric hospitalization. Although much has been written regarding women's mental health and psychiatric complications during pregnancy, there are no guidelines for the medical clearance for those patients. **Box 2** show the minimum testing the investigators recommend for pregnant patients.

GERIATRIC PATIENTS

Elderly patients presenting with psychiatric complaints are at high risk for underlying medical conditions. A study found that approximately 80% of the patients admitted to the geriatric unit of the mental hospital turned out to have a physical diagnosis relevant to the problem.[33] Another retrospective study of 489 consecutive elderly admissions to the psychiatry ward found that the main stressor associated with admissions was a change in medical status of the patient. At least 2 medical diagnoses were present in 70% of admissions, with many new physical illnesses being diagnosed.[34]

Infections, electrolyte abnormalities, and medication side effects are common causes of altered mental status that mimic psychiatric disease in the elderly. In recent years, polypharmacy in elderly patients has steadily increased, as has the incidence of adverse events. Nearly 20% of elderly patients brought for emergency psychiatric evaluation may be experiencing a drug reaction.[35]

Comprehensive history and examination are highly recommended for every geriatric patient presenting with primary psychiatric complaints. History should elicit any medical comorbidities, history of falls, functional capacity, and any change in living situation. Unlike the general adult population, the authors recommend routine laboratory testing in those geriatric patients with primary psychiatric complaints because of the higher incidence of medical disease in this population.[36] Our recommended minimum testing is noted in **Box 3**.

Extra caution should be taken with elderly patients with psychiatric complaints because they have a higher incidence of medical disease that might need to be addressed before being admitted to a psychiatric facility.

Box 2
Recommended ancillary testing for the medical clearance of pregnant patients

Complete blood count

ABO type and RH (if not already documented)

Comprehensive metabolic panel

TSH

Human immunodeficiency virus, RPR, Neisseria gonorrhoeae(GC)/Chlamydia urine antigen

Urine drug screen

Urinalysis

Dating ultrasonography with documented fetal heart tones

Box 3
Ancillary testing for geriatric populations

Urinalysis with culture

Complete blood count

Complete metabolic panel

Electrocardiogram

Cardiac panel

Urine drug screen (polypharmacy is a major issue in this population)

Alcohol level

TSH

Computed tomography of the head if any evidence of trauma or neurologic deficits (maintain a low threshold to scan)

SUMMARY

This article summarizes the challenges providers face when medically clearing patients with psychiatric complaints.

REFERENCES

1. Riba M, Hale M. Medical clearance: fact or fiction in the hospital emergency room. Psychosomatics 1990;31:400–4.
2. Stefan S. Emergency department treatment of the psychiatric patient: policy issues and legal requirements. New York: Oxford Press; 2006.
3. Newcomer JW. Metabolic considerations in the use of antipsychotic medications: a review of recent evidence. J Clin Psychiatry 2007;68(Suppl 1):20–7.
4. Jauregui-Garrido B, Jauregui-Lobera I. Sudden death in eating disorders. Vasc Health Risk Manag 2012;8:91–8.
5. Forney KJ, Buchman-Schmitt JM, Keel PK, et al. The medical complications associated with purging. Int J Eat Disord 2016;49(3):249–59.
6. Trent SA, Moreira ME, Colwell CB, et al. ED management of patient with eating disorders. Am J Emerg Med 2013;31:859–65.
7. Mascolo M, Trent S, Colwell C, et al. What the emergency department needs to know when caring for your patients with eating disorders. Int J Eat Disord 2012;45(8):977–81.
8. Dickstein LP, Franco KN, Rome ES, et al. Recognizing, managing medical consequences of eating disorders in primary care. Cleve Clinic J Med 2014;81(4): 255–63.
9. Academy for Eating Disorders (AED). Critical points for early recognition of medical risk management in the care of individuals with eating disorders. Available at: http://ww.aedweb.org/AM/Template.cfm?Section=Medical_Care_Standards&Template=/CM/ContentDisplay.cfm&contentID=2413. Accessed November 20, 2016.
10. Brown CA, Mehler PS. Medical complications of self induced vomiting. Eat Disord 2013;21:287–94.
11. Mehler PS, Walsh K. Electrolyte and acid-base abnormalities associated with purging behaviors. Int J Eat Disord 2016;49(3):311–8.

12. Gaudiani JL, Mehler PS. Rare manifestations of severe restricting and purging: "zebras," missed diagnosis and best practices. Int J Eat Disord 2016;49(3): 331–44.
13. Löwe B, Zipfel S, Buchholz C, et al. Long-term outcome of anorexia nervosa in a prospective 21-year follow-up study. Psychol Med 2001;31(5):881–90.
14. Sun D, Abraham I, Slack M, et al. Emergency department visits in the United States for pediatric depression: estimates of charges and hospitalizations. Acad Emerg Med 2014;21(9):1003–14.
15. Donofrio JJ, Santillanes G, McCammack BD, et al. Clinical utility of screening laboratory tests in pediatric psychiatric patients presenting to the emergency department for medical clearance. Ann Emerg Med 2014;63(6):666–75.
16. Santillanes G, Donofrio JJ, Lam CC, et al. Is medical clearance necessary for pediatric psychiatric patients? J Emerg Med 2014;46(6):800–6.
17. Baren JM, Mace SE, Hendry PL. Children's mental health emergencies-part: emergency department evaluation and treatment of children with mental health disorders. Pediatr Emerg Care 2008;24(7):485–98.
18. Karas S. Behavioral health emergencies: differentiating medical from psychiatric disease. Emerg Med Pract 2002;4(3):1–20.
19. Onigu-Otite E, Oyebadejo AO, Moukaddam N, et al. Like a prisoner in Azkaban: medical clearance of the pediatric psychiatric patient. Pediatr Emerg Care Med 2016; 1(1):1–9. Available at: http://pediatric-emergency-care.imedpub.com/archive.php. Accessed June 9, 2017.
20. Donofrio JJ, Horeczko T, Kaji A. Most routine laboratory testing of pediatric psychiatric patients in the emergency department is not medically necessary. Health Aff (Millwood) 2015;34(5):812–8.
21. Janiak BD, Atteberry S. Medical clearance if the psychiatric patient in the emergency department. J Emerg Med 2009;43(5):866–9.
22. Parmar P, Goolsby CA, Udompanyanan K, et al. Value of mandatory screening studies in emergency department patients cleared for psychiatric admission. West J Emerg Med 2012;13(5):388–93.
23. Shihabuddin BS, Hack CM, Sivitz AB. Role of urine drug screen in the medical clearance of pediatric: psychiatric patients is there one? Pediatr Emerg Care 2013;29(8):903–6.
24. Fortu JM, Kim K, Cooper A, et al. Psychiatric patients in the pediatric emergency department undergoing routine urine toxicology screens for medical clearance. Pediatr Emerg Care 2009;25(6):387–92.
25. Tucci V. Inpatient exclusionary criteria and the pediatric psychiatric patient. Int J Acad Med, in press.
26. Lee S, Tucci V, Moukaddam N, et al. Pregnant and virtually abandoned: the multiple hurdles of medically clearing and admitting a pregnant patient to an inpatient psychiatric unit. J Psychiatry Ment Health 2016;1(1).
27. Zolotor AJ, Carlough MC. Update on prenatal care. 2014. Available at: http://www.aafp.org/afp/2014/0201/p199.html. Accessed November 11, 2016.
28. American Academy of Pediatrics, American College of Gynecologists. Guidelines for perinatal care. 7th edition. Washington, DC: American Academy of Pediatrics; 2007. p. 105–17.
29. American College of Obstetricians and Gynecologists. Hypertension in pregnancy. 2013. Available at: http://www.acog.org/Resources-And-Publications/Task-Force-and-Work-Group-Reports/Hypertension-in-Pregnancy. Accessed November 27, 2016.

30. Cuero MR, Panayiotis NV. Neurologic complications in pregnancy. Crit Care Clin 2016;32:43–59.
31. Cline MK. Chronic medical conditions in pregnancy. In: Ratcliffe SD, Baxley EG, Cline MK, et al, editors. Family medicine obstetrics. 3rd edition. Philadelphia: Mosby Elsevier; 2008. p. 202–57.
32. American College of Obstetrics and Gynecologists. Anemia in pregnancy. Obstet Gynecol 2008;112(1):201–7.
33. Golüke-Willemse GA, Klijnsma PJ, Tuinier S, et al. Geriatric wards in a psychiatric and a general hospital: a comparison of problems leading to admission of the patient. Tijdschr Gerontol Geriatr 2001;32(5):194–9.
34. Draper B, Golüke-Willemse GA, Klijnsma PJ, et al. The elderly admitted to a general hospital psychiatry ward. Aust N Z J Psychiatry 1994;28(2):288–97.
35. Puryear DA, Lovitt R, Miller DA. Characteristics of elderly persons seen in an urban psychiatric emergency room. Hosp Community Psychiatry 1991;42(8): 802–7.
36. Kolman PB. The value of laboratory investigations of elderly psychiatric patients. J Clin Psychiatry 1984;45:112–6.

Behavioral Emergencies

Special Considerations in the Pregnant Patient

Awais Aftab, MD[a,*], Asim A. Shah, MD[b,c,d]

KEYWORDS

- Psychiatric emergencies • Pregnancy • Psychotropics • Teratogenicity
- Depression • Bipolar disorder • Psychosis • Suicide

KEY POINTS

- The perinatal period is a time of psychiatric vulnerability. Up to 1 in 6 pregnant women experience major depressive disorder, and 1 in 4 pregnant women with bipolar disorder experience mood exacerbation.
- Untreated psychiatric illness in pregnancy puts the mother and child at considerable risks, and discontinuation of psychotropics during pregnancy increases the risk of relapse of psychiatric disorders.
- Mood stabilizers (valproate, carbamazepine and lithium) have well-recognized teratogenic risks. There is risk of neonatal toxicity and withdrawal with benzodiazepine use. The association of paroxetine and cardiac malformations is of concern but remains controversial.
- Women during late pregnancy are at risk of developing vena cava syndrome with the use of mechanical restraints for agitation. Suicidality in pregnant women is substantial and warrants adequate screening and assessment of suicide risk.
- All efforts should be made to prevent alcohol and opioid withdrawal syndromes during pregnancy given risk of harm to the fetus.

Disclosure: All authors have no relevant conflicts of interest or disclosures.

[a] Department of Psychiatry, Case Western Reserve University, University Hospitals Cleveland Medical Center, 10524 Eucolid Avenue, 8th Floor, Cleveland, OH 44106, USA; [b] Menninger Department of Psychiatry, Baylor College of Medicine, 1977 Butler Boulevard, Houston, TX 77030, USA; [c] Menninger Department of Family and Community Medicine, Baylor College of Medicine, 3701 Kirby Drive, Suite 600, Houston, TX 77098, USA; [d] Mood Disorder Research Program at BT, Community Behavioral Health Program, Psychotherapy Services, Neuropsychiatric Center, Ben Taub Hospital, HHS, Room 2.125, 1502 Taub Loop, Houston, TX 77030, USA
* Corresponding author. 10524, Euclid Avenue, 8th Floor, Cleveland, OH 44106.
E-mail address: awaisaftab@gmail.com

Psychiatr Clin N Am 40 (2017) 435–448
http://dx.doi.org/10.1016/j.psc.2017.05.017 psych.theclinics.com
0193-953X/17/© 2017 Elsevier Inc. All rights reserved.

INTRODUCTION

It has been traditionally believed that pregnancy has a protective effect against mental illness and that gestation is a time of relative mental well-being. A body of literature over the past decades disproves this notion as a myth; the perinatal period is in fact a time of psychiatric vulnerability for many women, and presents its own unique challenges of management, given that the health of 2 lives is at stake. Mental disorders during pregnancy negatively affect maternal and neonatal outcomes. Management of psychiatric disorders in pregnancy therefore requires urgent and timely intervention. Psychiatric emergencies are clinical situations in which there is significant risk of harm to self or others in subjects with mental disorders, and these cases are likely to present in the emergency or acute inpatient setting for evaluation and management. Psychiatric emergencies in pregnant women constitutes the subject matter of this review. Although we base our discussion on the extensive literature that explores the management of psychiatric disorders during pregnancy, it is important to note that we are restricting ourselves to considerations that apply to behavioral emergencies, and this review is not intended to serve as an exhaustive resource for the general management of psychiatric disorders in peripartum.

SEVERE MENTAL ILLNESS IN PREGNANCY

The prevalence of major depression in pregnant women ranges from 7% to 16%, and rates of depression in pregnancy appear to be comparable, or slightly lower, than in nonpregnant women.[1–3] The onset of many depressive episodes occurs for the first time during pregnancy,[4] and major depression also may be more undiagnosed in pregnant women.[5] A prior history of depression, perinatal or otherwise, is the biggest factor predictive of future risk.[6] Severe depression, especially if untreated, can proceed to outcomes such as psychosis, catatonia, and suicide. Screening all pregnant women for depression is recommended, and several tools are available to screen for depression in perinatal populations. These include instruments that were developed for generic depression screening, such as the Beck Depression Inventory, General Health Questionnaire, and the Hospital Anxiety and Depression Scale, as well as instruments that were specifically developed for use in perinatal women, such as the Edinburgh Postnatal Depression Scale (EPDS) and Postpartum Depression Screening Scale.[7] EPDS is self-report, 10-item scale that is convenient and widely used in the perinatal population.[8] Antidepressants and psychotherapy remain the first line of treatment.[9] Electroconvulsive therapy (ECT) should be considered for patients with psychotic symptoms, catatonia, suicidality, severe psychomotor retardation, and lack of response to multiple antidepressant trials.[9]

Symptomatic mood episodes are reported to occur in approximately 25% to 30% of women with bipolar disorder during pregnancy.[10,11] Patients with active mania in pregnancy present challenges in management. Given the teratogenic risks of mood stabilizers, antipsychotics are preferred agents for psychopharmacological treatment of mania. First-generation antipsychotics, particularly haloperidol, have a long tracking record of safety, and are commonly used.[12] Second-generation antipsychotics are also reasonable alternatives.[12] For patients not responding to antipsychotics, lithium and ECT are options to consider.[12] Adjunctive benzodiazepines can be helpful as well. Valproate and carbamazepine should be avoided unless clinical benefits outweigh the teratogenic risks. For patients with bipolar depression in pregnancy, lamotrigine and quetiapine are first-line medications[13]; lithium and ECT can be considered for treatment-resistant cases.[13] Psychopharmacological considerations during pregnancy are discussed in detail later in this article.

Literature on schizophrenia during pregnancy is limited; however, there does not appear to be an increased risk of acute relapse, with only 0.3% of acute episodes occurring during pregnancy in a study of more than 900 women with schizophrenia.[14]

Untreated psychiatric illness in pregnancy puts the mother and child at considerable risk. For instance, neonates with mothers experiencing prenatal depression are at risk for premature delivery, low birth weight, and growth retardation.[15] Untreated maternal depression affects childhood development, with higher impulsivity, maladaptive social interactions, and cognitive, behavioral, and emotional difficulties.[16] Neonates of depressed mothers also exhibit a biochemical and physiologic profile that resembles the prenatal biochemical/physiologic profile of the depressed mother, with elements such as elevated cortisol, and lower levels of dopamine and serotonin.[15] Anxiety disorders are associated with increased risk of prolonged labor, fetal distress, preterm delivery, and spontaneous abortion.[3] Schizophrenia is reported to be associated with an increased risk of congenital malformations (independent of medication use), preterm delivery, low birth weight, placental abnormalities, and postnatal death.[3]

RELAPSE OF PSYCHIATRIC DISORDERS IN PREGNANCY

Rate of relapse of major depression in women who discontinue their antidepressant during pregnancy is 68% compared with 26% in women who maintain their medication during pregnancy.[17] The odds ratio may be as high as 8 for the incidence of deterioration and relapse with discontinuation of medication during pregnancy, compared with medication maintenance.[18]

In a prospective observational clinical cohort study, women with bipolar disorder who discontinued their mood stabilizer treatment during pregnancy experienced a twofold greater recurrence risk, fourfold shorter median time to first recurrence, and fivefold greater duration of illness compared with women who maintained mood stabilizer treatment. Time to recurrence was 11 times shorter with abrupt discontinuation compared with gradual discontinuation. Almost three-quarters of mood episodes were depressed or mixed, and almost half occurred during the first trimester.[19] Additionally, in women with bipolar disorder, postpartum relapse rates are significantly higher among those who are medication free during pregnancy (66%) compared with those who stayed on medication prophylactically (23%).[20]

In the general population, there is a two- to threefold greater risk of schizophrenia relapse with antipsychotic discontinuation,[21] and the risk of psychotic relapse with antipsychotic discontinuation during pregnancy has been described in case reports[22,23] (**Box 1**).

Box 1
Risk of psychiatric relapse in pregnancy with medication discontinuation

- Women who discontinue their antidepressant during pregnancy have a relapse rate that is 2.5 times higher compared with women who maintain their medication.[17]
- Women with bipolar disorder who discontinue their mood stabilizer treatment during pregnancy experience a twofold greater recurrence risk, fourfold shorter median time to first recurrence, and fivefold greater duration of illness.[19]
- Postpartum relapse rates of bipolar mood episodes are significantly higher among those who are not on mood stabilizer prophylaxis during pregnancy.[20]

PSYCHOPHARMACOLOGICAL CONSIDERATIONS DURING PREGNANCY

A qualitative study investigating the perspectives of women with severe mental illness concerning the use of psychotropic medicines while pregnant found that in nearly all cases, women felt that their providers had limited access to necessary information, leaving women to rely on experiential and common-sense evidence when making decisions about taking medicine during pregnancy.[24]

The Food and Drug Administration's (FDA's) new Pregnancy and Lactation Labeling Rule (PLLR) was implemented in June 2015, which supersedes the prior pregnancy and lactation categories of A, B, C, D, and X, given the limitations of these categories.[25] Instead of assigning a misleading risk category, the new labeling provides pertinent risk summary, clinical considerations, and available research data on the safety of medications in pregnancy and lactation. Medications approved after June 2015 follow the PLLR, and medications approved after June 2001 will be updated to PLLR within a span of 3 years.[25] Although we do refer to old pregnancy categories where pertinent, readers should be mindful of this change implemented by the FDA.

Antidepressants

Approximately 8% of pregnant women are prescribed antidepressants in the United States, with selective serotonin reuptake inhibitors (SSRIs) being the most commonly prescribed class of antidepressants.[26] This is despite that most women on antidepressants discontinue the medication before or during the first trimester of pregnancy.[27]

A large body of literature has consistently shown that SSRIs are not major teratogens, and whenever associations between SSRIs and congenital abnormalities are reported, the absolute magnitude of the risk remains small. A 2013 meta-analysis of 19 studies reported no association between antidepressant exposure and congenital malformations, as well as major malformations. The meta-analysis did find an increased risk for cardiovascular malformations (relative risk [RR] 1.36) and septal heart defects (RR 1.4).[28] However, the association between antenatal exposure to SSRIs and heart defects remains controversial and hotly contested, and the association has not been found in several large studies.[29,30] A relative risk increase of 1.4 would result in an absolute risk of 7 in 1000 live births. Although some evidence suggests that paroxetine may be associated with a small absolute increase in congenital heart defects, results across different observational studies are inconsistent. A 2014 large, population-based cohort study that included 949,504 pregnant women did not find an increased risk of cardiac malformations with antidepressant use during the first trimester. The study also did not found an association with the specific use paroxetine or sertraline and cardiac malformations.[31] While recent literature casts doubt on the association between paroxetine and cardiac defects, it is important to mention that when this concern was initially brought to light, FDA issued a public health advisory and changed paroxetine's pregnancy and lactation category from C to D based on preliminary epidemiological findings data from two epidemiological studies which were unpublished at that point, making paroxetine the only SSRI with a D category rating.[3,32,33]

The use of SSRIs during late pregnancy (eg, third trimester) appears to be associated with a small increased risk of persistent pulmonary hypertension of the newborn. A 2014 systematic review found an association between antenatal exposure and persistent pulmonary hypertension in late pregnancy, but not during the first trimester, with an odds ratio of 2.5. The baseline low incidence translates into the fact that the absolute increase with SSRI exposure is nonetheless low. Approximately 350 women would have to be treated with SSRIs in late pregnancy to cause 1 additional case of persistent pulmonary hypertension of the newborn.[34] A subsequent observational study found no association between persistent pulmonary hypertension and prenatal exposure.[35]

In utero exposure to antidepressants during the third trimester appears to be associated with poor neonatal adjustment syndrome.[36] The reported incidence varies widely, as the definitions for the syndrome vary widely as well. It is usually mild and transient in most cases, warranting only observation, but could potentially be severe and may lead to respiratory distress and seizures. Whether this is a form of neonatal antidepressant discontinuation syndrome or antidepressant toxicity remains unknown. Dose reduction or medication discontinuation before delivery does not appear to reduce the risk of the syndrome,[37] and is not clinically recommended.

Traditional Mood Stabilizers

Lithium's teratogenic risk is well-recognized; it has specifically been associated with Ebstein anomaly, which is a malformation of the tricuspid valve and right ventricle. With lithium exposure, the risk of Ebstein anomaly is believed to increase by approximately 20 times, from 1 in 20,000 live births to 1 in 1000, which is an absolute risk of still less than 1%.[38,39] This teratogenic risk is present with lithium use before week 12, as afterward the fetal heart has already formed. Risk ratio is reported to be 1.2 to 7.7 for all cardiac malformations and 1.5 to 3.0 for all congenital defects.[40] Lithium use is second, and the third trimester has been noted to result in neonatal complications, such as nephrogenic diabetes insipidus, goiter and hypothyroidism, floppy infant syndrome, and lithium toxicity.[3,32]

Sodium valproate is an established major teratogen with an FDA black box warning for neural tube defects and decreased IQ. Its risk of congenital malformations is approximately fourfold that of any other antiepileptic drug, and sevenfold that of the general population.[41] Approximately 1% to 2% of fetuses exposed to valproate during pregnancy develop neural tube defects, and this is a 10 to 20 times higher risk compared with the general population. Other congenital malformations also have been reported. These risks appear to be dose dependent,[42] and folate supplementation (although recommended) does not appear to protect again these risks.[43]

Like valproate, carbamazepine has established teratogenic effects, and includes neural tube defects, such as spina bifida, along with other congenital malformations.[3,32] The risk of neural tube defects with carbamazepine is significantly high but less than that of valproate. Fetal carbamazepine syndrome and developmental delays also are reported.[3,32] Approximately 1% of fetuses exposed to carbamazepine develop spina bifida, which is a 7 times higher risk compared with the general population.[44]

Benzodiazepines

There is controversy surrounding the teratogenic risks of benzodiazepines. Some studies have linked in utero benzodiazepine exposure with development of oral cleft; however, this association has not been replicated in other studies. A meta-analysis by Dolovich and colleagues[45] shows that although aggregated data from case-control studies show an association with an odds ratio of 1.8, cohort studies have not found this association, casting doubt on its validity. Even if valid, the magnitude of increased risk is 1 to 5 additional births with oral cleft per 10,000 births,[46,47] which is a small absolute risk. Although teratogenicity does not appear to be of major concern, neonatal benzodiazepine toxicity and neonatal benzodiazepine withdrawal following in utero exposure are of significant clinical concern, warranting close monitoring of the newborn.[3,32]

Antipsychotics

The literature shows that discontinuation of antipsychotics is common in pregnant women. Only 38% of women on atypical antipsychotics and 19% of women on typical antipsychotics before pregnancy are still receiving antipsychotic treatment at the start of the third trimester.[48]

Data from the Massachusetts General Hospital National Pregnancy Registry for Atypical Antipsychotics reveals that the absolute risk of major malformations is 1.4% for exposed infants and 1.1% for unexposed infants, with an odds ratio of 1.25 (95% confidence interval 0.13–12.19), which is not statistically significant. This indicates that second-generation antipsychotics are unlikely to raise the risk of major malformations more than 10-fold beyond that observed in the general population or among control groups using other psychotropic medications.[49]

A systematic review and meta-analysis reported that the use of second-generation antipsychotics during the first trimester of pregnancy was associated with a significant increased risk for major congenital malformations (odds ratio 2.03); however, no specific pattern of malformations was found.[50] Another systematic review and meta-analysis of case-control and cohort studies reported an increased risk of major malformations with an absolute risk difference of 0.03. There was no significant difference in the risk of major malformations between typical and atypical antipsychotic medications.[51]

In a recent study with the largest population of women exposed to antipsychotics published to date, the RR for major malformations and cardiac malformations with first-trimester antipsychotic exposure was not found to be significant for typical and atypical antipsychotics. On analysis of individual agents, a small significant increased risk in overall malformations (RR 1.26) was found for risperidone, the significance of which is unclear and requires confirmation in additional studies. Overall, this large study shows that the use of antipsychotics in the first trimester of pregnancy is not associated with a meaningful increase in risk of congenital malformations[52] (**Table 1**).

ACUTE AGITATION IN PREGNANT PATIENTS

Agitation in a pregnant woman can be a consequence of many different underlying conditions: acute psychosis, mania, catatonic agitation, delirious agitation, and intoxication/withdrawal from alcohol or other substances are some of the common psychiatric causes. Although definitive management depends on the identification of the underlying cause of agitation, immediate management generally applies to most cases of agitation. Verbal deescalation and behavioral redirection should be the first interventions.[53] The presence of pain or other physical distress should be ruled out. Any anxiety or fears vocalized by the patient should be addressed in an effort to calm the patient. If behavioral interventions fail and agitation continues, medications may be warranted. Diphenhydramine has no proven risk of humans in pregnancy, and is labeled category B per the FDA's former pregnancy and lactation category system.[53] In mild cases of agitation, oral or intramuscular administration of diphenhydramine may suffice. In severe cases, an antipsychotic agent, haloperidol being a common choice, can be used. Benzodiazepines can be avoided, given the possibility of harms as discussed previously; however, the risks of 1-time or limited doses administered in the context of agitation are unknown and are likely to be considerably less compared with regular use. Therefore, the severity of agitations may warrant appropriate clinical use of benzodiazepines after the risks and benefits of short-term administration have been weighed.

Table 1
Medications and fetal risks during pregnancy

Medication Group	Fetal Risks with Use in Pregnancy
Antidepressants (selective serotonin reuptake inhibitors [SSRIs])	• SSRIs are not major teratogens. • The association of paroxetine with cardiac malformations has been reported but remains controversial. • Use in third trimester: risk of persistent pulmonary hypertension of the newborn and poor neonatal adjustment syndrome.
Mood stabilizers	• Lithium use is associated with risk of Ebstein anomaly and lithium toxicity. • Sodium valproate is a major teratogen with a Food and Drug Administration black box warning for neural tube defects and decreased IQ. • Carbamazepine is also associated with significantly increased risk of neural tube defects (less than valproate).
Benzodiazepines	• Inconsistent evidence for a small increase in risk of oral cleft. • Use in late pregnancy is associated with risk of neonatal benzodiazepine toxicity and withdrawal.
Antipsychotics	• Antipsychotics do not appear to be associated with a meaningful increase in risk of congenital malformations.

Use of seclusion and restraints should be an intervention of last resort. Women in the second and third trimesters of pregnancy are vulnerable to the development of vena cava syndrome if mechanical restraints are used.[54] The inferior vena cava syndrome is caused by the compression of the inferior vena cava, blocking the flow of venous blood to the heart. This can result in hypotension, tachycardia, and peripheral edema, as well as fetal hypoxia and distress. This can happen in late pregnancy from lying supine or on the right side, as in this position the gravid uterus can compress the vein. This can easily occur if a pregnant woman is placed in 4-point restraints on her back, and the agitated state may even prevent timely recognition of the symptoms of the syndrome. The risk can be reduced by ensuring that restrained pregnant women have their bodies turned partway to the left with support under the right hip.[54] Pregnant women in restraints also should be monitored at short intervals for medical stability while they are in restraints.

SUICIDALITY IN PREGNANCY

Although it has been recognized that the rates of suicide attempts and completed suicides are lower during pregnancy and the postpartum period compared with the general population, suicidal ideation is experienced by a substantial number of pregnant women (ranging from 5%–14%), which in some cases progresses to a suicide attempt. Suicidal ideation experienced during pregnancy is also associated with a higher risk of developing postpartum depression.[55]

Data from the United Kingdom spanning 1997 to 2012 reveals that suicide in the perinatal period constitutes 2% of suicides in women aged 16 to 50 years, and 4% of suicides in the age group 20 to 35 years. The study also reported that women who died by suicide in the perinantal period were more likely to have a diagnosis of depression and were less likely to be receiving any active treatment.[56] A study from the United States looked at 2005 to 2010 data from enhanced pregnancy mortality surveillance, and reported that pregnancy-associated suicide risk ranged from 1.6 to 4.5 per 100,000 live births compared with 5.3 to 5.5 per 100,000 women aged 10 to 54 years among nonpregnant/nonpostpartum women. The RR of suicide among pregnant/postpartum women was calculated to be 0.62.[57]

A study investigating the prevalence of self-harm and its correlates in women with psychotic disorders and bipolar disorder during pregnancy reported that 24.5% of identified pregnant women with these disorders had a record of suicidal ideation during the first index pregnancy, with self-harm recorded in 7.9%.[58] A study that looked at pregnant women who had been admitted to the hospital due to suicidal attempts by drug ingestion reported that the peak period of suicide attempts was in the first postconceptual months, and it resulted in a very early fetal loss in most cases.[59] Although the prevalence of suicidal behavior is higher among those with depression diagnoses, more than 30% of hospitalizations are for suicidal behavior without depression diagnoses.[60]

Risk factors for perinatal suicidality include younger maternal age, unmarried status, prior suicidality and psychiatric disorders, family history of psychiatric disorders and suicidality, domestic violence, lack of social support, rejection of paternity by the partner, unwanted pregnancy and nulliparity, and abrupt discontinuation of psychotropic medications during pregnancy.[55] Suicidality also appears to be more likely to occur during pregnancy compared with the postpartum period.[55]

A thorough risk assessment in pregnant women involves consideration of all the same factors involved in risk assessment in the general population, additionally considering the specific risk factors for perinatal suicidality. It is important to recognize that a substantial proportion of women with suicidal ideation do not meet clinical thresholds of depression, and there is a susceptibility to suicidal behavior independent of depressive disorders, which indicates that screening for suicidal ideation should not simply be in the context of screening for depression.[61]

This literature points out the substantial burden and negative impact of suicidality during the perinantal period, and underscores the importance of a thorough screening and assessment of suicide risk during pregnancy. Individuals determined to be at high risk of suicide in the acute setting are generally best treated in an inpatient setting (**Box 2**).

CATATONIA IN PREGNANCY

Literature on catatonia during pregnancy is scarce, limited primarily to a handful of case reports, but there is no doubt that catatonia during pregnancy constitutes a

Box 2
Risk factors for perinantal suicidality

- Younger maternal age
- Unmarried status
- Prior suicidality and psychiatric disorders
- Family history of psychiatric disorders and suicidality
- Domestic violence
- Lack of social support
- Rejection of paternity by the partner
- Unwanted pregnancy and nulliparity
- Abrupt discontinuation of psychotropic medications during pregnancy

Adapted from Orsolini L, Valchera A, Vecchiotti R, et al. Suicide during perinatal period: epidemiology, risk factors, and clinical correlates. Front Psychiatry 2016;7:138.

psychiatric emergency, as it can result in neglect of pregnancy and prenatal care, reduced food and water intake can cause imminent harm to the fetus, and prolonged catatonia can cause various medical complications, for instance decubitus ulcers, aspiration pneumonia, and deep vein thrombosis. This warrants early and aggressive treatment of catatonia in pregnant patients. Benzodiazepines (lorazepam being the most commonly used agent) and ECT remain the standard first-line treatments in pregnancy as in the nonpregnant population. The potential risks of benzodiazepines have been discussed previously. ECT has been traditionally regarded as effective and safe for mother and fetus during pregnancy,[62] and in this light, some investigators have recommended considering ECT earlier during the treatment of catatonia in pregnancy. However, a recent systematic review of case reports highlights potential risks of ECT during pregnancy, including fetal heart rate reduction, uterine contractions, premature labor, and even child mortality.[63] As case reports naturally tend to overreport adverse outcomes compared with the absence of adverse outcomes, the interpretation of the results of the systematic review is debated. Clinicians should not shy from appropriate utilization of ECT in pregnant patients when it is clinically indicated to do so, for instance if catatonia fails to respond to benzodiazepines.

ALCOHOL USE DISORDER IN PREGNANCY

Although pregnant women consume less alcohol compared to nonpregnant women, the rates of alcohol intake in pregnant women remain substantial and significant. The 2012 National Survey on Drug Use and Health[64] reported that during the prior month, 8.5% of pregnant women in America had consumed at least 1 alcoholic drink, 2.7% had consumed 5 or more drinks during 1 episode ("binge drinking"), and 0.3% had 5 or more drinks on the same occasion 5 or more times ("heavy drinking"). Psychiatric practitioners, therefore, are likely to encounter pregnant women with alcohol use disorders.

The teratogenic properties of alcohol have been recognized since the 1960s. There is a well-described fetal alcohol syndrome consisting of craniofacial, limb, and cardiovascular defects along with growth deficiency and developmental delay associated with fetal exposure to alcohol.[65] A host of other pathologic consequences have also been reported, such as low birth weight, preterm birth, spontaneous abortions, cognitive deficits, and behavioral problems.[65] It is important, therefore, to minimize fetal exposure to alcohol as much as possible in women with alcohol use disorders.

Alcohol withdrawal even in the general population can cause severe, potentially fatal, phenomena, such as alcoholic hallucinosis, withdrawal seizures, and delirium tremens. In pregnant women, the risks of alcohol withdrawal are even greater due to possible adverse effects to the fetus.[66] Chronic heavy drinking disturbs the hypothalamic-pituitary-adrenal axis, and alcohol withdrawal particularly can lead to elevated levels of cortisol. The hypercortisol state in pregnancy can lead to preterm labor.[65] Alcohol withdrawal–related hypertension poses additional medical concerns. Placental abruption and fetal distress are also potential consequences.[66] The confusional state of delirium tremens also may lead to potential physical harm through accidents or injury. All efforts should be made to prevent the development of alcohol withdrawal in pregnant women. No specific studies on the treatment of alcohol withdrawal during pregnancy are available; therefore, current discussion in literature extrapolates existing knowledge to this situation.

Benzodiazepines are the medications of choice in treatment of alcohol withdrawal in the general population and by extrapolation in pregnant patients.[67] As discussed previously, there is controversy surrounding the teratogenic potential of benzodiazepine use during the first trimester. The risks with short-term administration of benzodiazepines, as is typical for alcohol detoxification, are likely to be even lower. The potential harms of untreated withdrawal to mother and infant must therefore be balanced against the potential risks of benzodiazepine use during pregnancy.[67] In many cases, the former is likely to outweigh the latter; however, clinicians should weigh these risks on a case-by-case basis.

Anticonvulsants also have been used in the treatment of withdrawal, to mediate withdrawal symptoms and prevent seizures; however anticonvulsants, such valproate and carbamazepine, are associated with a higher risk of fetal malformations, and cannot be considered as preferred agents over benzodiazepines in pregnant patients.[67] Gabapentin can be of benefit in managing mild alcohol withdrawal syndrome,[68] and may be a consideration, given its relative safety in pregnancy.[69]

OPIOID USE DISORDER DURING PREGNANCY

Maternal opioid withdrawal can lead to the development of an intrauterine abstinence syndrome, which could be potentially fatal for the fetus, and can have potential long-term effects on the development of the fetal brain.[70] Opioid detoxification without maintenance treatment also places women at a high risk of opioid relapse, with its own subsequent social, medical, and psychiatric risks. Given these considerations, opioid maintenance therapy is considered the standard of care for pregnant opioid-dependent women. Medically assisted opioid withdrawal is not recommended in pregnancy, and should be used only if the patient refuses opioid maintenance treatment.

Both methadone and buprenorphine have been demonstrated as safe and effective for opioid maintenance treatment in the pregnant population. A 2016 meta-analysis reported that moderately strong evidence indicates that buprenorphine treatment during pregnancy is associated with a lower risk of preterm birth, greater birth weight, and larger head circumference, compared with methadone treatment.[71] Buprenorphine also leads to a milder neonatal withdrawal syndrome in neonates born to mothers on maintenance therapy. However, these benefits must be balanced with the fact that buprenorphine inductions require that mothers already be in opioid withdrawal, which is undesirable in pregnant patients. Although methadone remains the current standard of care, buprenorphine is increasingly being preferred by many practitioners, given limited access to methadone maintenance treatment programs, similar efficacy, and other relatively favorable outcomes described in this article.[72]

REFERENCES

1. Mota N, Cox BJ, Enns MW, et al. The relationship between mental disorders, quality of life, and pregnancy: findings from a nationally representative sample. J Affect Disord 2008;109(3):300–4.
2. Vesga-Lopez O, Blanco C, Keyes K, et al. Psychiatric disorders in pregnant and postpartum women in the United States. Arch Gen Psychiatry 2008;65(7):805–15.
3. Bulletins–Obstetrics ACoP. ACOG practice bulletin: clinical management guidelines for obstetrician-gynecologists number 92, April 2008 (replaces practice bulletin number 87, November 2007). Use of psychiatric medications during pregnancy and lactation. Obstet Gynecol 2008;111(4):1001–20.
4. Patton GC, Romaniuk H, Spry E, et al. Prediction of perinatal depression from adolescence and before conception (VIHCS): 20-year prospective cohort study. Lancet 2015;386(9996):875–83.

5. Ko JY, Farr SL, Dietz PM, et al. Depression and treatment among U.S. pregnant and nonpregnant women of reproductive age, 2005-2009. J Womens Health (Larchmt) 2012;21(8):830–6.
6. Raisanen S, Lehto SM, Nielsen HS, et al. Risk factors for and perinatal outcomes of major depression during pregnancy: a population-based analysis during 2002-2010 in Finland. BMJ Open 2014;4(11):e004883.
7. Milgrom J, Gemmill AW. Screening for perinatal depression. Best Pract Res Clin Obstet Gynaecol 2014;28(1):13–23.
8. El-Den S, O'Reilly CL, Chen TF. A systematic review on the acceptability of perinatal depression screening. J Affect Disord 2015;188:284–303.
9. Grigoriadis S. Severe antenatal unipolar major depression: treatment. In: Roy-Byrne PP, Lockwood CJ, editors. UpToDate. Waltham (MA): UpToDate; 2016. Available at: https://www.uptodate.com/contents/severe-antenatal-unipolar-major-depression-treatment. Accessed October 31, 2016.
10. Viguera AC, Tondo L, Koukopoulos AE, et al. Episodes of mood disorders in 2,252 pregnancies and postpartum periods. Am J Psychiatry 2011;168(11): 1179–85.
11. Yonkers KA, Vigod S, Ross LE. Diagnosis, pathophysiology, and management of mood disorders in pregnant and postpartum women. Obstet Gynecol 2011; 117(4):961–77.
12. Hendrick V. Bipolar disorder in pregnant women: treatment of mania and hypomania. In: Keck P, Wilkins-Haug L, editors. UpToDate. Waltham (MA): UpToDate; 2016. Available at: https://www.uptodate.com/contents/bipolar-disorder-in-pregnant-women-treatment-of-mania-and-hypomania. Accessed October 31, 2016.
13. Hendrick V. Bipolar disorder in pregnant women: treatment of major depression. In: Keck P, editor. UpToDate. Waltham (MA): UpToDate; 2016. Available at: https://www.uptodate.com/contents/bipolar-disorder-in-pregnant-women-treatment-of-major-depression. Accessed October 31, 2016.
14. Trixler M, Gati A, Tenyi T. Risks associated with childbearing in schizophrenia. Acta Psychiatr Belg 1995;95(3):159–62.
15. Field T, Diego M, Hernandez-Reif M. Prenatal depression effects on the fetus and newborn: a review. Infant Behav Dev 2006;29(3):445–55.
16. Chan J, Natekar A, Einarson A, et al. Risks of untreated depression in pregnancy. Can Fam Physician 2014;60(3):242–3.
17. Cohen LS, Altshuler LL, Harlow BL, et al. Relapse of major depression during pregnancy in women who maintain or discontinue antidepressant treatment. JAMA 2006;295(5):499–507.
18. Suzuki S, Kato M. Deterioration/relapse of depression during pregnancy in Japanese women associated with interruption of antidepressant medications. J Matern Fetal Neonatal Med 2017;30(10):1129–32.
19. Viguera AC, Whitfield T, Baldessarini RJ, et al. Risk of recurrence in women with bipolar disorder during pregnancy: prospective study of mood stabilizer discontinuation. Am J Psychiatry 2007;164(12):1817–24 [quiz: 1923].
20. Wesseloo R, Kamperman AM, Munk-Olsen T, et al. Risk of postpartum relapse in bipolar disorder and postpartum psychosis: a systematic review and meta-analysis. Am J Psychiatry 2016;173(2):117–27.
21. Robinson GE. Treatment of schizophrenia in pregnancy and postpartum. J Popul Ther Clin Pharmacol 2012;19(3):e380–6.
22. Ifteni P, Moga MA, Burtea V, et al. Schizophrenia relapse after stopping olanzapine treatment during pregnancy: a case report. Ther Clin Risk Manag 2014; 10:901–4.

23. Wakil L, Perea E, Penaskovic K, et al. Exacerbation of psychotic disorder during pregnancy in the context of medication discontinuation. Psychosomatics 2013; 54(3):290–3.
24. Stevenson F, Hamilton S, Pinfold V, et al. Decisions about the use of psychotropic medication during pregnancy: a qualitative study. BMJ Open 2016;6(1):e010130.
25. Ramoz LL, Patel-Shori NM. Recent changes in pregnancy and lactation labeling: retirement of risk categories. Pharmacotherapy 2014;34(4):389–95.
26. Andrade SE, Raebel MA, Brown J, et al. Use of antidepressant medications during pregnancy: a multisite study. Am J Obstet Gynecol 2008;198(2)(194):e191–5.
27. Hayes RM, Wu P, Shelton RC, et al. Maternal antidepressant use and adverse outcomes: a cohort study of 228,876 pregnancies. Am J Obstet Gynecol 2012; 207(1)(49):e41–9.
28. Grigoriadis S, VonderPorten EH, Mamisashvili L, et al. Antidepressant exposure during pregnancy and congenital malformations: is there an association? A systematic review and meta-analysis of the best evidence. J Clin Psychiatry 2013; 74(4):e293–308.
29. Furu K, Kieler H, Haglund B, et al. Selective serotonin reuptake inhibitors and venlafaxine in early pregnancy and risk of birth defects: population based cohort study and sibling design. BMJ 2015;350:h1798.
30. Reis M, Kallen B. Combined use of selective serotonin reuptake inhibitors and sedatives/hypnotics during pregnancy: risk of relatively severe congenital malformations or cardiac defects. A register study. BMJ Open 2013;3(2) [pii:e002166].
31. Huybrechts KF, Palmsten K, Avorn J, et al. Antidepressant use in pregnancy and the risk of cardiac defects. N Engl J Med 2014;370(25):2397–407.
32. Shah AA, Khawaja IS, Aftab A. Are psychotropic drugs safe to use during pregnancy? Psychiatr Ann 2015;45(2):71–6.
33. FDA. Public Health Advisory: Paroxetine. Available at: https://www.fda.gov/Drugs/DrugSafety/PostmarketDrugSafetyInformationforPatientsandProviders/ucm051731.htm. Accessed June 17, 2017.
34. Grigoriadis S, Vonderporten EH, Mamisashvili L, et al. Prenatal exposure to antidepressants and persistent pulmonary hypertension of the newborn: systematic review and meta-analysis. BMJ 2014;348:f6932.
35. Huybrechts KF, Bateman BT, Palmsten K, et al. Antidepressant use late in pregnancy and risk of persistent pulmonary hypertension of the newborn. JAMA 2015; 313(21):2142–51.
36. Grigoriadis S, VonderPorten EH, Mamisashvili L, et al. The effect of prenatal antidepressant exposure on neonatal adaptation: a systematic review and meta-analysis. J Clin Psychiatry 2013;74(4):e309–20.
37. Warburton W, Hertzman C, Oberlander TF. A register study of the impact of stopping third trimester selective serotonin reuptake inhibitor exposure on neonatal health. Acta Psychiatr Scand 2010;121(6):471–9.
38. Cohen LS. Treatment of bipolar disorder during pregnancy. J Clin Psychiatry 2007;68(Suppl 9):4–9.
39. Correa-Villasenor A, Ferencz C, Neill CA, et al. Ebstein's malformation of the tricuspid valve: genetic and environmental factors. The Baltimore-Washington Infant Study Group. Teratology 1994;50(2):137–47.
40. Cohen LS, Friedman JM, Jefferson JW, et al. A reevaluation of risk of in utero exposure to lithium. JAMA 1994;271(2):146–50.
41. Wyszynski DF, Nambisan M, Surve T, et al. Increased rate of major malformations in offspring exposed to valproate during pregnancy. Neurology 2005;64(6): 961–5.

42. Artama M, Auvinen A, Raudaskoski T, et al. Antiepileptic drug use of women with epilepsy and congenital malformations in offspring. Neurology 2005;64(11): 1874–8.
43. Hernandez-Diaz S, Werler MM, Walker AM, et al. Folic acid antagonists during pregnancy and the risk of birth defects. N Engl J Med 2000;343(22):1608–14.
44. Rosa FW. Spina bifida in infants of women treated with carbamazepine during pregnancy. N Engl J Med 1991;324(10):674–7.
45. Dolovich LR, Addis A, Vaillancourt JM, et al. Benzodiazepine use in pregnancy and major malformations or oral cleft: meta-analysis of cohort and case-control studies. BMJ 1998;317(7162):839–43.
46. Altshuler LL, Cohen L, Szuba MP, et al. Pharmacologic management of psychiatric illness during pregnancy: dilemmas and guidelines. Am J Psychiatry 1996; 153(5):592–606.
47. Yonkers KA, Wisner KL, Stowe Z, et al. Management of bipolar disorder during pregnancy and the postpartum period. Am J Psychiatry 2004;161(4):608–20.
48. Petersen I, McCrea RL, Osborn DJ, et al. Discontinuation of antipsychotic medication in pregnancy: a cohort study. Schizophr Res 2014;159(1):218–25.
49. Cohen LS, Viguera AC, McInerney KA, et al. Reproductive safety of second-generation antipsychotics: current data from the Massachusetts General Hospital National Pregnancy Registry for atypical antipsychotics. Am J Psychiatry 2016; 173(3):263–70.
50. Terrana N, Koren G, Pivovarov J, et al. Pregnancy outcomes following in utero exposure to second-generation antipsychotics: a systematic review and meta-analysis. J Clin Psychopharmacol 2015;35(5):559–65.
51. Coughlin CG, Blackwell KA, Bartley C, et al. Obstetric and neonatal outcomes after antipsychotic medication exposure in pregnancy. Obstet Gynecol 2015; 125(5):1224–35.
52. Huybrechts KF, Hernandez-Diaz S, Patorno E, et al. Antipsychotic use in pregnancy and the risk for congenital malformations. JAMA Psychiatry 2016;73(9): 938–46.
53. Wilson MP, Nordstrom K, Shah AA, et al. Psychiatric emergencies in pregnant women. Emerg Med Clin North Am 2015;33(4):841–51.
54. Henshaw E, Marcus S. Psychiatric emergencies during pregnancy and postpartum and review of gender issues in psychiatric emergency medicine. In: Glick RL, Berlin JS, Fishkind A, editors. Emergency psychiatry: principles and practice. Philadelphia: Lippincott Williams & Wilkins; 2008. p. 313–43.
55. Orsolini L, Valchera A, Vecchiotti R, et al. Suicide during perinatal period: epidemiology, risk factors, and clinical correlates. Front Psychiatry 2016;7:138.
56. Khalifeh H, Hunt IM, Appleby L, et al. Suicide in perinatal and non-perinatal women in contact with psychiatric services: 15 year findings from a UK national inquiry. Lancet Psychiatry 2016;3(3):233–42.
57. Wallace ME, Hoyert D, Williams C, et al. Pregnancy-associated homicide and suicide in 37 US states with enhanced pregnancy surveillance. Am J Obstet Gynecol 2016;215(3):364.e1–10.
58. Taylor CL, van Ravesteyn LM, van denBerg MP, et al. The prevalence and correlates of self-harm in pregnant women with psychotic disorder and bipolar disorder. Arch Womens Ment Health 2016;19(5):909–15.
59. Czeizel AE, Timar L, Susanszky E. Timing of suicide attempts by self-poisoning during pregnancy and pregnancy outcomes. Int J Gynaecol Obstet 1999;65(1): 39–45.

60. Zhong QY, Gelaye B, Miller M, et al. Suicidal behavior-related hospitalizations among pregnant women in the USA, 2006-2012. Arch Womens Ment Health 2016;19(3):463–72.
61. Gelaye B, Kajeepeta S, Williams MA. Suicidal ideation in pregnancy: an epidemiologic review. Arch Womens Ment Health 2016;19(5):741–51.
62. Anderson EL, Reti IM. ECT in pregnancy: a review of the literature from 1941 to 2007. Psychosom Med 2009;71(2):235–42.
63. Leiknes KA, Cooke MJ, Jarosch-von Schweder L, et al. Electroconvulsive therapy during pregnancy: a systematic review of case studies. Arch Womens Ment Health 2015;18(1):1–39.
64. Substance Abuse and Mental Health Services Administration. Results from the 2012 National Survey on Drug Use and Health: summary of national findings. NSDUH Series H-46, HHS Publication No. (SMA) 13-4795. Rockville (MD): Substance Abuse and Mental Health Services Administration; 2013.
65. DeVido J, Bogunovic O, Weiss RD. Alcohol use disorders in pregnancy. Harv Rev Psychiatry 2015;23(2):112–21.
66. Bhat A, Hadley A. The management of alcohol withdrawal in pregnancy–case report, literature review and preliminary recommendations. Gen Hosp Psychiatry 2015;37(3)(273):e271–3.
67. Heberlein A, Leggio L, Stichtenoth D, et al. The treatment of alcohol and opioid dependence in pregnant women. Curr Opin Psychiatry 2012;25(6):559–64.
68. Leung JG, Hall-Flavin D, Nelson S, et al. The role of gabapentin in the management of alcohol withdrawal and dependence. Ann Pharmacother 2015;49(8):897–906.
69. Fujii H, Goel A, Bernard N, et al. Pregnancy outcomes following gabapentin use: results of a prospective comparative cohort study. Neurology 2013;80(17):1565–70.
70. McCarthy JJ. Intrauterine abstinence syndrome (IAS) during buprenorphine inductions and methadone tapers: can we assure the safety of the fetus? J Matern Fetal Neonatal Med 2012;25(2):109–12.
71. Zedler BK, Mann AL, Kim MM, et al. Buprenorphine compared with methadone to treat pregnant women with opioid use disorder: a systematic review and meta-analysis of safety in the mother, fetus and child. Addiction 2016;111(12):2115–28.
72. Wilder CM, Winhusen T. Pharmacological management of opioid use disorder in pregnant women. CNS Drugs 2015;29(8):625–36.

Behavioral Emergencies

Special Considerations in the Geriatric Psychiatric Patient

Awais Aftab, MD[a,*], Asim A. Shah, MD[b,c,d,e]

KEYWORDS

- Geriatric psychiatry • Emergency psychiatry • Delirium • Dementia • Agitation
- Suicide

KEY POINTS

- As a result of multiple physiological and pharmacokinetic changes, the elderly are more vulnerable to the side-effects of medications, and require lower doses of medications and slower rates of titration.
- Geriatric population is a high-risk group for suicide, with more serious intent, fewer warning signs, and more lethality. Suicide risk assessment should be part of a standard emergency psychiatric assessment.
- Prompt diagnosis and treatment of delirium in emergency settings is essential given the association with worse outcomes such as prolonged hospital stay, risk of cognitive decline, and increased mortality.
- Behavioral interventions for agitation in dementia are the first-line measure before pharmacologic interventions. Pharmacologic options with demonstrable efficacy are mostly limited to antipsychotics, the use of which is problematic, as all antipsychotics increase the risk of mortality in dementia.

INTRODUCTION

It is estimated that by the year 2030 about 72 million US citizens will be age 65 or older, making up about 20% of the US population.[1] A total of 15.4% of visits to the

Disclosure: All authors have no relevant conflicts of interest or disclosures.
[a] Department of Psychiatry, University Hospitals Cleveland Medical Center, Case Western Reserve University, 10524 Euclid Avenue, 8th Floor, Cleveland, OH 44106, USA; [b] Psychiatric Residency Education, Menninger Department of Psychiatry, Baylor College of Medicine, 1977 Butler Boulevard, Houston, TX 77030, USA; [c] Menninger Department of Family and Community Medicine, Baylor College of Medicine, 3701 Kirby Drive Suite 600, Houston, TX 77098, USA; [d] Mood Disorder Research Program at BT, Neuropsychiatric Center, Ben Taub Hospital/HHS, Room 2.125, 1502 Taub Loop, Houston, TX 77030, USA; [e] Community Behavioral Health Program, Psychotherapy Services, Neuropsychiatric Center, Ben Taub Hospital/HHS, Room 2.125, 1502 Taub Loop, Houston, TX 77030, USA
* Corresponding author.
E-mail address: awaisaftab@gmail.com

Psychiatr Clin N Am 40 (2017) 449–462
http://dx.doi.org/10.1016/j.psc.2017.05.010
0193-953X/17/© 2017 Elsevier Inc. All rights reserved.

emergency department are by the elderly,[2] and the visit rates by older adults have had the highest increase among all age groups in the last decades.[2]

Emergency psychiatric presentations in the elderly are often challenging, given the lack of well-defined presenting complaints, multiple medical and neurologic comorbidities, and the complex nature of presentations. Psychiatric symptoms can often be the result of a medical disorder in the elderly, and particularly new-onset psychiatric symptoms should warrant a thorough medical and neurological work-up. Evaluation of cognitive status and suicide risk assessment should be essential components of any emergency psychiatric assessment of the elderly. Review of medications for polypharmacy and medication side effects are also important. Substance use is often overlooked in the geriatric population and warrants careful history taking and urine toxicology. Geriatric patients are sometimes unreliable historians, and collateral history taking in many cases is warranted. Common disorders like depression can also have atypical presentations in the elderly compared with adults.

This report provides an overview of special psychiatric considerations in the geriatric population and common psychiatric emergencies of specific relevance in the elderly that warrant prompt assessment and management.

GENERAL PSYCHOPHARMACOLOGIC CONSIDERATIONS IN THE ELDERLY

Geriatric subjects are more vulnerable to the side effects of medications. This increased susceptibility is a result of several physiologic changes associated with aging that lead to pharmacokinetic changes. For instance, decreased concentration of plasma albumin can lead to increased plasma concentration of free drugs, decreased glomerular filtration rate results in decreased renal clearance of medications and active metabolites, reduction in hepatic blood flow can cause decreased hepatic clearance, and increase in body fat can lead to increase in elimination half-life of lipid soluble drugs.[3,4] Furthermore, elderly patients are frequently subjected to polypharmacy, leading to an increased burden of side effects.[3,4]

Homeostatic mechanisms (eg, orthostatic circulation, postural control, and thermoregulation) are also less vigorous in the aged, which can lead to additional vulnerabilities, such as increased risk of falls and hip fractures with psychotropics.[4] The elderly are also more vulnerable to the development of the syndrome of inappropriate antidiuretic hormone secretion.[4] Neurotransmitter changes such as reduction in dopamine and acetylcholine function mean that elderly have increased sensitivity to extrapyramidal symptoms with antipsychotics and cognitive impairment with anticholinergic medications[4] (**Table 1**).

As a general rule, physicians should use lower doses of medications and slower rates of titration in the elderly compared with the younger adult population.

As a result of reduced renal clearance and decreased total body water, the elderly are more susceptible to lithium toxicity. This vulnerability is present even with therapeutic serum lithium levels, in particular to neurological adverse effects such as tremor and ataxia.[5] Elderly patients therefore generally are best maintained on serum levels lower than those recommended in adults—in the range of 0.4 to 0.8 mEq/L.[5]

Benzodiazepines are best avoided in the geriatric population. Even short-term use can lead to impairments in cognition and psychomotor functioning.[3,5] These drugs increase the risk of falls and hip fractures.[3,5] These negative effects are in addition to the general risk of abuse and dependence that exists with benzodiazepine use. If benzodiazepines are clinically necessitated, lorazepam may be preferred given that it does not undergo phase I hepatic metabolism, it has no active metabolites, the half-life does not vary as much with age, and it is well absorbed intramuscularly.[5]

Table 1
Physiologic and pharmacokinetic changes in the elderly and their consequences

Physiologic and Pharmacokinetic Changes	Consequences
Decreased concentration of plasma albumin	Increased plasma concentration of free drug
Decreased glomerular filtration rate	Reduced renal clearance and accumulation of medication in the body
Reduction in hepatic blood flow	Reduced hepatic clearance and accumulation of medication in the body
Increase in body fat	Increase in half-life of lipid-soluble drugs
Reduced homeostatic integrity	Increased risk of falls and hip fractures
Reduced dopamine function	Increased sensitivity to extrapyramidal symptoms
Reduced cholinergic function	Increased sensitivity to anticholinergic medications
Reduced total body water	Vulnerability to medication toxicity

Data from Mulsant BH, Pollock BG. Psychopharmacology. In: Steffens DC, Blazer DG, Thakur ME, editors. The American psychiatric publishing textbook of geriatric psychiatry. 5th edition. Arlington (VA): American Psychiatric Publishing; 2015; and Roose SP, Pollock BG, Devanand DP. Treatment during late life. In: Schatzberg AF, Nemeroff CB, editors. The American psychiatric publishing textbook of psychopharmacology. 4th edition. Arlington (VA): American Psychiatric Publishing; 2009.

The increased risk of mortality with use of antipsychotics in individuals with dementia is addressed later in this review.

GERIATRIC SUICIDALITY

Geriatric patients are among the highest-risk epidemiologic groups for suicide. Worldwide rates of completed suicide generally increase as a function of age for both men and women.[6] In elderly suicides, there is often more serious intent and fewer warning signs, and suicides are more lethal when compared with the younger population.[7,8] Additionally, depressed geriatric patients with suicidality are more difficult to treat with higher relapse rates.[9] The ratio between suicide attempts and completed suicides progressively decreases with age: the ratio in United States is 36:1 in the youths, 8:1 in the general population, and 4:1 in the elderly.[10]

A Swedish study that identified the characteristics of suicide attempters 70 years and older compared with the general population comparison group reported that elderly suicide attempters were more likely to be unmarried, to be living alone, have low level of education, have a history of psychiatric treatment, and have prior suicide attempts.[11] Death of spouse is another risk factor for suicide in older subjects.[12] In a British survey of suicides in individuals 60 or older, hanging was the most common method for men, with overdose most common method for women.[13]

Clinical risk factors include depression, alcohol use disorders, schizophrenia, personality disorders, and medical comorbidities.[14] Psychiatric disorders are found on psychological autopsies in 71% to 97% of elderly suicides subjects, with mood disorders being the most widely reported.[6] A study from Canada found that elderly patients with 3 physical illnesses had an approximately 3-fold increase in estimated relative risk for suicide compared with subjects who had no diagnosis, and the relative risk increased to 9-fold when the number of physical illnesses was 7.[15] Loss of independence and financial problems are additional social risk factors.[6,14]

Elderly individuals may not be forthcoming about suicidal thoughts unless they are directly queried about it. Assessing for suicidality should therefore be part of a standard emergency psychiatric assessment. An evaluation of a geriatric patient with suicidality centers around the identification of the risk factors. Unfortunately, the predictive value of these risk factors at the individual level remains poor, making determination of suicide risk in a specific case a matter of clinician's judgment. Patients determined to be at high risk for suicide in the short term are best managed in the inpatient psychiatric setting. If the risk is elevated, involuntary psychiatric admission may be necessary, keeping in mind the applicable legal statues related to involuntary civil commitment. If hospitalization against will is being pursued, it should be presented to the patient as a means of helping them recover from a state of crisis by keeping them in a supervised, safe setting. Patients with vague suicidal ideation with no intent or plan, strong social support, and no ready access to means of suicide can generally be managed closely on an outpatient basis.

It is crucial to investigate the presence of a suicide plan and availability of means to carry out the plan, personal and family history of suicidal behavior, degree of available social support, concurrent psychiatric and medical disorders, and presence of suicide warning signs. Many behaviors in the elderly may be warning signs and precursors leading to a suicide attempt. These behaviors include neglect of personal care; intentional self-starvation; finalizing a will; distributing personal belongings to friends, family, or charities; giving up positions of responsibility; and purchase of a gun.[16–18] (**Box 1**).

Addressing the underlying factors related to suicidality remains the primary modality of management. In most patients, suicidality would be present in the context of psychiatric disorders, which is best addressed by the relevant pharmacotherapy (antidepressants, mood stabilizers, antipsychotics) and psychotherapy. For depressive episodes with acute suicidality, electroconvulsive therapy remains an effective and underutilized treatment in the geriatric patient population.

DELIRIUM AND AGITATION IN DELIRIUM

Delirium is a neurocognitive disorder characterized by disturbances in attention, awareness (orientation to the surrounding environment), and various aspects of cognition (memory, language, visuospatial ability, perception), which develops over a relatively short period and represents a significant change from baseline status. There is commonly a waxing and waning fluctuation in the degree of confusion during the day. Delirium can also be described as a neurobehavioral syndrome caused by dysregulation of baseline neuronal activity secondary to systemic disturbances.[19] It is an acute, usually temporary, psychiatric disorder caused by an underlying medical condition, substance intoxication/withdrawal, or medication adverse effect. Delirium is associated with several worse outcomes such as prolonged hospital stay, need for

Box 1
Suicide warning signs and precursors in the elderly

Neglect of personal care

Intentional self-starvation

Finalizing a will

Distribution of personal belongings

Giving up positions of responsibility

Purchase of a gun

Data from Refs.[16–18]

institutional postacute care, risk of cognitive decline, and increased cost of medical care.[20,21] Prompt diagnosis of delirium in the emergency room is also critical, as mortality for undiagnosed delirious patients in the emergency department is significantly higher than that of patients with a diagnosis of delirium.[22]

Epidemiology

Although the prevalence of delirium in the general population is low (1%–2%), the prevalence increases steeply in the geriatric population—reported to be around 14% in subjects 85 or older.[23] Delirium is highly prevalent in the hospital settings. The overall occurrence rates (sum of incidence and prevalence) of delirium in the general medical and geriatric wards are 29% to 64%.[21] Delirium is present in 8% to 17% of elderly patients and 40% of nursing home residents on presentation to the emergency room.[21] It is also very common postoperatively, in intensive care units, in nursing homes, and in postacute care settings.

Risk Factors

There are risk factors that increase the baseline vulnerability of delirium development, and there are others that serve as precipitating factors.

The vulnerability factors include advanced age, sensory impairment, and neurologic conditions such as dementia, stroke, and Parkinson disease. Delirium superimposed on dementia is highly prevalent (ranging from approximately 20%–90%).[24] In many cases, it is the presence of delirium that brings attention to the underlying dementia that had been hitherto undiagnosed. It is also important to note that in cases of delirium without prior dementia, a significant percentage of these patients will go on to have dementia over the next 5 years compared with controls (69% vs 20%).[25]

The list of precipitating factors is long and includes broad categories of medications and toxins, substance intoxications and withdrawals, infections (systemic and central nervous system), metabolic disturbances, systemic organ failures (eg, cardiac, hepatic, pulmonary, renal), and extensive physical trauma such as burns.[21,26] Conditions such as seizures and psychiatric disorders (psychosis, mania, catatonia) can mimic the clinical syndrome of delirium.[21,26] Polypharmacy is a significant risk factor in the elderly, and review of medications (both prescribed and over the counter) should be an essential first step.

Clinical Features

A decrease in the level of awareness and deficit in attention are usually the earliest signs of delirium. Initially, they may be subtle, picked up only by the family members, and may be missed by clinicians who are not familiar with the patients (caregiver reports therefore should not be summarily dismissed). Distractibility can progress to frank drowsiness and lethargy, with further progression to a semicomatose condition in severe cases. The sedation may be punctuated by episodes of psychomotor agitation. Perceptual disturbances ranging from illusions to frank hallucinations are common. Unlike primary psychotic disorders, visual hallucinations are more common than auditory, and hallucinations may range from simple to complex. Sleep disturbances, emotional lability, anxiety, and low mood are all commonly seen. Hypoactive delirium may be mistaken for depression, and it is a common experience in consultation-liaison psychiatry to be consulted for depression on patients with unrecognized delirium.

Delirium has a characteristic waxing and waning course, with interspersed periods of lucidity. Once developed, delirium can linger on for days to months, even after the underlying causes have been addressed.[26] Delirium can be the first manifestation of an acute medical illness in the elderly.[26]

Diagnosis

Delirium remains a diagnosis based on clinical evaluation, although a medical workup is essential. In cases where symptoms are subtle, cognitive screening measures are helpful. Simple tests of attention such as serial subtraction, spelling a word (such as *world*) backwards, repeating a sequence of random numbers, are highly useful in bedside clinical practice and often suffice for clinical diagnosis. Confusion Assessment Method has emerged as the standard clinical tool for screening of delirium.[27] It is valid across different settings, has a sensitivity approaching 100% and specificity of 90% to 95%, and has been found superior to Mini-Mental State Examination.[28] Cognitive screening tools developed for dementia such as Mini-Mental State Examination and Montreal Cognitive Assessment are often cumbersome in the emergency settings for use in delirium.

Evaluation

Because delirium is the consequence of an underlying medical disturbance, uncovering the disease process is a priority. A comprehensive physical examination and routine laboratory tests (complete blood count with differential, comprehensive metabolic panel, urinalysis, urine toxicology, serum creatinine kinase if indicated) should be undertaken. If the results show no obvious cause, neuroimaging and electroencephalogram (EEG) should be conducted. Lumbar puncture may be indicated if a neurologic process such as meningitis is suspected. Some authors consider lumbar puncture to be mandatory when the cause of delirium is not obvious,[26] as meningitis in the elderly may present only with delirium and without classic features. EEG can be helpful in ruling out seizures (EEG is the only definitive method of diagnosing nonconvulsive status epilepticus) and finding the presence of metabolic encephalopathy. EEG can also help differentiate delirium tremens from other causes of encephalopathy. Metabolic encephalopathies will show diffuse background slowing. Triphasic waves, classically associated with hepatic encephalopathy, may be seen. In contrast, delirium tremens will show fast EEG activity (**Box 2**).

Management

One aspect of the management of delirium directly springs from evaluation, and that is to correct the underlying medical etiology of delirium. This correction should

Box 2
Common medical workup of delirium

- Comprehensive physical examination
- Complete blood count with differential
- Comprehensive metabolic panel
- Urinalysis
- Urine toxicology
- Serum creatinine kinase
- Neuroimaging
- EEG
- Lumbar puncture

accompany general medical supportive measures, such as ensuring the patient remains hydrated, minimizing prolonged inactivity and immobilization, reducing distracting stimuli in the environment, frequent reorientation, bedside sitters, and addressing any comorbid pain. Physical restraints should be avoided, as they may worsen delirium[29] and should be used only when necessary as a last resort.

Severe agitation is often the most problematic behavioral manifestation of delirium and usually the reason for psychiatric involvement as well. Evidence of efficacy is limited, but among the available psychopharmacologic options, antipsychotic agents are the medications of choice in addressing agitation in the context of delirium.[20] Haloperidol has traditionally been used as the pharmacologic agent of choice. In recent years, psychiatrists have relied more on atypical antipsychotic agents, which seem to have similar efficacy to haloperidol in the management of agitation in delirium. Lower doses of haloperidol (0.5 mg to 5 mg/d) are recommended, and it may be used via oral or intramuscular routes. Intravenous administration remains commonly used in intensive care unit settings. Although the intravenous route is not approved by the US Food and Drug Administration (FDA), it can be a reasonable alternative if the patient has electrocardiographic monitoring for QT prolongation and torsade, as patients in an intensive care unit setting typically have.

General adult literature suggests that around 75% of delirious patients receiving short-term treatment with low-dose antipsychotics experience clinical response, with response rates consistent across different settings.[30] However, robust and generalizable evidence regarding the use of antipsychotics in delirium is sorely lacking, even for haloperidol, the use of which is backed by decades of clinical experience.[31]

With regard to controlled studies in the elderly population, studies have severe methodologic limitations, and evidence of efficacy is further limited. Studies either do not find an improvement in delirium or there is no impact on clinical outcomes such as hospital length of stay or mortality. This has led some authors to state that pharmacologic approaches to treatment of delirium are not currently recommended.[21,32] Nonetheless, in cases of severe agitation, which either disrupts essential medical therapy or poses a danger for the safety of patients, or involves severe, distressing psychotic symptoms, pharmacologic treatment with antipsychotics is often a necessary clinical strategy.

Valproic acid may be a viable treatment of hyperactive or mixed delirium but requires further investigation.[33] Benzodiazepines can worsen confusion and have a limited role in the treatment of delirium; unfortunately, they still are commonly prescribed by many clinicians.[34] Benzodiazepines remain preferred agents in delirium treatment, and may be required in emergency situations where antipsychotics are contraindicated and acute sedative effect is needed.

Many geriatric hospitalized individuals have evidence of thiamine deficiency, and history of alcoholism is often missed in the elderly. As thiamine supplementation is cheap and virtually without side effects, some authors recommend it as a consideration in all cases of delirium.[20]

Patients with delirium typically lack decision-making capacity, and it is essential to defer medical decision to next of kin/medical power of attorney/guardian in such situations. Nonetheless, the mere presence of delirium should not preclude a capacity evaluation, as patients may have enough intact cognition to make some decisions.

Adverse Outcomes

Delirium is associated with an increased risk of subsequent mortality. A meta-analysis looking at studies with follow-up ranging from 3 to 48 months found that the risk of death was elevated with a hazard ratio of 1.95.[35] The mortality rate may be as high as 14% and 22% at 1 and 6 months, respectively.[36]

Delirium frequently leads to persistent cognitive dysfunction and increase in the risk of subsequent dementia. In a meta-analysis, delirium was associated with an increased rate of incident dementia over 3 to 5 years of follow-up with an odds ratio of 12.52.[35] In patients with pre-existing dementia, delirium increases the rate of future cognitive decline. For instance, in a study of patients with Alzheimer disease, after an episode of delirium, subsequent cognitive deterioration was at twice the rate, and this higher rate was noted even after 5 years from the delirium.[37]

AGITATION AND NEUROPSYCHIATRIC SYMPTOMS IN DEMENTIA

Neuropsychiatric symptoms (NPS) are frequently reported and observed in patients with neurocognitive disorders. These disorders include psychotic symptoms (delusions, hallucinations), agitation and aggression, depression, anxiety, apathy, disinhibition, and wandering. Prevalence of these symptoms reported in literature ranges from 60% to 90%, and generally greater prevalence is seen with greater severity of dementia.[38,39] Agitation and aggression in Alzheimer disease are reported to be prevalent with respective ranges of 20% to 80% and 11% to 46%.[40]

Psychotic symptoms have been reported with broad ranges in the literature, around 10% to 70% for delusions and 4% to 75% for hallucinations in Alzheimer disease.[41,42] Dementia patients tend to be preoccupied with certain delusional themes, with delusions of theft being the most common. Other delusions include phantom boarder syndrome, misidentification syndromes (such as Capgras delusion), persecutory delusions, and delusions of infidelity. Psychotic symptoms increase with progression of dementia; although they seem to plateau after 3 years,[43] they are often persistent and associated with poor prognosis.[42]

Nonpharmacologic Management

Authors and guidelines universally recommend nonpharmacologic interventions for agitation in major neurocognitive disorder as the first-line measure before pharmacologic interventions. Randomized, controlled trials (RCTs) are limited currently, but research is accumulating over time. Person-centered care, communication skills training, and adapted dementia care mapping were behavioral interventions shown to reduce agitation immediately and in the long term (up to 6 months) in a systematic review of RCTs.[44] Group activities and music therapy decreased agitation immediately but had no long-term effect. Aroma therapy and light therapy were ineffective in controlled trials.

It is also crucial to assess and exclude sources of distress, for instance pain, hunger, thirst, and constipation. Educating the caregivers is also important. A behavioral plan that identifies the environmental triggers and calming influences for the patient is vital. Other helpful measures include redirecting the patient, adjusting the routine to the patient's schedule, regular toileting, and avoiding stimulants such as coffee in the evening.[45]

Approved Pharmacologic Agents and Off-Label Prescribing

No pharmacologic agent has approval from the FDA for the treatment of NPS in dementia in the United States; therefore, all treatment with medications is off label. Although off-label prescribing increases risk of liability, this should not hinder judicious use when risks and benefits have been carefully weighed and consent has been obtained.

USE OF ANTIPSYCHOTIC DRUGS IN DEMENTIA

Efficacy

More than a dozen RCTs investigating typical antipsychotics (haloperidol, thioridazine, thiothixene, chlorpromazine, trifluoperazine, acetophenazine, perphenazine) show that their efficacy in the management of NPS is small at best.[46] A Cochran review found haloperidol to be effective for the treatment of aggression but not agitation.[47]

RCTs of olanzapine and risperidone examined in 2 systematic reviews generally show modest efficacy for treatment of NPS, with the trials mostly being conducted in nursing home residents with moderate-to-severe dementia.[46,48] A meta-analysis[49] looking at aripiprazole, olanzapine, quetiapine, and risperidone found aripiprazole and olanzapine to be efficacious with small effect sizes. Two CATIE-AD studies have been conducted[50,51] investigating olanzapine, quetiapine, and risperidone. In the first CATIE-AD study, time to discontinuation owing to lack of efficacy favored olanzapine and risperidone, but on other outcomes there was no difference from placebo.[50] In the second CATIE-AD study, olanzapine and risperidone again showed efficacy on various neuropsychiatric rating scales compared with placebo, but quetiapine was not significantly different from placebo.[51]

Risk of Mortality

In 2003, the FDA updated the prescribing information for risperidone with a warning for increased cerebrovascular adverse events, including stroke, in elderly patients with dementia.[52] In 2005, the FDA issued a black box warning for the entire class of atypical antipsychotics, with a reported 1.6- to 1.7-fold increase in mortality in placebo-controlled trials performed with olanzapine, aripiprazole, risperidone, and quetiapine.[52] Most of the causes of death were heart-related events (eg, heart failure, sudden death) or infections events (mostly pneumonia).[24] In 2008, the black box warning was also applied to typical antipsychotic drugs.[52]

The increased risk of mortality with the use of both typical and atypical antipsychotics has consistently been reproduced in subsequent studies. A meta-analysis of RCTs by Schneider and colleagues[53] found that there was increased mortality in dementia patients treated with atypical antipsychotics with an odds ratio of 1.54 (95% confidence interval, 1.06–2.23). The mortality risk increases with the duration of treatment and has been studied up to 36 months.[54]

Typical antipsychotics seem to have a significantly higher adjusted risk of death compared with atypical antipsychotics with relative risk of 1.37 (95% confidence interval, 1.27–1.49).[55] Studies[56–58] reported a higher risk of mortality with haloperidol (hazard ratio, ~1.5) and a lower risk of mortality with quetiapine (hazard ratio, ~0.8) compared with risperidone. Aripiprazole and olanzapine seem to have similar risk. Higher doses of antipsychotics are associated with a higher mortality risk. A study published in 2015 indicated that the mortality risk may be even higher than what had been reported in the prior studies.[59]

Risk of Cerebrovascular Events and Stroke

Studies also indicate that antipsychotics carry an increased risk of cerebrovascular events such as stroke. One study reported that odds of stroke were 1.8 times higher when exposed to antipsychotics than when unexposed.[60] In a systematic review of

RCTs and observational studies, a 2- to 3-fold increased risk of all cerebrovascular events was reported with atypical antipsychotics compared with placebo, but no association with serious stroke that required hospitalization was discovered.[61] These studies, however, have methodologic limitations, and some studies have reported no associations.[62]

American Psychiatric Association Guidelines

The American Psychiatric Association (APA) has recently issued practice guidelines on the use of antipsychotics in the treatment of agitation or psychosis in patients with dementia.[63] The guidelines mostly reflect existing recommendations such as using nonpharmacologic interventions before nonemergency use of antipsychotics, assessing for modifiable contributing factors such as pain, using the lowest effective dose, and attempting to taper after stabilization of symptoms. Some points, however, stand out. The APA recommends that response to treatment be determined with a quantitative measure in patients with dementia with agitation or psychosis, something that is not commonly used currently in clinical settings. The APA also recommends that in the absence of delirium and in nonemergency situations, haloperidol should not be used as a first-line agent. The APA also recommends against using a long-acting injectable antipsychotic medication (unless it is indicated for a comorbid chronic psychotic disorder). Readers are referred to the guidelines for additional information.

Other Pharmacologic Agents

Evidence regarding the use of cholinesterase inhibitors for treatments of NPS is limited. A systematic review reported that only 3 of 14 studies had statistically significant but modest differentiation from placebo.[64] The authors, however, recommended that given the absence of alternative safe and effective options, the use of cholinesterase inhibitors is an appropriate pharmacologic strategy. A systematic review and meta-analysis by Wang and colleagues[65] showed no efficacy of memantine for treatment of NPS in Alzheimer disease.

Anticonvulsants have no proven efficacy in NPS of dementia. A Cochrane review looking at the use of valproate for agitation in dementia concluded that it is ineffective for treatment of agitation in dementia and that it is associated with unacceptable rates of adverse effects.[66] There is some small and limited evidence for use of carbamazepine.[67] Other newer anticonvulsants require further investigation.

There are limited and mixed results regarding efficacy of antidepressants. In a Cochrane review, 2 small studies found some benefit with citalopram and sertraline in treatment of NPS compared with placebo, whereas multiple other studies with antidepressants found none.[68] In a 12-week RCT in nondepressed patients with dementia comparing citalopram and risperidone, no statistical difference was found in the efficacy of citalopram and risperidone for the treatment of either agitation or psychotic symptoms.[69] Use of citalopram should be cautious because of concerns for QTc prolongation and arrhythmias at higher doses over 40 mg. The maximum recommended dose in the geriatric population is 20 mg/d.

Benzodiazepines are associated with cognitive decline and contribute to increased falls and hip fractures, and should be avoided.[41] Multiple studies found negative effects of benzodiazepines of cognitive function in dementia, and despite recommendations against their use, the use of benzodiazepines in dementia remains prevalent.[70] Studies on the use of benzodiazepines for NPS show inconsistent results and generally suggest a positive effect in less than half of agitated patients in the short term[70] (**Table 2**).

Table 2
Pharmacologic treatment of agitation and neuropsychiatric symptoms in dementia

Treatment	Efficacy
Typical antipsychotics	Modest efficacy at best; possibly higher risk of mortality compared with atypical antipsychotics
Atypical antipsychotics	Modest efficacy at best; risperidone, olanzapine and aripiprazole have some support from evidence; quetiapine seems to have minimal efficacy; increased risk of mortality
Valproic acid	No demonstrable efficacy
Carbamazepine	Very limited evidence of efficacy
Cholinesterase inhibitors	Minimal efficacy at best
Memantine	No proven efficacy
Antidepressants	Limited evidence of benefit with citalopram and sertraline
Benzodiazepines	Possible short-term benefit; not recommended because of demonstrated negative effects on cognition

REFERENCES

1. The state of aging and health in America 2013. Atlanta (GA): Centers for Disease Control and Prevention, US Dept of Health and Human Services; 2013.
2. McCaig LF, Burt CW. National hospital ambulatory medical care survey: 2003 emergency department summary. Advance Data 2005;358:5.
3. Mulsant BH, Pollock BG. Psychopharmacology. In: Steffens DC, Blazer DG, Thakur ME, editors. The American psychiatric publishing textbook of geriatric psychiatry. 5th edition. Arlington (VA): American Psychiatric Publishing; 2015.
4. Roose SP, Pollock BG, Devanand DP. Treatment during late life. In: Schatzberg AF, Nemeroff CB, editors. The American psychiatric publishing textbook of psychopharmacology. 4th edition. Arlington (VA): American Psychiatric Publishing; 2009.
5. Mulsant BH, Pollock BG. Psychopharmacology. In: Thakur ME, Blazer DG, Steffens DC, editors. Clinical manual of geriatric psychiatry. Arlington (VA): American Psychiatric Publishing; 2014.
6. Conwell Y, Van Orden K, Caine ED. Suicide in older adults. Psychiatr Clin North Am 2011;34(2):451–68, ix.
7. Conwell Y, Duberstein PR, Cox C, et al. Age differences in behaviors leading to completed suicide. Am J Geriatr Psychiatry 1998;6(2):122–6.
8. Salib E, Rahim S, El-Nimr G, et al. Elderly suicide: an analysis of coroner's inquests into two hundred cases in Cheshire 1989-2001. Med Sci Law 2005; 45(1):71–80.
9. Szanto K, Mulsant BH, Houck PR, et al. Treatment outcome in suicidal vs. non-suicidal elderly patients. Am J Geriatr Psychiatry 2001;9(3):261–8.
10. Minayo MC, Cavalcante FG. Suicide in elderly people: a literature review. Rev Saude Publica 2010;44(4):750–7 [in English, Portuguese].
11. Wiktorsson S, Runeson B, Skoog I, et al. Attempted suicide in the elderly: characteristics of suicide attempters 70 years and older and a general population comparison group. Am J Geriatr Psychiatry 2010;18(1):57–67.
12. Duberstein PR, Conwell Y, Cox C. Suicide in widowed persons. A psychological autopsy comparison of recently and remotely bereaved older subjects. Am J Geriatr Psychiatry 1998;6(4):328–34.

13. Harwood DM, Hawton K, Hope T, et al. Suicide in older people: mode of death, demographic factors, and medical contact before death. Int J Geriatr Psychiatry 2000;15(8):736–43.
14. Ajilore OA, Kumar A. Suicide in late life. In: Dwivedi Y, editor. The neurobiological basis of suicide. Boca Raton (FL): CRC Press/Taylor & Francis; 2012.
15. Juurlink DN, Herrmann N, Szalai JP, et al. Medical illness and the risk of suicide in the elderly. Arch Intern Med 2004;164(11):1179–84.
16. Bruce ML, Ten Have TR, Reynolds CF 3rd, et al. Reducing suicidal ideation and depressive symptoms in depressed older primary care patients: a randomized controlled trial. JAMA 2004;291(9):1081–91.
17. Conwell Y, Brent D. Suicide and aging. I: patterns of psychiatric diagnosis. Int Psychogeriatr 1995;7(2):149–64.
18. Montross L, Mohamed S, Kasckow J, et al. Preventing late-life suicide: 6 steps to detect the warning signs. Current Psychiatry 2003;2(8):15–26.
19. Maldonado JR. Neuropathogenesis of delirium: review of current etiologic theories and common pathways. Am J Geriatr Psychiatry 2013;21(12):1190–222.
20. Francis J. Delirium and acute confusional states: prevention, treatment, and prognosis. In: Aminoff MJ, Schmader KE, editors. UpToDate. Waltham (MA): UpToDate; 2016. Available at: https://www.uptodate.com/contents/delirium-and-acute-confusional-states-prevention-treatment-and-prognosis. Accessed November 11, 2016.
21. Inouye SK, Westendorp RG, Saczynski JS. Delirium in elderly people. Lancet 2014;383(9920):911–22.
22. Kakuma R, du Fort GG, Arsenault L, et al. Delirium in older emergency department patients discharged home: effect on survival. J Am Geriatr Soc 2003; 51(4):443–50.
23. Inouye SK. Delirium in older persons. N Engl J Med 2006;354(11):1157–65.
24. Fick DM, Agostini JV, Inouye SK. Delirium superimposed on dementia: a systematic review. J Am Geriatr Soc 2002;50(10):1723–32.
25. Lundstrom M, Edlund A, Bucht G, et al. Dementia after delirium in patients with femoral neck fractures. J Am Geriatr Soc 2003;51(7):1002–6.
26. Francis J, Young GB. Diagnosis of delirium and confusional states. In: Aminoff MJ, Schmader KE, editors. UpToDate. Waltham (MA): UpToDate; 2016. Available at: https://www.uptodate.com/contents/diagnosis-of-delirium-and-confusional-states. Accessed November 11, 2016.
27. Wei LA, Fearing MA, Sternberg EJ, et al. The confusion assessment method: a systematic review of current usage. J Am Geriatr Soc 2008;56(5):823–30.
28. Wong CL, Holroyd-Leduc J, Simel DL, et al. Does this patient have delirium?: value of bedside instruments. JAMA 2010;304(7):779–86.
29. Inouye SK, Zhang Y, Jones RN, et al. Risk factors for delirium at discharge: development and validation of a predictive model. Arch Intern Med 2007;167(13): 1406–13.
30. Meagher DJ, McLoughlin L, Leonard M, et al. What do we really know about the treatment of delirium with antipsychotics? Ten key issues for delirium pharmacotherapy. Am J Geriatr Psychiatry 2013;21(12):1223–38.
31. Schrijver EJ, de Graaf K, de Vries OJ, et al. Efficacy and safety of haloperidol for in-hospital delirium prevention and treatment: a systematic review of current evidence. Eur J Intern Med 2016;27:14–23.
32. Flaherty JH, Gonzales JP, Dong B. Antipsychotics in the treatment of delirium in older hospitalized adults: a systematic review. J Am Geriatr Soc 2011; 59(Suppl 2):S269–76.

33. Sher Y, Miller Cramer AC, Ament A, et al. Valproic acid for treatment of hyperactive or mixed delirium: rationale and literature review. Psychosomatics 2015; 56(6):615–25.
34. Carnes M, Howell T, Rosenberg M, et al. Physicians vary in approaches to the clinical management of delirium. J Am Geriatr Soc 2003;51(2):234–9.
35. Witlox J, Eurelings LS, de Jonghe JF, et al. Delirium in elderly patients and the risk of postdischarge mortality, institutionalization, and dementia: a meta-analysis. JAMA 2010;304(4):443–51.
36. Cole MG, Primeau FJ. Prognosis of delirium in elderly hospital patients. CMAJ 1993;149(1):41–6.
37. Fong TG, Jones RN, Shi P, et al. Delirium accelerates cognitive decline in Alzheimer disease. Neurology 2009;72(18):1570–5.
38. Lyketsos CG, Lopez O, Jones B, et al. Prevalence of neuropsychiatric symptoms in dementia and mild cognitive impairment: results from the cardiovascular health study. JAMA 2002;288(12):1475–83.
39. Lyketsos CG, Steinberg M, Tschanz JT, et al. Mental and behavioral disturbances in dementia: findings from the Cache County Study on Memory in Aging. Am J Psychiatry 2000;157(5):708–14.
40. Jeste DV, Blazer D, Casey D, et al. ACNP White Paper: update on use of antipsychotic drugs in elderly persons with dementia. Neuropsychopharmacology 2008; 33(5):957–70.
41. Bassiony MM, Lyketsos CG. Delusions and hallucinations in Alzheimer's disease: review of the brain decade. Psychosomatics 2003;44(5):388–401.
42. Ropacki SA, Jeste DV. Epidemiology of and risk factors for psychosis of Alzheimer's disease: a review of 55 studies published from 1990 to 2003. Am J Psychiatry 2005;162(11):2022–30.
43. Paulsen JS, Salmon DP, Thal LJ, et al. Incidence of and risk factors for hallucinations and delusions in patients with probable AD. Neurology 2000;54(10):1965–71.
44. Livingston G, Kelly L, Lewis-Holmes E, et al. Non-pharmacological interventions for agitation in dementia: systematic review of randomised controlled trials. Br J Psychiatry 2014;205(6):436–42.
45. Cummings JL. The black book of Alzheimer's disease, part 2. Prim Psychiatry 2008;15(3):69.
46. Sink KM, Holden KF, Yaffe K. Pharmacological treatment of neuropsychiatric symptoms of dementia: a review of the evidence. JAMA 2005;293(5):596–608.
47. Lonergan E, Luxenberg J, Colford J. Haloperidol for agitation in dementia. Cochrane Database Syst Rev 2002;(2):CD002852.
48. Lee PE, Gill SS, Freedman M, et al. Atypical antipsychotic drugs in the treatment of behavioural and psychological symptoms of dementia: systematic review. BMJ 2004;329(7457):75.
49. Schneider LS, Dagerman K, Insel PS. Efficacy and adverse effects of atypical antipsychotics for dementia: meta-analysis of randomized, placebo-controlled trials. Am J Geriatr Psychiatry 2006;14(3):191–210.
50. Schneider LS, Tariot PN, Dagerman KS, et al. Effectiveness of atypical antipsychotic drugs in patients with Alzheimer's disease. N Engl J Med 2006;355(15): 1525–38.
51. Sultzer DL, Davis SM, Tariot PN, et al. Clinical symptom responses to atypical antipsychotic medications in Alzheimer's disease: phase 1 outcomes from the CATIE-AD effectiveness trial. Am J Psychiatry 2008;165(7):844–54.
52. Shah AA, Aftab A. Should physicians prescribe antipsychotics in Dementia? Psychiatr Ann 2016;46(2):97–102.

53. Schneider LS, Dagerman KS, Insel P. Risk of death with atypical antipsychotic drug treatment for dementia: meta-analysis of randomized placebo-controlled trials. JAMA 2005;294(15):1934–43.
54. Ballard C, Hanney ML, Theodoulou M, et al. The dementia antipsychotic withdrawal trial (DART-AD): long-term follow-up of a randomised placebo-controlled trial. Lancet Neurol 2009;8(2):151–7.
55. Wang PS, Schneeweiss S, Avorn J, et al. Risk of death in elderly users of conventional vs. atypical antipsychotic medications. N Engl J Med 2005;353(22): 2335–41.
56. Gerhard T, Huybrechts K, Olfson M, et al. Comparative mortality risks of antipsychotic medications in community-dwelling older adults. Br J Psychiatry 2014; 205(1):44–51.
57. Huybrechts KF, Gerhard T, Crystal S, et al. Differential risk of death in older residents in nursing homes prescribed specific antipsychotic drugs: population based cohort study. BMJ 2012;344:e977.
58. Kales HC, Kim HM, Zivin K, et al. Risk of mortality among individual antipsychotics in patients with dementia. Am J Psychiatry 2012;169(1):71–9.
59. Maust DT, Kim HM, Seyfried LS, et al. Antipsychotics, other psychotropics, and the risk of death in patients with dementia: number needed to harm. JAMA Psychiatry 2015;72(5):438–45.
60. Wang S, Linkletter C, Dore D, et al. Age, antipsychotics, and the risk of ischemic stroke in the Veterans Health Administration. Stroke 2012;43(1):28–31.
61. Pratt N, Roughead EE, Salter A, et al. Choice of observational study design impacts on measurement of antipsychotic risks in the elderly: a systematic review. BMC Med Res Methodol 2012;12:72.
62. Barnett MJ, Wehring H, Perry PJ. Comparison of risk of cerebrovascular events in an elderly VA population with dementia between antipsychotic and nonantipsychotic users. J Clin Psychopharmacol 2007;27(6):595–601.
63. Reus VI, Fochtmann LJ, Eyler AE, et al. The American Psychiatric Association Practice Guideline on the use of antipsychotics to treat agitation or psychosis in patients with dementia. Am J Psychiatry 2016;173(5):543–6.
64. Rodda J, Morgan S, Walker Z. Are cholinesterase inhibitors effective in the management of the behavioral and psychological symptoms of dementia in Alzheimer's disease? A systematic review of randomized, placebo-controlled trials of donepezil, rivastigmine and galantamine. Int Psychogeriatr 2009;21(5):813–24.
65. Wang J, Yu JT, Wang HF, et al. Pharmacological treatment of neuropsychiatric symptoms in Alzheimer's disease: a systematic review and meta-analysis. J Neurol Neurosurg Psychiatry 2015;86(1):101–9.
66. Lonergan E, Luxenberg J. Valproate preparations for agitation in dementia. Cochrane Database Syst Rev 2009;(3):CD003945.
67. Gallagher D, Herrmann N. Antiepileptic drugs for the treatment of agitation and aggression in dementia: do they have a place in therapy? Drugs 2014;74(15): 1747–55.
68. Seitz DP, Adunuri N, Gill SS, et al. Antidepressants for agitation and psychosis in dementia. Cochrane Database Syst Rev 2011;(2):CD008191.
69. Pollock BG, Mulsant BH, Rosen J, et al. A double-blind comparison of citalopram and risperidone for the treatment of behavioral and psychotic symptoms associated with dementia. Am J Geriatr Psychiatry 2007;15(11):942–52.
70. Defrancesco M, Marksteiner J, Fleischhacker WW, et al. Use of Benzodiazepines in Alzheimer's disease: a systematic review of literature. Int J Neuropsychopharmacol 2015;18(10):pyv055.

Special Considerations in the Pediatric Psychiatric Population

Genevieve Santillanes, MD[a,*], Ruth S. Gerson, MD[b]

KEYWORDS

- Pediatric behavioral health • Pediatric mental health • Pediatric psychiatry
- Psychiatric emergency • Suicidal ideation • Agitation • Aggression

KEY POINTS

- Psychiatric and behavioral complaints account for a significant proportion of emergency department visits for children and adolescents.
- Multidisciplinary evidence-based guidelines on best practices in evaluation and management of youth in psychiatric crisis are needed for emergency settings.
- Available evidence does not support routine laboratory testing in pediatric patients undergoing medical clearance examinations.
- Risk assessment of youth with suicidal ideation is challenging; suicide screening tools may be helpful.
- De-escalation techniques may decrease emergent mediation administration and restraint use in agitated and aggressive patients.

INTRODUCTION

Emergency department (ED) visits for youth in psychiatric or behavioral crisis have risen significantly over the past 20 years, with mental health diagnoses accounting for approximately 5% of ED visits for children.[1] Suicide remains a leading cause of death among children and adolescents. In the past year, 17% of high school students seriously considered suicide; 13.6% made a suicide plan, and 8% attempted suicide. 2.7% of high school students made a serious attempt requiring medical attention within the past year.[2] Yet when these youth present to the ED, they encounter a

The authors have nothing to disclose.
[a] Department of Emergency Medicine, Keck School of Medicine of University of Southern California, 1200 North State Street, GH Room 1011, Los Angeles, CA 90033, USA; [b] Bellevue Hospital Children's Comprehensive Psychiatric Emergency Program, Department of Child and Adolescent Psychiatry, New York University School of Medicine, 462 1st Avenue, New York, NY 10016, USA
* Corresponding author.
E-mail address: genevieve.santillanes@usc.edu

Psychiatr Clin N Am 40 (2017) 463–473
http://dx.doi.org/10.1016/j.psc.2017.05.009
0193-953X/17/© 2017 Published by Elsevier Inc.

system poorly equipped to care for them. Most youth presenting to EDs in psychiatric crisis are seen in general (or less commonly, pediatric) EDs lacking specialized mental health staff (psychiatrists, child psychiatrists, social work, or nursing).[3] They are frequently seen only by emergency medicine or pediatric emergency physicians who generally lack comfort and training in assessing and managing pediatric behavioral health emergencies. For example, less than a third of emergency medicine physicians feel comfortable briefly counseling suicidal patients or making a safety plan.[4] As a result, many youth receive suboptimal evaluation and treatment in the ED. Bridge and colleagues[5] reported that only half of youth presenting to EDs nationwide after a suicide attempt received any mental health assessment, and those who did not had higher rates of later self-harm. Gairin and colleagues[6] found that 39% of people who committed suicide were seen in the ED in the prior year, suggesting that opportunities for life-saving intervention are being missed.

Lack of ED-based psychiatric staff contributes to longer wait times, longer lengths of stay, and higher rates of admission and boarding for youth with psychiatric complaints compared with youth with medical complaints.[7–10] Many youth admitted from the ED could be discharged with brief ED stabilization and referral to immediate, acute outpatient services, were such services available.[11] Youth presenting with chief complaints of aggression, anxiety, or agitation are often exacerbated by the ED environment, leading to restraint and administration of intramuscular (IM) medication.

This article will address how EDs can better care for 2 groups: first, children with psychiatric chief complaints in need of assessment and medical clearance, and second, children with comorbid medical and psychiatric needs. The article also discusses management of agitation and systems changes needed to improve ED care for psychiatrically ill youth.

SPECIAL CONSIDERATIONS IN MEDICAL CLEARANCE

Otherwise healthy patients with psychiatric complaints frequently present to the ED for medical clearance prior to psychiatric evaluation and placement. The term medical clearance may have different meanings to providers, so it is important to be clear when using the term. Emergency medicine providers generally intend medically cleared to mean that presenting symptoms are not due to an underlying medical cause and that active medical issues are stabilized. They generally do not intend for medical clearance to rule out nonurgent medical issues. Rather than documenting that a patient is medically cleared, communicating that the patient is medically stable for admission to psychiatry is more accurate and less likely to lead to misunderstanding.

One issue in medical clearance is whether laboratory testing is required. No national guideline has been published on medical clearance of pediatric psychiatric patients. The American College of Emergency Physicians' clinical policy for medical clearance of adult psychiatric patients states that laboratory testing is not necessary in awake, alert patients with normal histories and physical examinations, but excluded discussion of pediatric patients.[12,13] American Association for Emergency Psychiatry guidelines state that routine laboratory testing is not indicated in the evaluation of agitated patients, but did not specifically address pediatric patients.[14] Medical clearance evaluations tend to vary by provider and facility. Many psychiatric inpatient facilities require a battery of tests before accepting patients from EDs; required tests vary between institutions.[15] Multiple studies have found that routine laboratory evaluation, including toxicology screening, is not medically indicated in pediatric patients with normal histories and physical examinations.[16–19]

ED evaluation should consist of a thorough history and mental status, physical, and neurologic examinations. Although tachycardia may be due to agitation or anxiety, abnormal vital signs should not be ignored, as they may indicate serious medical pathology. The medical evaluation is critical to determining that the symptoms are caused by a psychiatric illness, not a medical illness. Patients with disorientation or waxing and waning mental status should be presumed to have a medical disorder. Visual hallucinations, new-onset psychosis, and sudden, drastic changes in behavior should be investigated thoroughly. Conditions such as head trauma, hypoglycemia, postictal state, thyrotoxicosis, infectious encephalitis, anti-N-Methyl-D-aspartic acid or N-Methyl-D-aspartate (NMDA) receptor encephalitis, brain tumors, intoxications, and withdrawal syndromes can present with agitation or other psychiatric symptoms, but should be suspected based on a thorough history and physical examination. Ancillary testing, subspecialty consultation, and medical admission may be required if an organic etiology is suspected. Patients should also be evaluated for evidence of self-harm or other traumatic injury and signs of abuse and ingestion. Any medical complaints or active medical issues should be stabilized prior to transfer to a psychiatric facility.

Abuse screening is another important component of the medical evaluation. Victims of child maltreatment are at increased risk of a variety of mental health problems.[20,21] As child maltreatment and mental health disorders often co-exist, children presenting with mental health emergencies should be screened for neglect and emotional, physical and sexual abuse. Children with disabilities and special health care needs are also known to be at increased risk of maltreatment and should likewise be screened for abuse.

ASSESSING PSYCHIATRICALLY ILL YOUTH: SUICIDE

Youth presenting with depression, suicidal ideation, or self-harming behaviors can be challenging to assess. Although suicidal ideation and self-harming behavior are not uncommon during adolescence, and completed suicides are relatively uncommon, every suicide threat must be taken seriously. An overall assessment of suicide risk factors is necessary. Youth with suicidal ideation should be questioned about their plans. Suicide plans with high lethality and patient access to guns, dangerous medications, or other highly lethal means are particularly concerning. Patients should be queried about past suicide attempts and risk factors such as drug and alcohol abuse and social isolation. In addition, the patient's thought patterns should be probed. Patients with distorted thoughts and perceptions or black-and-white thinking and perceived narrowed options represent a high risk.[22] It is concerning if the patient minimizes events or cannot calmly discuss the acute precipitants. Protective factors such as identifying reasons to continue living, engagement with school and friends, and strong coping mechanisms should also be sought.

Family support and stability are key. Family turmoil such as domestic violence, parental marital problems, or substance abuse should be investigated. If the home environment seems to be causing or exacerbating the child's suicidal ideation, hospitalization is likely indicated.[23] A family history of psychiatric disorders and violence is important. Family history of completed or attempted suicide is a risk factor for future suicide attempts.[23,24] The family should be asked if guns or other dangers are available in the home. Parents should be interviewed to determine their understanding of the severity of symptoms. If discharge is planned, the ability and motivation of the patient and parent to access outpatient care must be assured. Responsible caretakers must be available to closely monitor the child and return for care if necessary, and the caretakers must be comfortable with the plan.

In addition to the patient's family members, others may be able to provide important collateral information. Existing outpatient mental health providers should be involved, especially if discharge is contemplated. If social services are involved, the child's case worker or social worker may be able to provide valuable information. If the patient disclosed suicidal ideation to a friend, teacher, or other individual, that person should be contacted to corroborate the story, if possible.

Suicide screening tools should be used in conjunction with clinical interview in patient evaluation. ASQ is a 4-question suicide screening tool developed for ED use in youth.[25] It is available online (https://www.nimh.nih.gov/news/science-news/ask-suicide-screening-questions-asq.shtml). The SAFE-T reminds clinicians of questions to ask about risk factors, protective factors, and suicidal thoughts, and based on responses suggests risk level and potential interventions. It is also available for free download (http://www.integration.samhsa.gov/images/res/SAFE_T.pdf). One tool specifically studied in adolescents with psychiatric emergencies is the Columbia-Suicide Severity Rating Scale (C-SSRS).[26] A pediatric version can be downloaded at http://www.cssrs.columbia.edu/scales_practice_cssrs.html.[27] The C-SSRS requires training to administer and includes questions on suicidal ideation and intensity of ideation, preparatory behavior, and past suicide attempts, including aborted attempts, medical consequences, and potential lethality of past attempts. Intensity of suicidal ideation on the C-SSRS and a past history of nonsuicidal self-injury predicted return visits for psychiatric emergencies including suicide attempts.[26]

ASSESSING PSYCHIATRICALLY ILL YOUTH: AGGRESSION AND PSYCHOSIS

EDs are increasingly seeing violent youth, who are often frequent fliers and may carry multiple diagnoses including cognitive impairments. Juvenile justice and child welfare systems are often involved, adding legal complications. Patients with aggressive or agitated behavior pose management, diagnostic, and disposition challenges.

Techniques including verbal intervention, medication, and, when required, seclusion or restraint can be useful in de-escalating and containing aggressive behavior. Diagnostic evaluation and risk assessment start with the presentation of the aggression and response to interventions. Aggression can range from overblown tantrums to psychotic lashing out to premeditated, purposeful assault. An adolescent who is screaming and threatening staff, unable to respond to verbal de-escalation, who seems disorganized or paranoid may be psychotic or intoxicated. A child brought by police and school officials cursing and kicking but able to speak calmly to clinicians may be an impulsive child with attention deficit hyperactivity disorder (ADHD) or post-traumatic stress disorder (PTSD) who became agitated due to a stressor without true intent to harm anyone.

Once the child is calm, the clinician must attempt to understand the aggressive behavior, always assuming that there is a reason for the behavior. The reason may not be immediately obvious to the clinician or even to the child, but patient, empathic questioning can uncover the triggers. These may be external (such as teasing from peers, being told "no," a disruption of routine, confrontation with staff or police) or internal (frustration, anxiety, paranoia, intoxication, command hallucinations, trauma flashbacks), or both (an anxious child confronted by school staff, or a paranoid teen interacting with police). Aggressive acts can be reactive (in response to a trigger or perceived insult) or instrumental (planned with intent to harm or use aggression to get something). Reactive aggression may be triggered by events that appear benign to adults, like a school staff putting a hand on the child's shoulder to calm her but which feels threatening due to the child's history. Children with autism, intellectual disability, and learning disabilities may become aggressive when frustrated, because they lack the verbal skills to problem solve and express themselves. These children, and young children in general, may have difficulty expressing why they lashed out, and may even describe "a voice in my head" telling them to hit or break things. Young children and those with cognitive or emotional delays may describe hallucinations that are not truly psychotic, because they are misinterpreting their own thoughts and urges or trying to externalize blame.

After addressing the initial agitation, the clinician must determine whether the risk of future violence warrants inpatient admission. Risk depends in part on the nature of the violence, past history of violence, and on the presence or absence of underlying psychiatric illness. Youth with psychiatric illnesses such as ADHD, PTSD, and anxiety disorders can be prone to reactive aggression, and the treatment must be targeted to the illness or symptoms present. Understanding from the child's perspective the triggers for reactive aggression can also provide a therapeutic opportunity, as the ED clinician can help the child and family identify ways to avoid or cope with such triggers in the future. Instrumental aggression is seen in conduct disorder and substance use disorders. Treatment involves setting clear consequences, often in collaboration with parents and law enforcement, while promoting prosocial behavior with positive reinforcements; the inpatient unit may be less effective than intensive outpatient care for these youth. For example, a boy with ADHD who strikes out impulsively when he is frustrated, or a girl with PTSD who becomes agitated each time she sees the peers who "jumped" her, bear a chronically increased risk for future violence due to their psychiatric symptoms, but they do not have intent or plan to harm anyone. They need treatment, but can likely be safely discharged with appropriate outpatient care and increased supports and monitoring at school. By comparison, a teen who brings a knife to school due to paranoid psychosis remains at acute risk for violence and requires hospitalization, while another teen who is gang involved but without underlying psychiatric symptoms may also be at high risk for violence but may not be well served by hospitalization.

ASSESSMENT OF YOUTH WITH COMORBID MEDICAL AND SEVERE PSYCHIATRIC SYMPTOMS

Youth with chronic or severe psychiatric symptoms, such as schizophrenia or autism spectrum disorder (ASD), are not only at increased risk for acute medical problems but may also be unable to express what is wrong. Minor ailments such as ear infections, tooth pain, hunger, or fatigue can trigger psychiatric or behavioral symptoms including aggression, self-injury, inappropriate sexual behaviors, sleep cycle reversal, or running away. These cases can be difficult, because youth with ASD or schizophrenia can be medically and psychiatrically complicated and on multiple medications, and also because they often have a difficult time in the ED due to the unpredictability, unfamiliarity, noise, bright lights, blood draws, and physical examinations.

ED clinicians should not assume that physical symptoms are delusional in patients with schizophrenia, or that new problematic behaviors such as head banging are simply part of autism. Dismissing such symptoms is dangerous. New behaviors in youth with ASD are often triggered by physical discomforts including seasonal allergies, pain, fatigue, sedation due to polypharmacy, and adverse effects from medication. They can also be set off by changes in routine or home or school environment. Long-standing behavior that is now bringing the patient to the ED may indicate that community treatments are insufficient or ineffective and require reevaluation.

A careful medical examination is crucial, and cannot be skipped because the patient is difficult or agitated. Keeping patients with ASD calm requires removal of unnecessary stimuli, clear communication (simple, concrete, and written or picture-based if possible), attention to physical comfort, and use of soothing activities or family members when possible. The team should ask the caregivers what works at home, including preferred toys and caregivers, communication tools (such as picture communication tools and sign language), and soothing techniques. Understanding what typically triggers negative behaviors at home will also help the to avoid outbursts in the ED. Sedating patients with ASD is dangerous, as they may have paradoxic reactions to medications such as diphenhydramine and benzodiazepines, yet have little positive effect from antipsychotics. Behavioral interventions are much more likely to be effective.

Many youth with ASD can be stabilized quickly if the medical or physical etiology of their distress is discovered and resolved. Pain control, dental care, management of insomnia and constipation, and resolution of polypharmacy and medication adverse effects can be accomplished in the ED and provide great relief to patients and families. Often when these problems are resolved, the child who had been increasingly aggressive or difficult to manage is now calm and comfortable.

As few inpatient units accept youth with ASD (particularly if they are aggressive or engage in self-injurious behaviors), the ED clinician should familiarize himself or herself with available community services. Often home-based and respite services are available to patients who qualify, although families may need help from social work staff to access these services.

MANAGEMENT OF AGITATION

Severe agitation must be controlled to prevent patients from hurting themselves or others. Approach varies based on the patient's level of agitation and aggression, potential for violence, and developmental level. The least restrictive and least coercive method safe for the situation should be employed. Providers should recognize that agitated patients are doing their best under the circumstances. Failure to cooperate may be due to the underlying psychiatric or developmental disorder or lack of skills in getting needs met.[28] Maintaining an empathic, calm attitude can diffuse the situation and help patients to calm themselves.[28] Whenever possible, de-escalation attempts should be made before medication or physical restraint; this may include removing the patient from a sensory-overloaded environment, removing agitating family members or police, providing comfort needs such as food and warmth, and talking the patient down.[29] Relaxed, nonconfrontational body language, a soft voice, slow movements, allowing personal space, a nonjudgmental attitude, and reassurance that you are there to help may also help to de-escalate the situation.[29] Providers should be concise and clear, set limits, but also identify patients' wants and needs and offer choices.[28] Repetition may be necessary to assure patients that they are being heard and to communicate limits to agitated patients.[28]

The American Association of Emergency Psychiatry developed Best Practices in Evaluation and Treatment of Agitation (Project BETA) for acute care settings.[28,30,31] Although these guidelines are not specific to pediatric patients, many suggestions in the Project BETA guidelines are applicable to children. The guidelines acknowledge that while restraint events likely cannot be completely eliminated because of the acuity of patients and the hectic nature of the ED, verbal de-escalation, medications, and a seclusion room might decrease the need for restraint events.[31]

If the patient remains agitated despite these strategies, oral medications should be offered. Prior diagnoses and medications should guide the choice of medication used in a crisis. For example, an adolescent with a known anxiety disorder on a benzodiazepine or alpha-agonist medication (such as guanfacine or clonidine) might respond well to a small oral dose of the same medication, while a teen with schizophrenia may require an extra dose of his antipsychotic medication. The ED clinician must be careful if giving new medications, as the medications commonly used for agitation in adults can have significant adverse effects in children. Benzodiazepines are often disinhibiting and can cause paradoxic agitation, particularly in young children and those with ASD or intellectual disability. Antipsychotics, particularly high-potency antipsychotics, carry a high risk of extrapyramidal side effects in antipsychotic-naïve youth, particularly those who are not psychotic or manic. Often diphenhydramine is the safest medication choice, particularly for young children (though in those with intellectual disability or autism diphenhydramine can be disinhibiting). Guanfacine or other alpha-agonist medications may be useful in youth who are agitated due to ADHD or anxiety, although monitoring blood pressure is important when these medications are used. Oral medication should be offered before IM medication, as many youth become more agitated when approached with an injection. Often, an injection will require a physical hold or restraint, so this should be a last resort for safety after all other interventions have failed.

As with oral medications, the choice of IM medication in children is more complicated than the standard "5, 2, and 1" cocktail typically used in adult psychiatric patients. If the child is already on an antipsychotic or benzodiazepine, the same medication may be used to avoid the risks of polypharmacy. If the child is not on a standing medication that is available in immediate-release injectable form, the choice of medication should be based on the child's age, size, recent medication administration, medical conditions, and ideally some consideration of the psychological cause of his or her agitation. As with oral medications, the IM medication choice for an agitated adolescent who is psychotic should be different than that for one who is anxious, targeting the underlying cause of agitation, not just providing sedation. Diphenhydramine IM may be used for younger children, as it is calming, anxiolytic, and generally well tolerated, although total daily dose should be monitored, as overmedication can lead to disinhibition, confusion, or delirium. For adolescents who are agitated because of anxiety, benzodiazepines such as lorazepam or sedating lower-potency antipsychotics such as chlorpromazine may be effective, while patients who are manic or psychotic will likely require haloperidol or another high-potency antipsychotic. If first-generation antipsychotics are given, they should be given with diphenhydramine or benztropine to prevent acute dystonic adverse effects, particularly if the patient is antipsychotic naive or if his or her agitation is not secondary to psychosis or mania. Olanzapine and ziprasidone should be used with caution, as olanzapine can cause acute respiratory depression if combined with benzodiazepines, and ziprasidone may be dangerous in patients with cardiac arrythmias. In general, dosing of IM medications is half of the oral dose used. For example, 50 mg of oral diphenhydramine or chlorpromazine corresponds to 25 mg IM (**Table 1**).

Physical (by staff) or mechanical (cloth or leather cuffs) restraint is sometimes necessary to prevent injury to the patient or others. Restraints should never be employed as punishment, for staff convenience or because of inadequate staffing.[32] In patients with a history of trauma, restraint should be avoided whenever possible.[32] Although restraint use has been studied in pediatric residential treatment facilities and psychiatric inpatient facilities, there is little research on restraints in pediatric patients in acute care settings. Physical restraint use in pediatric ED patients with psychiatric complaints seems to vary

Table 1
Medications commonly utilized for agitation

Medication administration should follow and be accompanied by verbal and environmental de-escalation. Medication choices should be based on child's history and the etiology of agitation. See text for common adverse effects.

Drug	*Child (5–11 y or up to 90 pounds)*	*Teen (12 y and over or >90 pounds)*
Diphenhydramine	12.5–25 mg by mouth or IM every 4-6 h; TDD 100 mg	25–50 mg by mouth or IM every 4-6 h; TDD 150 mg
Chlorpromazine	12.5–25 mg by mouth every 4-6 h, IM dose is half of oral dose; TDD 50 mg	25–50 mg by mouth every 4-6 h, IM dose is half of the oral dose; TDD 100 mg
Lorazepam	Not recommended given disinhibition	0.5-2 mg by mouth or IM every 4-6 h; TDD 4-6 mg
Haloperidol	Not recommended given EPS risk	0.5 mg-10 mg by mouth or 1-5 mg IM; TDD 20 mg (10 mg if antipsychotic naïve)
Risperidone	0.25mg-0.5 mg by mouth every 4-6 h; TDD 3 mg	0.5-2 mg by mouth every 4-6 h; TDD 6 mg (3 mg if antipsychotic naive)
Olanzapine[a]	1.25–2.5 mg by mouth or IM every 4-6 h; TDD 7.5 mg (5 mg if antipsychotic naive)	2.5-5 mg by mouth or IM every 4-6 h; TDD 15 mg (10 mg if antipsychotic naive)
Guanfacine	0.5 mg-1 mg by mouth every 6-8 h	0.5 mg-2 mg by mouth every 6-8 h

Abbreviation: TDD, total daily dose.
[a] Do not administer within 2 h of benzodiazepines because of risk of respiratory depression.

greatly between facilities, with EDs reporting that 0.1% to 18% of patients presenting for mental health complaints are physically restrained.[9,33,34] One ED reported significantly decreasing the use of restraints in pediatric patients with mental health complaints after implementing a dedicated mental health team.[33]

Joint Commission requirements for physical or mechanical restraint of pediatric patients are more stringent than for adults. A physician or other licensed independent practitioner must conduct a face-to-face evaluation of patients as soon as possible and within 1 hour of initiation of restraints in Medicare/Medicaid-funded programs and within 2 hours in other programs, and patients must have a face-to-face re-evaluation by a physician or other licensed independent practitioner. Restraint orders are limited by federal regulation to 1 hour in children under the age of 9 years and 2 hours in children between 9 and 17 years of age, and may be further restricted by state or local regulation. After that period, a new order for continuation of restraints is necessary if the patient still requires restraint. The patient must be continually monitored by appropriately trained staff while restrained.

EQUIPPING EMERGENCY DEPARTMENTS TO BETTER SERVE PSYCHIATRICALLY ILL YOUTH

Truly improving emergency psychiatric care for youth requires an investment not only by individual EDs but by the fields of child psychiatry and emergency medicine to identify best practice guidelines, standards for care and staffing, and strategies for collaboration, training, and extension of scarce resources.

Emergency and pediatric emergency physicians have been leaders in the idea of best practice standards, such as for pediatric head injury, with research networks collaborating to develop and study standardized care pathways and implement best practices nationwide. Unfortunately, this innovation has not been extended to pediatric behavioral or psychiatric emergencies. There are few standards for assessment, management, or treatment, and little collaboration between child psychiatry and emergency medicine to develop or study such standards of care. A collaboration between child psychiatry and the Pediatric Emergency Care Research Network (PECARN) could provide the groundwork for research and standards development.

Collaboration between child psychiatry and EM is also needed to address deficits in child psychiatric staffing in the ED. Given the national shortage of child psychiatrists, EDs will never be fully staffed with around-the-clock child psychiatric specialists, yet training for emergency medicine and pediatric emergency medicine physicians includes little teaching in management of child psychiatric emergencies. Child psychiatry must play a larger role in emergency and pediatric emergency training programs, although as child psychiatric crises are relatively low-frequency events in many EDs, opportunities for ongoing support and consultation will be needed as well. Telepsychiatry and consultation networks for child psychiatry, similar to networks developed in some states for primary care physicians, would assist ED clinicians in providing better care to youth in psychiatric crisis.

SUMMARY

Given the lack of adequate outpatient mental health resources, youth with psychiatric and behavioral health complaints will continue to seek treatment in general and pediatric EDs. Emergency providers must provide the best care possible for youth with psychiatric and behavioral emergencies despite significant systems limitations. Techniques outlined in the article and collaboration with mental health professionals can help emergency and pediatric emergency physicians who feel inadequately prepared to care for youth in psychiatric crisis. Psychiatric health professionals can work collaboratively with EDs to develop evaluation and treatment protocols and identify community resources. Multidisciplinary collaboration is also needed to advance research and develop evidence-based guidelines to guide best practices in evaluation and treatment of pediatric mental health emergencies. Improved outpatient resources are needed to prevent patients with psychiatric conditions from decompensating to the point of requiring ED management and to provide follow-up options, potentially preventing the need for admission of low-risk patients.

REFERENCES

1. Grupp-Phelan J, Harman JS, Kelleher K. Trends in mental health and chronic condition visits by children presenting for care at U.S. emergency departments. Public Health Rep 2007;122:55–61.
2. Kann L, Kinchen S, Shanklin SL, et al. Youth risk behavior surveillance—United States, 2013. MMWR Suppl 2014;63(4):1–168.
3. Baraff LJ, Janowicz N, Asarnow JR. Survey of California emergency departments about practices for management of suicidal patients and resources available for their care. Ann Emerg Med 2006;48(4):452–8.
4. Betz ME, Sullivan AF, Manton AP, et al. Knowledge, attitudes, and practices of emergency department providers in the care of suicidal patients. Depress Anxiety 2013;30(10):1005–12.
5. Bridge JA, Marcus SC, Olfson M. Outpatient care of young people after emergency treatment of deliberate self-harm. J Am Acad Child Adolesc Psychiatry 2012;51(2):213–22.e1.

6. Gairin I, House A, Owens D. Attendance at the accident and emergency department in the year before suicide: retrospective study. Br J Psychiatry 2003;183:28–33.
7. Case SD, Case BG, Olfson M, et al. Length of stay of pediatric mental health emergency department visits in the United States. J Am Acad Child Adolesc Psychiatry 2011;50(11):1110–9.
8. Mahajan P, Alpern ER, Grupp-Phelan J, et al. Epidemiology of psychiatric-related visits to emergency departments in a multicenter collaborative research pediatric network. Pediatr Emerg Care 2009;25(11):715–20.
9. Grupp-Phelan J, Mahajan P, Foltin GL, et al. Referral and resource use patterns for psychiatric-related visits to pediatric emergency departments. Pediatr Emerg Care 2009;25:217–20.
10. Mepelli E, Black T, Doan Q. Trends in pediatric emergency department utilization for mental health-related visits. J Pediatr 2015;167(4):905–10.
11. Havens JF. Making psychiatric emergency services work better for children and families. J Am Acad Child Adolesc Psychiatry 2011;50(11):1093–4.
12. Lukens TW, Wolf SJ, Edlow JA, et al. Clinical policy: critical issues in the diagnosis and management of the adult psychiatric patient in the emergency department. Ann Emerg Med 2006;47(1):79–99.
13. Wiler JL, Brown NA, Chanmugam AS, et al. Care of the psychiatric patient in the emergency department—a review of the literature. 2014. Available at: https://www.acep.org/uploadedFiles/ACEP/Clinical_and_Practice_Management/Resources/Mental_Health_and_Substance_Abuse/Psychiatric%20Patient%20Care%20in%20the%20ED%202014.pdf Accessed June 10, 2016.
14. Nordstrom K, Zun LS, Wilson MP, et al. Medical evaluation and triage of the agitated patient: Consensus statement of the American Association for emergency psychiatry project BETA medical evaluation workgroup. West J Emerg Med 2012;13(1):3–10.
15. Onigu-Otite E, Oyebadejo OA, Moukaddam N, et al. Like a prisoner in Azkaban: medical clearance of the pediatric psychiatric patient. Pediatr Emerg Care Med Open Access 2016;1(1):6.
16. Santiago LI, Tunik MG, Foltin GL, et al. Children requiring psychiatric consultation in the pediatric emergency department: epidemiology, resource utilization, and complications. Pediatr Emerg Care 2006;22:85–9.
17. Donofrio JJ, Santillanes G, McCammack BD, et al. Clinical utility of screening laboratory tests in pediatric psychiatric patients presenting to the emergency department for medical clearance. Ann Emerg Med 2014;63(6):666–75.
18. Fortu JM, Kim IK, Cooper A, et al. Psychiatric patients in the pediatric emergency department undergoing routine urine toxicology screens for medical clearance: results and use. Pediatr Emerg Care 2009;25(6):387–92.
19. Shihabuddin BS, Hack CM, Sivitz AB. Role of urine drug screening in the medical clearance of pediatric psychiatric patients: is there one? Pediatr Emerg Care 2013;29(3):903–6.
20. Gilbert R, Widom CS, Browne K, et al. Burden and consequences of child maltreatment in high-income countries. Lancet 2009;373(9657):68–81.
21. Afifi TO, MacMillan HL, Boyle M, et al. Child abuse and mental disorders in Canada. CMAJ 2014;186(9):E324–32.
22. Copelan R. Assessing the potential for violent behavior in children and adolescents. Pediatr Rev 2006;27(5):e36–41.

23. Tishler CL, Reiss NS, Rhodes AR. Suicidal behavior in children younger than twelve: a diagnostic challenge for emergency department personnel. Acad Emerg Med 2007;14(9):810–8.
24. Stowell KR, Florence P, Harman HJ, et al. Psychiatric evaluation of the agitated patient: consensus statement of the American Association for emergency psychiatric project BETA psychiatric evaluation workgroup. West J Emerg Med 2012; 13(1):11–6.
25. Horowitz LM, Bridge JA, Teach SJ, et al. Ask suicide-screening questions (ASQ). A brief instrument for the pediatric emergency department. Arch Pediatr Adolesc Med 2012;166(12):1170–6.
26. Gipson PY, Agarwala P, Opperman KJ, et al. Columbia-Suicide Severity Rating Scale. Predictive validity with adolescent psychiatric emergency patients. Pediatr Emerg Care 2015;31:88–94.
27. Posner K, Brent D, Lucas C, et al. Columbia-Suicide Severity Rating Scale (C-SSRS) pediatric/cognitively impaired—lifetime recent–clinical. Available at: http://www.cssrs.columbia.edu/scales_practice_cssrs.html. Accessed June 16, 2016.
28. Richmond JS, Berlin JS, Fishkind AB, et al. Verbal de-escalation of the agitated patient: Consensus statement of the American Association for emergency psychiatry project BETA de-escalation workgroup. West J Emerg Med 2012;13(1): 17–25.
29. Marzullo LR. Pharmacologic management of the agitated child. Pediatr Emerg Care 2014;30(4):269–75.
30. Holloman GH Jr, Zeller SL. Overview of project BETA: best practices in evaluation and treatment of agitation. West J Emerg Med 2012;13(1):1–2.
31. Knox DK, Holloman GH Jr. Use and avoidance of seclusion and restraint: statement of the American Association for emergency psychiatry project BETA seclusion and restraint workgroup. West J Emerg Med 2012;13(1):35–40.
32. Masters KJ, Bellonci C, Bernet W, et al. Practice parameter for the prevention and management of aggressive behavior in child and adolescent psychiatric institutions, with special reference to seclusion and restraint. J Am Acad Child Adolesc Psychiatry 2002;41(Suppl 2):4S–25S.
33. Uspal NG, Rutman LE, Kodish I, et al. Use of a dedicated, non-physician-led mental health team to reduce pediatric emergency department lengths of stay. Acad Emerg Med 2016;23(4):440–7.
34. Sheridan DC, Spiro DM, Fu R, et al. Mental health utilization in a pediatric emergency department. Pediatr Emerg Care 2015;31(8):555–9.

Addictive Disorders in Adolescents

Anh Truong, MD*, Nidal Moukaddam, MD, PhD, Alexander Toledo, MD, Edore Onigu-Otite, MBBS

KEYWORDS

• Adolescence • Addiction • Substance use disorders • Gambling • Internet gaming • Video games

KEY POINTS

- Addictive disorders in adolescents show continuously changing patterns owing to increased availability, shifts in adolescent perceptions of available drugs, new psychoactive substances, and new technologies.
- Treatment recommendations should be personalized based on the assessment and needs of the adolescent.
- Attention to underlying mental health and medical conditions and severity of symptoms help to determine the optimal treatment setting.
- Emerging trends show legitimate use of prescription pain medication in adolescence increases risk of opioid use disorder with a significant increase in heroin addiction and overdose deaths in young adulthood.

EPIDEMIOLOGY

Addictive disorders include substance-related and non–substance-related disorders. Substance-related disorders are a leading cause of morbidity and mortality in the United States and are becoming increasingly pervasive in the adolescent population. Data from national surveys show a changing pattern of substance use in teens, with the prevalence of marijuana use decreasing at a slower rate than alcohol or cigarettes. Recent data shows the prevalence of electronic tobacco is steadily increasing, whereas opioids, and particularly nonprescription pain medications in youth, have increased to epidemic levels.[1,2] Recent surveys show use of any illicit substances to be 15% by the time teens reach 8th grade, 28% by 10th grade, 39% by 12th grade, and 41% by the time adolescents reach college. With the recent legalization of marijuana use in many states, there are now concerns that there may be an increase in the use of illicit substances among adolescents in the coming years.[1]

1977 Butler Boulevard, #E4400, Houston, TX 77030, USA
* Corresponding author.
E-mail address: altruong@bcm.edu

Psychiatr Clin N Am 40 (2017) 475–486
http://dx.doi.org/10.1016/j.psc.2017.05.012

0193-953X/17/© 2017 Elsevier Inc. All rights reserved.

Recreational drug use is a significant cause of mortality and morbidity in children and adolescents.[3] Delivery systems have changed to provide novel ways to use substances, including vaporization and electronic cigarettes.[1] Common drugs of abuse have also continued to evolve and now contain a variety of designer drugs, including synthetic marijuana, synthetic stimulants, synthetic cathinones ("bath salts"), and other new psychoactive substances.

Although novel drugs continue to come into the market, opioid use remains rampant in adolescents. There are now an estimated 26 million to 36 million individuals abusing opioids worldwide, with 2.1 million people in the United States suffering from abuse of prescription opioid pain relievers. The nonmedical use of opioids is especially problematic, with overdose deaths involving prescription opioids having quadrupled since 1999 in the United States.[4] In contrast with prior studies, recent literature highlights the potential risk of legitimate prescription opioid use with future misuse in adolescents.[5,6] Recent findings show legitimate opioid prescription use by 12th grade significantly predicts future opioid misuse after high school in individuals with little to no history of drug use or a strong disapproval of drug use. Those who were provided legitimate opioid prescriptions were 33% more likely to have opioid misuse after high school compared with those who had never received an opioid prescription.[5] This association is thought to be mediated by an individual's initial experience with the substance, which can be pleasurable, seemingly safe, and with limited perceived risk or consequence.[7]

Non–substance-related disorders include gambling disorder and Internet gaming disorder: gambling and problematic Internet use are becoming more of a concern with the spread of Internet and online access for youth. Currently, 0.2% to 12.3% of youth meet criteria for problematic gambling.[8] The prevalence of Internet gaming disorder is estimated to be 6% to 11% in adolescents, with a 2:1 male predominance.[9,10] The popularity of Internet gaming may be attributed in part to the social aspects of Internet gaming, including increased social relationships, communication between friends, team building with coordination or leadership of teams of players to advance in a game, and continued character development.[11] One genre of Internet gaming that has received particular attention is massive multiplayer online role playing games, which have been found to be particularly addictive owing to social networks and never-ending game play in a detailed virtual world.[12]

SUBSTANCE USE DISORDERS

Substance use disorders fundamentally involve a cluster of cognitive, behavioral, and physiologic symptoms associated with ongoing use of a substance despite significant substance-related dysfunction. The brain's circuitry is thought to undergo an underlying change that may persist after detoxification, especially in severe cases. Diagnosis is based on a pathologic pattern of behavior related to substance use, which is divided into 4 basic categories of criteria in the *Diagnostic and Statistical Manual of Mental Disorders*, 5th edition (DSM-5): impaired control, social impairment, risky use, and pharmacologic criteria (**Box 1**). In general, the presence of 2 to 3 criteria indicates a mild substance use disorder, 4 to 5 criteria indicate a moderate disorder, and 6 or more criteria indicate a severe disorder.

Substance-Induced Disorders

Substance-induced disorders include intoxication, withdrawal, and substance-induced mental disorders. The essential feature of intoxication is development of a reversible substance-related syndrome owing to the recent ingestion of a substance. Withdrawal is a substance-specific syndrome owing to cessation or reduction in heavy

Box 1
Risk factors for adolescent substance abuse

Individual
- Genetic predisposition
- Prenatal drug exposure
- Temperament
- Lack of behavioral self-control and regulation

Family
- Parent and sibling modeling of drug and alcohol abuse
- Permissive parenting
- Parental hostility
- Harsh discipline
- Parent–child conflict
- Low parental warmth
- Child abuse, maltreatment, and neglect

School and peers
- Failure in school
- Peer rejection and alienation
- Peer involvement in substance abuse

Neighborhood and community
- Accessibility and availability of illicit substances
- Poverty
- Social norms that favor use

Data from National Research Council and Institute of Medicine. 2009. *Preventing Mental, Emotional, and Behavioral Disorders Among Young People: Progress and Possibilities*. Washington, DC: The National Academies Press.

and prolonged substance use that causes significant distress or functional impairment. For both intoxication and withdrawal conditions, symptoms must not be due to another medical condition or mental disorder. Substance-induced mental disorders are disorders that develop within 1 month or during substance intoxication or withdrawal and are not better explained by an independent mental disorder. They must precede the onset of intoxication, withdrawal, or exposure to a substance or medication, and persist for more than 1 month after cessation of acute withdrawal or severe intoxication. They cannot cause significant distress or functional impairment exclusively during the course of delirium.

Risk factors for adolescent substance abuse include individual, family, peer, and community risk factors.

SCREENING

Screening measures are typically used in outpatient primary care settings and psychiatric practices to identify those at risk or who have developed a substance use disorder. There are few screening tools validated for use in adolescents, which include the CRAFFT (**Table 1**) and AUDIT.[13–15] Despite recent changes in the criteria for substance use from the DSM-IV to the DSM-5, there is evidence that the CRAFFT remains sensitive and specific in identifying substance use disorders in the adolescent population.[16] Other commonly used scales include the Drug Abuse Screening Test, the Drug Abuse Screening Test for Adolescents, and the Adolescent Alcohol and Drug Involvement Scale.[17–21] Additionally, there are combination tools that include

Table 1
Client assessment treatment recommendations

Use Pattern	Treatment Recommendations
No history of use No current use	Primary prevention
History of use No current use	Anticipatory guidance and support
Problems resulting from use Low to moderate use	Brief office intervention Outpatient treatment
Problems resulting from use Moderate to heavy use	Intensive outpatient treatment Day treatment Partial hospitalization Inpatient rehabilitation

Data from Treatment Improvement Protocol (TIP) Series 32, Treatment of Adolescents with Substance Use Disorders. Winters K, Botzet A, Anderson N, et al. Screening and Assessment Study, Wisconsin Division of Juvenile Corrections, Alcohol and Other Drug Abuse. University of Minnesota. Minneapolis (MN): Center for Adolescent Substance Abuse Research. 2001; Available at: http://162.99.3.213/products/tools/keys/pdfs/KK_31_32.pdf.

screening with brief intervention and referral to treatment, the SBIRT (Screening, Brief Intervention and Referral to Treatment), designed for adolescent patients.

DRUG TESTING

Uses and Limitations

Toxicologic testing can be used to identify drug use as part of a clinical assessment. It can also be used to detect or deter substance use in a variety of clinical situations, or as part of a treatment program for substance use disorders. Drug screening of urine, blood, saliva, or hair can be used to detect use of substances. A false-positive result may result from cross-reactivity with another substance in the urine. Confirmatory testing is much less likely to yield a false-positive result, but cannot distinguish between appropriate use of prescribed medications and illicit substance use. False-negative urine drug tests can result from an adolescent intentionally manipulating the urine sample, either by dilution, addition of a “masking” agent that interferes with the test, or use of another person’s urine. False-negative results can also occur if the substance is detected at an amount lower than the cutoff concentration for a positive result. A limitation of drug testing is the increasing use of newer designer drugs that are not included in the standard test panel.[22]

Usefulness in Adolescents

Drug use by teenagers often presents with nonspecific signs and symptoms. When a family member or clinician suspects drug use, voluntary drug testing can be useful as an adjunct to a thorough history. Drug testing of a competent adolescent without their consent is not only impractical, but also unethical and illegal. However, consent may be inferred and drug testing may be appropriate in an emergent situation, such as after an accident, suicide attempt, unexplained seizure, arrhythmia, or in the case of a toxidrome. Emerging research also suggests that drug testing is effective in adolescents participating in drug abuse treatment programs. This testing typically includes random urine screening. Because of the low sensitivity for detecting drug use in the general population, drug testing is generally not considered a useful screening tool.[23,24]

TREATMENT

Given the morbidity and mortality associated with adolescent addictive disorders, adolescent substance use needs to be identified and addressed as soon as possible. Adolescents can benefit from substance use intervention even when they are not addicted to a substance. Family pressure and legal consequential interventions can play a central role in getting adolescents to enter, stay in, and complete treatment, all of which could be critical in the adolescent's life. It is worth noting that, owing to the unique needs of adolescents, adult-based treatment approaches often do not meet the treatment needs of adolescents. Substance use treatment should be customized to the unique needs of the adolescent. Treatment planning should begin with a comprehensive assessment to identify the adolescent's strengths and weaknesses that need to be addressed. Appropriate treatment considers an adolescent's level of development including biological, psychological, and social development including school performance, family and peer relationships, gender, cultural factors, and any physical or mental health issues. It is crucially important to identify any cooccurring mental health conditions and treat optimally.

Treatment recommendations should be personalized based on the assessment and needs of the individual adolescent.[25] The best treatment programs provide a combination of therapies and other services to meet the specific needs of the individual adolescent. Components of a comprehensive substance use program includes mental health, educational, legal, family, vocational services, and medical services including for infectious diseases.

Treatment setting recommendations are also based on the individual client's severity of symptoms (**Table 2**).[25] Other factors affecting treatment setting include the adolescent's level of intoxication and potential for withdrawal, presence of other mental health or medical conditions, readiness or motivation to change, risk of relapse, and recovery environment.

Table 2
Types of family therapy

Therapy	Description
Multidimensional family therapy	Views adolescent drug use in terms of a network of influences (individual, family, peer, community). Treatment includes individual and family sessions held in the clinic, in the home, or with family members at the family court, school, or other community locations.
Brief strategic family therapy	Targets family interactions that are thought to maintain or exacerbate adolescent drug abuse and other cooccurring problem behaviors.
Functional family therapy	Another treatment based on a family systems approach, in which an adolescent's behavior problems are seen as being created or maintained by a family's dysfunctional interaction patterns.
Adolescent community reinforcement approach	Another comprehensive substance abuse treatment intervention that involves the adolescent and his or her family. It seeks to support the individual's recovery by increasing family, social, and educational/vocational reinforcers.
Assertive continuing care	Home-based continuing care approach to preventing relapse. Weekly home visits take place over a 12- to 14-week period after an adolescent is discharged from residential, intensive outpatient, or regular outpatient treatment.

Medications

Medications approved by the US Food and Drug Administration to treat addictive disorders are currently available for nicotine, alcohol, and opioid use disorders in individuals aged 18 and older. As of yet, relatively little research has been done on the use of these medications in adolescents. Nevertheless, some providers use these medications "off-label" for adolescents, especially older adolescents and youth.[24]

Nicotine use disorders

The available treatments include nicotine replacement therapy, bupropion, and varenicline. Nicotine replacement therapy seems not to be dangerous for adolescents and does not seem to have much abuse potential.[26,27] Various formulations exist including nicotine gum (Nicorette), patch (Nicoderm CQ), nasal spray (Nicotrol NS), inhaler (Nicotrol), and lozenge (Commit). Although there is currently 1 double-control, placebo-controlled trial showing efficacy of bupropion (Wellbutrin SR) in 312 adolescents aged 14 to 17 years, bupropion currently has no US Food and Drug Administration label for smoking cessation in adolescents. Varenicline (Chantix) has not been assessed as a treatment modality in adolescents.[28,29]

Alcohol use disorders

The available treatments for alcohol use disorders include disulfiram (Antabuse), The available treatments for alcohol use disorders include disulfiram (Antabuse), naltrexone (Revia), naltrexone depot (Vivitrol), and acamprosate (Campral). These medications are currently approved for use in individuals aged 18 and older.

Opioid use disorders

The available treatments for opioid use disorders include naltrexone (Revia), naltrexone depot (Vivitrol), naloxone autoinjection (Evzio), buprenorphine (Subutex), buprenorphine/naltrexone (Suboxone), and methadone. These medications are currently approved for use in individuals aged 18 and older. However, in some states, given the severity of symptoms in conjunction with strict regulations, some of these medications are allowed for use in younger patients, usually 16 and older, with opioid use disorders.

Psychosocial Treatments

Evidence-based psychosocial treatments available for adolescent addictive disorders include the following.

1. Cognitive–Behavioral Therapy: This strategy helps patients to recognize, avoid, and cope with the situations in which they are most likely to abuse drugs.
2. Contingency Management: This method uses positive reinforcement, and provides rewards or privileges for remaining drug free and engaging in treatment.
3. Motivational Enhancement Therapy: This therapy uses motivational interviewing strategies to evoke internally inspired behavior change to stop drug use and engage in treatment. Motivational interviewing is a directive, client-centered counseling style for eliciting behavior change by helping clients to explore and resolve ambivalence.[30]
4. Brief Motivational Interventions: When delivered to adolescents by primary care physicians, this modality has been found to be effective.[31,32]
5. Group Therapy: With the support of peers, this intervention helps patients to face their drug abuse realistically and boosts their motivation to stay drug free. Patients learn effective ways to resolve their emotional and interpersonal problems without resorting to drugs.

6. Family Therapies: These strategies have been found to be effective in decreasing symptoms in adolescents with addictive disorders.

NON–SUBSTANCE-RELATED DISORDERS

Non–substance-related disorders, sometimes called behavioral addictions, include gambling disorder and Internet gaming disorder.

Gambling Disorder

The lifetime prevalence rate of gambling disorder is about 0.2% for females and 0.6% for males. Although the onset can be in adolescence, adolescents are less likely to meet full criteria for this disorder. Gambling during childhood or early adolescence is associated with a higher risk of developing gambling disorder. Among adolescents, gambling is more prevalent in males than in females. Adolescent gambling can include sports betting, poker playing, bets with friends, free online gambling simulations, and lottery purchases. Increased accessibility, convenience, and anonymity may make gambling more attractive to adolescents.[33] Sports-related gambling is particularly popular among adolescents. One study of 6000 high school students revealed that regular involvement in sports betting and fantasy sports betting was associated with higher risk of a gambling problem. The risk is higher in older adolescents ages 16 to 19 compared with younger adolescents.[34] Families and peers may also influence gambling behavior in adolescents. Several studies have shown that adolescents are more at risk of developing a gambling problem when they have a parent, older siblings, or peers who gamble.[35–37] Adolescents were found to have a lower risk of gambling if any of the following were present: parental knowledge of problematic gambling in siblings, perception by adolescents that their parents were aware of their whereabouts and companions, and increased parental support.[38,39] A longitudinal study showed that early adolescent gambling behavior may lead to worsening behavior into adulthood.[40]

Gambling disorder is defined as gambling behavior that causes clinically significant impairment or distress. The individual must meet at least 4 of the DSM-5 diagnostic criteria over a 12-month period, and the gambling behavior cannot be better explained by a manic episode (**Table 3**). Severity is based on the number of criteria endorsed, with 4 to 5 criteria seen in individuals with mild gambling disorder, 6 to 7 in those with moderately severe gambling disorder, and 8 to 9 in those with more severe gambling disorder. Individuals presenting for treatment of gambling disorder tend to fall into the moderate to severe categories.

There are multiple instruments that measure at-risk and problem gambling among youth, including the South Oaks Gambling Screen Revised for Adolescents, Canadian

Table 3
CRAFFT screening tool

C	Have you ever ridden in a Car driven by someone (including self) who was high, drunk, or has been using drugs?
R	Have you ever used drugs or alcohol to Relax?
A	Do you ever use Alone?
F	Do you ever Forget things that you did while using?
F	Do Family or Friends tell you to cut down?
T	Have you ever gotten into Trouble when using?

Adolescent Gambling Inventory, and the Gambling Addictive Behavior Scale for Adolescents. The most commonly used instrument is the South Oaks Gambling Screen Revised for Adolescents. However, none of these methods has been rigorously evaluated.[41]

Internet Gaming Disorder

Internet gaming has been found to have some similarities to substance use and gambling disorders. Internet gaming disorder is a pattern of excessive and prolonged Internet gaming that results in symptoms analogous to the symptoms of substance use disorders, including loss of control, tolerance, and withdrawal symptoms. Individuals with Internet gaming disorder engage in Internet gaming despite neglect of other activities, typically devoting 8 to 10 hours or more per day to this pursuit. They can become irritated or angry if they are prevented from using a computer, and often go for long periods without food or sleep. The prevalence of this disorder is highest in male adolescents and in Asian countries. There seems to be a weak association with depressive disorders, attention deficit hyperactivity disorder, and obsessive–compulsive disorder. Like gambling disorder, Internet gaming disorder can lead to poor performance at school or work, as well as relationship problems.[42]

There is currently no consensus on the definition of Internet gaming addiction. However, Internet gaming disorder has now been included in the DSM-5 as a disorder requiring further empirical inquiry owing to growing concern and research in the area of Internet gaming addiction. Similar to other addictive disorders, Internet gaming disorder is characterized by excessive use despite negative consequences. Adolescents may devote as much as 8 to 10 hours or more per day to this activity and at least 30 hours per week. The criteria includes a persistent and recurrent use of the Internet to engage in games, often with other players, leading to clinically significant impairment or distress as indicated by 5 or more of nine symptoms in a 12-month period:

- Preoccupation with Internet video games until they become the dominant activity of daily life;
- Loss of interest in activities or leisure pursuits with the exception of Internet video gaming;
- Irritability, anxiety, or sadness when Internet video gaming is reduced or ceased;
- The need to increase Internet video gaming to attain the same effects on arousal or mood;
- Unsuccessful attempt to control or reduce Internet video gaming;
- Deception of family members, therapists, or others over the amount of time spent Internet video gaming;
- Continued excessive Internet video gaming despite knowledge of the psychosocial problems it is causing;
- Use of Internet video gaming to escape a negative mood; and
- Loss of a significant relationship, job, educational or career opportunity owing to Internet video gaming (DSM-5).

The Internet Addiction Test is the most commonly used diagnostic instrument to identify those with gaming addiction.[43] It is a 20-item self-report assessment that measures Internet addiction based on characteristics of use, neglect of every day life, and negative consequences. Based on scores, individuals are categorized into mild, moderate, or severe levels of Internet addiction. It has been validated in multiple languages, including English, Greek, Spanish, and Italian.[44–47]

SPECIAL CONSIDERATIONS

Video Game Addiction

Video game addiction, although currently not a DSM diagnosis, has become a topic of increasing research interest over the past decade with multiple studies evaluating the characteristics, diagnosis, and treatment of video game addictions. Video game addiction refers to the persistent and maladaptive pattern of video game playing behavior. It may be subcategorized into technological addictions and may include Internet gaming addiction. Video game usage may include games played on home console systems (Nintendo Wii, Xbox, PlayStation), handheld consoles (Nintendo DS), arcade game machines, mobile phones, or tablets. In a national sample of youth ages 8 to 18, 8.5% of video game players exhibited pathologic patterns of play. Those with video game addiction spent twice as much time playing video games, and were more likely to have video game systems in their bedroom.[48] Excessive use may also result in psychosocial and medical consequences. Psychosocial consequences involve problems at work, poor education, loss of hobbies, increased stress, decreased sense of well-being, and maladaptive coping.[49] Medical consequences can include epileptic seizures, motion sickness, headaches, dry eyes, obesity, tenosynovitis, and auditory hallucinations. More commonly, individuals may experience irregular sleep pattern and impaired attention and concentration.[50]

REFERENCES

1. Miech RA, Johnston LD, O'Malley PM, et al. Monitoring the future national survey results on drug use, 1975–2014: Volume I, Secondary school students. Ann Arbor (MI): Institute for Social Research, The University of Michigan; 2015. Available at: http://monitoringthefuture. Accessed July 25, 2017.
2. O'Connell ME, Boat T, Warner KE, editors. Preventing mental, emotional, and behavioral disorders among young people: progress and possibilities. Washington (DC): National Academies Press; 2009.
3. Califano JA. The National Center on addiction and substance abuse. 2005. Available at: https://www.nap.edu/download/12480. Accessed November 24, 2016.
4. United Nations office on drugs and crime. 2012. Available at: http://www.unodc.org/unodc/en/data-and-analysis/WDR-2012.html. Accessed November 24, 2016.
5. Miech R, Johnston L, O'malley PM, et al. Prescription opioids in adolescence and future opioid misuse. Pediatrics 2015;136(5):e1169–77.
6. Hoppe JA, Kim H, Heard K. Association of emergency department opioid initiation with recurrent opioid use. Ann Emerg Med 2015;65(5):493–9.e4.
7. Lynskey MT, Heath AC, Bucholz KK, et al. Escalation of drug use in early-onset cannabis users vs co-twin controls. JAMA 2003;289(4):427–33.
8. Calado F, Alexandre J, Griffiths MD. Prevalence of adolescent problem gambling: a systematic review of recent research. J Gambl Stud 2017;33(2):397–424.
9. Park SK, Kim JY, Cho CB. Prevalence of Internet addiction and correlations with family factors among South Korean adolescents. Adolescence 2008;43(172):895–909.
10. Rehbein F, Kleimann M, Mössle T. Prevalence and risk factors of video game dependency in adolescence: results of a German nationwide survey. Cyberpsychol Behav Soc Netw 2010;13(3):269–77.

11. Loton D, Lubman DI. Just one more level: identifying and addressing internet gaming disorder within primary care. Aust Fam Physician 2016; 45(1):48–52.
12. Chappell D, Eatough V, Davies MN, et al. EverQuest—it's just a computer game right? An interpretative phenomenological analysis of online gaming addiction. Int J Ment Health Addict 2006;4(3):205–16.
13. Knight JR, Sherritt L, Shrier LA, et al. Validity of the CRAFFT substance abuse screening test among adolescent clinic patients. Arch Pediatr Adolesc Med 2002;156(6):607–14.
14. Kandemir H, Aydemir Ö, Ekinci S, et al. Validity and reliability of the Turkish version of CRAFFT substance abuse screening test among adolescents. Neuropsychiatr Dis Treat 2015;11:1505–9.
15. Hall W, Saunders JB, Babor TF, et al. The structure and correlates of alcohol dependence: WHO collaborative project on the early detection of persons with harmful alcohol consumption–III. Addiction 1993;88(12):1627–36.
16. Mitchell SG, Kelly SM, Gryczynski J, et al. The CRAFFT cut-points and DSM-5 criteria for alcohol and other drugs: a reevaluation and reexamination. Subst Abus 2014;35(4):376–80.
17. Skinner HA. The drug abuse screening test. Addict Behav 1982;7(4):363–71.
18. Martino S, Grilo CM, Fehon DC. Development of the drug abuse screening test for adolescents (DAST-A). Addict Behav 2000;25(1):57–70.
19. Mayer J, Filstead WJ. The adolescent alcohol involvement scale. An instrument for measuring adolescents' use and misuse of alcohol. J Stud Alcohol 1979; 40(3):291–300.
20. Moberg DP, Hahn L. The adolescent drug involvement scale. J Child Adolesc Subst Abuse 1991;2(1):75–88.
21. Winters K, Botzet A, Anderson N, et al. Screening and assessment study, Wisconsin division of juvenile corrections, alcohol and other drug abuse. University of Minnesota. Minneapolis (MN): Center for Adolescent Substance Abuse Research; 2001.
22. Levy S, Siqueira LM, Ammerman SD, et al. Testing for drugs of abuse in children and adolescents. Pediatrics 2014;133(6):e1798–807.
23. Schwartz RH, Clark HW, Meek PS. Laboratory tests for rapid screening of drugs of abuse in the workplace: a review. J Addict Dis 1993;12(2):43–56.
24. Hammett-Stabler CA, Pesce AJ, Cannon DJ. Urine drug screening in the medical setting. Clin Chim Acta 2002;315(1–2):125–35.
25. National Institute of Health, National Institute of Drug Abuse (2014). Principles of adolescent substance use disorder treatment: a research-based guide. Available at: https://www.drugabuse.gov/sites/default/files/podata_1_17_14.pdf. Accessed November 26, 2016.
26. Smith TA, House RF, Croghan IT, et al. Nicotine patch therapy in adolescent smokers. Pediatrics 1996;98(4 Pt 1):659–67.
27. Moolchan ET, Robinson ML, Ernst M, et al. Safety and efficacy of the nicotine patch and gum for the treatment of adolescent tobacco addiction. Pediatrics 2005;115(4):e407–14.
28. Muramoto ML, Leischow SJ, Sherrill D, et al. Randomized, double-blind, placebo-controlled trial of 2 dosages of sustained-release bupropion for adolescent smoking cessation. Arch Pediatr Adolesc Med 2007;161(11):1068–74.
29. Karpinski JP, Timpe EM, Lubsch L. Smoking cessation treatment for adolescents. J Pediatr Pharmacol Ther 2010;15(4):249–63.

30. Rollnick S, Butler CC, Kinnersley P, et al. Motivational interviewing. BMJ 2010; 340:c1900.
31. Jensen CD, Cushing CC, Aylward BS, et al. Effectiveness of motivational interviewing interventions for adolescent substance use behavior change: a meta-analytic review. J Consult Clin Psychol 2011;79(4):433–40.
32. Spirito A, Monti PM, Barnett NP, et al. A randomized clinical trial of a brief motivational intervention for alcohol-positive adolescents treated in an emergency department. J Pediatr 2004;145(3):396–402.
33. King DL, Delfabbro PH, Griffiths MD. Video game addiction. In: Principles of addiction: comprehensive addictive behaviors and disorders. San Diego (CA): Academic Press; 2013. p. 819–25.
34. Marchica L, Zhao Y, Derevensky J, et al. Understanding the relationship between sports-relevant gambling and being at-risk for a gambling problem among American adolescents. J Gambl Stud 2017;33(2):437–48.
35. Canale N, Vieno A, Griffiths MD, et al. "I am becoming more and more like my eldest brother!": the relationship between older siblings, adolescent gambling severity, and the attenuating role of parents in a large-scale nationally representative survey study. J Gambl Stud 2017;33(2):425–35.
36. Ladouceur R, Jacques C, Ferland F, et al. Parents' attitudes and knowledge regarding gambling among youths. J Gambl Stud 1998;14(1):83–90.
37. Sheela PS, Choo WY, Goh LY, et al. Gambling risk amongst adolescents: evidence from a school-based survey in the Malaysian setting. J Gambl Stud 2016;32(2):643–59.
38. Canale N, Vieno A, Ter bogt T, et al. Adolescent gambling-oriented attitudes mediate the relationship between perceived parental knowledge and adolescent gambling: implications for prevention. Prev Sci 2016;17(8):970–80.
39. Räsänen T, Lintonen T, Tolvanen A, et al. The role of social support in the association between gambling, poor health and health risk-taking. Scand J Public Health 2016;44(6):593–8.
40. Carbonneau R, Vitaro F, Brendgen M, et al. Trajectories of gambling problems from mid-adolescence to age 30 in a general population cohort. Psychol Addict Behav 2015;29(4):1012–21.
41. Edgren R, Castrén S, Mäkelä M, et al. Reliability of instruments measuring at-risk and problem gambling among young individuals: a systematic review covering years 2009-2015. J Adolesc Health 2016;58(6):600–15.
42. American Psychiatric Association. Diagnostic and statistical manual of mental disorders: DSM-5. Washington (DC): American Psychiatric Association; 2013.
43. Young KS. Internet addiction: the emergence of a new clinical disorder. Cyberpsychol Behav 1998;1(3):237–44.
44. Widyanto L, McMurran M. The psychometric properties of the internet addiction test. Cyberpsychol Behav 2004;7(4):443–50.
45. Fernández-villa T, Molina AJ, García-Martín M, et al. Validation and psychometric analysis of the internet addiction test in Spanish among college students. BMC Public Health 2015;15:953.
46. Tsimtsiou Z, Haidich AB, Kokkali S, et al. Greek version of the Internet addiction test: a validation study. Psychiatr Q 2014;85(2):187–95.
47. Fioravanti G, Casale S. Evaluation of the psychometric properties of the Italian internet addiction test. Cyberpsychol Behav Soc Netw 2015;18(2):120–8.
48. Gentile D. Pathological video-game use among youth ages 8 to 18: a national study. Psychol Sci 2009;20(5):594–602.

49. Griffiths MD, Kuss DJ, King DL. Video game addiction: past, present and future. Curr Psychiatry Rev 2012;8(4):308–18.
50. King D, Delfabbro P, Griffiths M. The convergence of gambling and digital media: implications for gambling in young people. J Gambl Stud 2010;26(2):175–87.

Intensive Care and its Discontents

Psychiatric Illness in the Critically Ill

Ali M. Hashmi, MD[a,*], Jin Y. Han, MD[b], Vishal Demla, MD[c]

KEYWORDS

- Intensive care • Critical illness • Delirium • Depression • Anxiety • Sleep problems • Pain

KEY POINTS

- Psychiatric illness, including delirium, substance withdrawal, depression, anxiety, and posttraumatic stress disorder, frequently complicate intensive care unit admissions.
- These illnesses can adversely affect recovery from critical illness and quality of life after discharge.
- Early recognition and management can ameliorate the negative impact of these illnesses both during a critical illness and after.

INTRODUCTION

More than 5 million patients are treated in intensive care units (ICUs) annually in the United States.[1] It is increasingly being recognized that simply preventing mortality should no longer be considered an optimal outcome of an ICU stay. Critically ill patients can develop a host of cognitive and psychiatric complaints during their ICU stay, many of which (sleep problems, anxiety, posttraumatic stress disorder (PTSD), depression, cognitive problems) can persist for weeks or months following discharge from the ICU and can seriously affect the person's quality of life, including the ability to return to work.[2] These problems have collectively been called post–intensive care syndrome (PICS).[3] Given how common these morbidities can be, it is essential that clinicians recognize the onset of some of these syndromes during the patient's ICU stay so that

Disclosure: The authors have nothing to disclose.
[a] Department of Psychiatry and Behavioral Sciences, King Edward Medical University/Mayo Hospital, Neela Gumbad, Lahore-54700, Pakistan; [b] Menninger Department of Psychiatry and Behavioral Sciences, Department of Family and Community Medicine, Baylor College of Medicine, 1502 Taub Loop NPC 2nd Floor, Houston, TX 77030, USA; [c] Division of Critical Care Medicine, Department of Internal Medicine, University of Texas Health Science Center, 6431 Fannin, MSB 1.150, Houston, TX 77030, USA
* Corresponding author.
E-mail address: ahashmi39@gmail.com

http://dx.doi.org/10.1016/j.psc.2017.05.011

0193-953X/17/© 2017 Elsevier Inc. All rights reserved.

appropriate measures may be taken to ameliorate their incidence in the ICU and prevent their occurrence after discharge. This article describes some of the most common psychiatric problems encountered by clinicians in the ICU. It reviews basic principles of assessment and management, including both pharmacologic and nonpharmacologic interventions. As mentioned earlier, research into outcomes of ICU treatment has traditionally focused on physical health, length of hospital stay, and mortalities. As this article makes clear, a more comprehensive approach is needed in order to decrease patient suffering, improve morbidity and mortality, and ensure that critically ill patients can return to the highest quality of life after their ICU stay.

ASSESSMENT AND MANAGEMENT OF DELIRIUM IN THE CRITICALLY ILL

Delirium is characterized by a disturbance of consciousness with accompanying change in cognition. It typically manifests as a constellation of symptoms with an acute onset and a fluctuating course.[4] Delirium is associated with increased mortality in ICU patients, prolonged ICU and hospital lengths of stay, and cognitive impairment after discharge.[5] The differential diagnosis for a patient experiencing altered sensorium is broad and this article focuses on delirium in ICU patients only.

Delirium occurs in up to 80% of critically ill patients, especially those who are mechanically ventilated. Its 3 subtypes are:

- Hyperactive
- Hypoactive
- Mixed

Its diagnosis is often missed unless screening tools are used.[6] One of the most frequently used screening tools for this is the Confusion Assessment Method for use in the ICU (CAM-ICU). It evaluates 4 features: (1) an acute change in mental status, (2) inattention, (3) disorganized thinking, and (4) altered level of consciousness. This test can be completed in 2 to 3 minutes with a sensitivity and specificity greater than 90%.[7] Other screening tools include Intensive Care Delirium Screening Checklist (ICDSC), Nursing Delirium Screening Scale, Delirium Detection Score, and Cognitive Test for Delirium.[8] Only CAM-ICU and ICDSC are recommended by Society of Critical Care Medicine (SCCM) guidelines.[5] A recent meta-analysis found the ICDSC to have 74% sensitivity and 81.9% specificity, whereas CAM-ICU was 80% sensitive and 95.9% specific.[9]

Risk factors for delirium in the ICU include a history of alcohol abuse, previous history of neurocognitive disorder (dementia), severity of illness, endotracheal or tracheostomy tube, no visible daylight, isolation, no visitors,[10] and benzodiazepine (BZD) use.[5]

No pharmacologic intervention is recommended for prevention of delirium.[5] If medication is needed, dexmedetomidine is recommended instead of benzodiapines.[5] An analgesia-first strategy should be used in mechanically ventilated patients[5] and adequate pain control must be maintained (discussed later). Early deep sedation in the ICU has been associated with delayed time to extubation; increased ICU length of stay; increased mortality; and, in turn, higher prevalence of delirium in these patients.[11] Nonpharmacologic techniques that have shown benefit include daily awakening trials, daily spontaneous breathing trials, early mobility and exercise,[8] music, reorientation and cognitive stimulation, [12] promoting sleep by controlling light and noise, opening and closing blinds at appropriate times, and decreasing stimuli at night.[5] There are no recommendations regarding mode of mechanical ventilation.[5]

When considering pharmacologic treatment, note that there is no evidence that haloperidol reduces duration of delirium.[5] Although atypical psychotics may reduce duration of delirium in the ICU,[5] exercising caution is advised for patients with a prolonged corrected QT interval. There is growing evidence that olanzapine is a safe and effective drug to treat agitation and delirium.[13]

ASSESSMENT AND MANAGEMENT OF SLEEP AND SLEEP PROBLEMS IN THE CRITICALLY ILL

Sleep disturbance and fatigue are two of the commonest problems in critically ill adults regardless of the type of hospital acute care unit or disease process.[14] Multiple factors can contribute including:

- Preexisting sleep problems
- The specific illness for which the patient is admitted to an ICU
- Therapeutic interventions, including medications, and the ICU environment[14–17]

Sleep disturbances and associated fatigue can cause or worsen diminished physical and cognitive functioning, mood instability, emotional distress, and amplification of concurrent symptoms and can adversely affect recovery and survival.[14,18–20] These symptoms start during illness and persist into recovery.[21] Sleep problems during critical illness include:

- Fragmented sleep.
- Long latency to both sleep onset and rapid eye movement (REM) sleep. Sleep duration is divided over 24 hours, including daytime.
- Increased arousals.
- Increased stage I sleep and reduced stage 2, 3, and 4 and REM sleep.

Sleep disruption is the second most stressful event reported by patients in ICU for cancer. The most distressing is being unable to communicate, as reported by those on mechanical ventilation.[22] It can persist for months after hospital discharge; more than half of ICU survivors (n = 39) continued to experience worse interrupted sleep or altered sleep patterns compared with their prehospital patterns.[23] Older patients may be particularly vulnerable to sleep problems in the ICU. Patients more than 65 years of age make up more than half of all hospital days in the ICU.[24]

The many causes of ICU-related sleep disturbance include preexisting sleep disorders, like obstructive sleep apnea, central sleep apnea, parasomnias, and circadian rhythm sleep disorders. Underlying illness and injury, including respiratory, renal, endocrine, infectious, cardiovascular, and neurologic illnesses, are known contributors.[25]

Many ICU interventions and the ICU environment also play a role because both diagnostic and therapeutic interventions can disrupt sleep in the ICU. Medications can play a significant role in sleep disturbance.[25] Multiple factors can disturb sleep in mechanically ventilated patients, including dyssynchronous breathing and endotracheal discomfort.[21] The ICU environment can also contribute to sleep disruption through factors like excessive nocturnal noise and lighting, diagnostic and therapeutic procedures (eg, blood draws, radiographs), and patient care activities.[21] Disruption in sleep in turn has potential multiple adverse consequences, including altered immune function and neurocognitive deterioration, possibly increasing the risk of delirium and reduced overall quality of life.

Polysomnography is the gold standard for assessment of sleep disturbance but may not be accessible in the ICU setting. Actigraphic monitoring has been shown to be effective.[25] Subjective evaluation methods, including clinician observation and patient self-reports (sleep diaries, visual analogue scales, questionnaires), may be useful.

A 2-pronged pharmacologic approach is recommended. Medications that may disrupt sleep should be reviewed and discontinued. These medications may include agents to support blood pressure, urine or cardiac output, or oxygen delivery. Others may include gastric agents, sedatives and opioids, antidepressants, and anticonvulsants.[16] Judicious use of sleep-promoting agents may be helpful, although before starting any new medicines a thorough review of existing medications should be done. Benzodiazepines may be helpful, although they can alter sleep architecture. Shorter-acting non-BZD agents, such as zaleplon and zolpidem may be preferred. Other potential sleep-enhancing agents, such as trazodone, ramelteon, or melatonin, can also be used.

Recommended nonpharmacologic approaches include cognitive-behavioral interventions including cognitive behavior therapy for insomnia. Complementary approaches include music, massage, relaxation, and therapeutic touch. Environmental modifications include light and noise control and scheduling uninterrupted time for sleep.[25]

ASSESSMENT AND MANAGEMENT OF PAIN IN THE CRITICALLY ILL

Approximately 50% of all critically ill patients experience moderate to severe pain during an ICU stay.[26] Risk factors for pain in critically ill patients in the ICU include (but are not limited to) the primary disease process, invasive procedures (both diagnostic and therapeutic: eg, intravenous lines, biopsies, aspirations, mechanical ventilation), administration of certain medications, mobilization of patients, and tissue damage. Unrecognized and untreated pain can have a significant negative impact on patient outcomes through stress-created imbalances in the levels of catecholamines, cortisol, and other chemicals.[27]

Pain assessment in ICU patients is complicated. Verbal or numerical scales such as the Visual Analogue Scale or the Numeric Rating Scale may be inapplicable if patients have altered mental status, are sedated, or are on mechanical ventilation. Observation of behavioral and physiologic signs alone may not be reliable enough. Most clinical practice guidelines recommend using either the Behavioral Pain Scale or the Critical-care Pain Observation Tool.[28]

Management of pain in the ICU requires adopting a pain-first approach because pain can be a major contributor to agitation and delirium.[28] Nonpharmacologic strategies for pain management include using pain management protocols, optimizing patient-ventilator synchrony, inclusion of family members during all invasive procedures, music and relaxation techniques, hypnosis, and relaxation exercises. The mainstay of pharmacologic treatment of pain in the ICU is opioids, with continuous IV infusion being the preferred route of administration. Commonly used agents include morphine, hydromorphone, fentanyl, and remifentanil. Selection of a specific agent needs to take into account multiple factors, such as presence of any organ dysfunction, expected duration of treatment, changes in volume of distribution, and concomitant medications. Nonopioids such as nonsteroidal antiinflammatory agents, acetaminophen, low-dose ketamine, GABAergic agents, and regional anesthetics, can be used to reduce opioid consumption and opioid-related adverse effects. The use of an analgesic for both pain and sedation, known as analgosedation, has been shown to reduce exposure to sedative medications, the duration of mechanical ventilation and ICU stay, and overall ICU mortality. Opioids are the usual agents used for analgosedation. Prolonged exposure requires careful weaning and continuous pain assessment for optimal outcomes.

ASSESSMENT AND MANAGEMENT OF DEPRESSION AND ANXIETY IN THE CRITICALLY ILL

Critically ill patients frequently develop cognitive and psychiatric symptoms during and after hospital stay, including impaired memory and executive functioning, delirium, acute stress disorder and PTSD, anxiety, and depression.[29] These symptoms may persist for months or years after discharge and may result in inability to return to work and increased health care use.

Acute stress disorder and PTSD resulting from multiple ICU-specific factors, such as endotracheal intubation, inability to speak/communicate, pain, lack of sleep, and physical restraints, is reported in up to 60% of ICU survivors, similar to that documented in survivors of a natural disaster.[30] Acute stress symptoms predict poor cognitive functioning, depression, and excessive alcohol use at 12 months.[29] The Intensive Care Psychological Assessment Tool has recently been studied and validated to detect acute distress in critically ill patients.[31]

ICU patients frequently experience anxiety. It is especially common in mechanically ventilated patients.[29] It can occur in up to 85% of critically ill patients and up to 62% still experience it a year after discharge. Persistent anxiety symptoms and post-ICU depression are associated with poor physical functioning and lower health-related quality of life.[32]

Depression is common among ICU patients, especially those who require prolonged mechanical ventilation.[33] It leads to longer ICU stays, more days on mechanical ventilation, and greater number of days on sedatives.[34] It often persists after discharge.

Pathogenesis of psychiatric illness in critically ill patients is poorly understood. Multiple risk factors are involved, including preexisting illness, acquired brain injury, hypoxia/hypotension/anemia/glycemic impairments, sleep deprivation, and use of medications that disrupt sleep and/or affect mood or cognitive functioning.[29] Older patients, those with chronic illness, women with young children, and the unemployed are especially at risk.

There is scant evidence to support the use of antidepressant or other psychotropic medicines for critically ill patients. Emerging evidence indicates that psychological counseling including psychological support, education, and coping techniques can help reduce symptoms of PTSD, anxiety, and depression.[34,35] Other interventions that have been shown to be helpful include sleep enhancement, sedation minimization (which helps reduce the consolidation of delusional memories and can help reduce the incidence of PTSD), and early physical rehabilitation.

ASSESSMENT AND MANAGEMENT OF ALCOHOL WITHDRAWAL IN THE CRITICALLY ILL

Alcohol withdrawal syndrome (AWS), like other withdrawal syndromes, is a physiologic response to abrupt withdrawal or reduced use of alcohol.[36] In the year 2015, approximately 65.7% of Americans used alcohol,[37] and it is the third leading cause of death in the United States.[36] Diagnosis, management, and rehabilitation vary according to different settings. This article focuses on substance use and withdrawal in critically ill patients admitted in the ICU. Between 16% and 31% of patients admitted to the ICU have a history of alcohol use disorder, putting them at increased risk for AWS,[38] which is associated with a doubling of mortality.[39]

AWSs often complicate the management of critically ill patients in the ICU. Prophylactic assessment and management is advised.[40] A detailed substance abuse history from the patient and the family is critical. Physical examination and biomarkers can provide further clues. Screening tests include urine toxicology for drugs, blood alcohol level, breathalyzer for alcohol, and liver function tests. Common clinical signs include irritability, dysphoria, anxiety, nausea, agitation, tachycardia, and hypertension.

Early detection and prevention of most severe symptoms in high-risk patients is crucial, including those with a history of prior withdrawal, seizures, and delirium tremens (DT), and those consuming alcohol while being treated for alcohol use disorder.[41]

Note that blood alcohol levels at admission do not reliably reflect the likelihood of developing AWS.[42] Symptoms are variable, ranging from no symptoms, to mild symptoms such as insomnia, to more severe features including DTs (**Fig. 1**), which may lead to death. Recommended screening tools include the CAGE questionnaire, Alcohol Use Disorders Identification Test, or the Short Michigan Alcoholism Screening Test as part of the admission assessment.[40,43]

Long-acting BZDs like chlordiazepoxide or diazepam are the mainstay of AWS management. No BZD is superior to another.[44] Once AWS is established, frequent assessments combining Clinical Institute Withdrawal Assessment for Alcohol Scale (CIWA-Ar) with the Riker Sedation-Agitation Scale to titrate BZDs for agitation symptoms are recommended.[42] The Richmond Agitation-Sedation Scale can also be used to titrate BZDs. For BZD-resistant AWS, a trial of rescue medications including phenobarbital, propofol, or dexmedetomidine is recommended.[44]

PSYCHIATRIC ILLNESS AFTER SERIOUS MEDICAL COMPLICATIONS

The interface of mental health and severe medical illnesses is well documented in the literature. There is growing evidence of better health outcomes when medical and psychiatric conditions are comanaged. It is imperative to recognize psychiatric comorbidities (eg, depression, anxiety, PTSD) after serious medical complications, including but not limited to sepsis, acute respiratory distress, myocardial infarction (MI), and cerebrovascular accidents (CVAs), which are frequently managed in ICU settings.[45–49] Many of these patients experience mental health issues as well as physical and cognitive impairments after being discharged from the ICU. This condition has been termed PICS.[50]

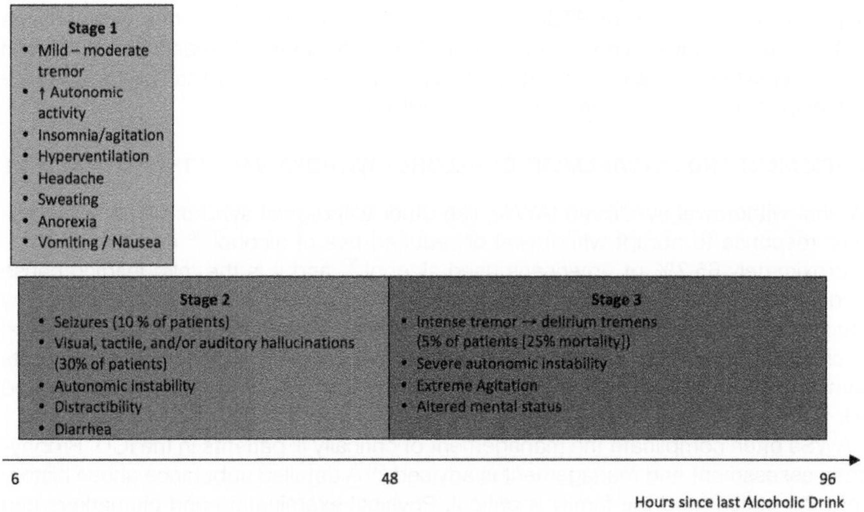

Fig. 1. Stages, signs, and symptoms of alcohol withdrawal.

According to the prospective BRAIN-ICU (Bringing to Light the Risk Factors and Incidence of Neuropsychological Dysfunction in ICU Survivors) study (2013), patients in medical and surgical ICU settings are at high risk for long-term cognitive impairment. Out of the 821 initially enrolled patients, only 6% had cognitive impairment at baseline but delirium developed in 74% during the hospital stay. At 3 months, 40% of patients had global cognition scores that were similar to scores for patients with moderate traumatic brain injury (TBI), and 26% had scores similar to patients with mild Alzheimer disease. At 12 months, 34% and 24% of all patients' scores were similar to those of patients with moderate TBI and mild Alzheimer disease, respectively.[51]

A population-based cohort study in Denmark of critically ill patients published in 2014 concluded that, among survivors of critical illness, new psychiatric diagnoses and psychoactive medication use increased after discharge.[52] Several risk factors have been identified as contributory to developing PICS, including previous neurocognitive impairment, duration of delirium, sepsis, acute respiratory distress, cardiac arrest, hypotension, hypoglycemia, and prolonged mechanical ventilation.[52–57] Preexisting psychiatric disorders are also considered risk factors for PICS.[45,48,58] PICS is essentially a constellation of neuropsychosomatic symptoms with the most common psychiatric features being depression, anxiety, and PTSD, which frequently lead to lower quality of life.[52,59]

An interdisciplinary team approach (the primary medical or surgical team as well as consultants from psychiatry and physical rehabilitation) can provide relevant information to identify PICS and coordinate care in order to accomplish better clinical outcomes.[60] The Mini Mental Status Examination is widely used in different clinical settings but the Montreal Cognitive Assessment seems to provide better sensitivity overall.[61] There are several screening tools for depression, anxiety, and PTSD that can be used in hospital settings, including Patient Health Questionnaire (PHQ-2)/PHQ-9, PCL-S (Post-Traumatic Stress Disorder [PTSD] Check-list), Beck or Zung Depression and Anxiety Inventories/Scales, PTSS-10 (Post-Traumatic Stress Syndrome Questionnaire), and the Hospital Anxiety and Depression Scale. Psychiatrists or psychologists can provide assistance with the initial assessment.[62] Some studies recommend an integrated, interdisciplinary strategy to decrease the risk of PICS, known as the ABCDE (awakening and breathing coordination with daily sedative interruption and ventilator liberation practices, effective management of delirium, and early ambulation in the ICU when feasible) bundle for ventilated patients.[63,64] Other studies highlight the benefits of using ICU diaries in order to fill patients' memory gaps, minimizing potential PTSD symptoms.[65]

Treatment should continue on an outpatient basis because some PICS symptoms persist over time. An integrated, interdisciplinary treatment approach (mental health, physical and occupational therapy, medical follow-up care) can improve the quality of life of these patients.[66,67] According to a systematic review and meta-analysis published in 2015, follow-up consultations can reduce symptoms of PTSD at 3 to 6 months after ICU discharge.[68]

In addition, this article briefly reviews some common medical conditions encountered in the ICU setting that are frequently comorbid with psychiatric illness.

TRAUMATIC BRAIN INJURY

TBI can present with a constellation of neuropsychosomatic symptoms called postconcussion syndrome. Many patients with TBI experience a wide variety of psychiatric symptoms, including but not limited to irritability, change in personality, depression, anxiety, poor impulse control, and decreased concentration.

According to a study conducted by US Army Medical Research, TBI was strongly associated with PTSD among soldiers deployed to Iraq.[69] Another study published in 2011 concluded that stressful events before head injury could also predict poorer outcomes after TBI, emphasizing the importance of screening and offering appropriate psychotherapeutic and psychopharmacologic treatments.[70,71]

CEREBROVASCULAR ACCIDENT

A systemic review and meta-analysis published in 2013 found the prevalence of depression after CVA to be close to 30%. Several risk factors were identified, including disability, preexisting depressive disorder, cognitive impairment, stroke severity, and anxiety. This study also emphasized the need for appropriate identification and treatment of psychiatric illness because it is linked to quality of life as well as morbidity and mortality in these patients.[72]

A cohort study from Denmark found that patients with stroke had a higher incidence of depression during the first 3 months after hospitalization. Depressed patients with stroke seem to have a higher mortality risk so it is imperative for clinicians to identify and treat the depression.[73] There is growing evidence that psychotherapy and/or antidepressants are helpful treatment interventions.[74–77]

MYOCARDIAL INFARCTION AND CORONARY ARTERY DISEASE

Approximately 1 out of 6 patients with MI meets criteria for major depressive disorder, which by itself is considered an independent risk factor for higher cardiac mortality.[77,78] The American Heart Association recommends screening for depression in patients with coronary artery disease so timely recognition can lead to appropriate treatment, which in turn is likely to improve compliance with medical treatment and provide better clinical outcomes.[79,80] A Danish population-based case-control study concluded that the risk of suicide was high among patients with MI, emphasizing again the importance of screening and intervention.[81] The treatment of depression in this population is similar to other clinical scenarios but tricyclic antidepressants should be avoided because of possible adverse effects like orthostatic hypotension, prolonged QT interval, and arrhythmias.[78] The US Food and Drug Administration has also recently advised against the use of citalopram in this population despite proven efficacy because of concerns about arrhythmia.[82] The large SADHEART (Sertraline Antidepressant Heart Attack Randomized Trial) study concluded that sertraline was a safe and effective selective serotonin reuptake inhibitor for recurrent major depression in patients with recent MI.[83]

A single-blind randomized clinical trial published in 2014 found that collaborative care models for mental health disorders in high-risk cardiac patients provide improvement in mental health–related quality of life.[84]

ORGAN TRANSPLANT AND CANCER

Depression and anxiety are common comorbidities of chronic medical conditions, especially when dealing with the need for an organ donation/transplant to sustain life. A retrospective observational study based on the US Renal Data System found that depression was associated with several identifiable factors and a 2-fold greater risk of graft failure and death with a functioning graft.[85] Another cohort study found that patients with end-stage renal disease are more likely to commit suicide than the general population.[86] The prevalence of depression and anxiety are high in patients with cancer. An observational cohort study found that nearly 50% of women with early breast cancer had depression, anxiety, or both in the year after diagnosis; 25% in the second, third, and fourth years; and 15% in the fifth year.[87] The National Comprehensive Cancer Network has recommended routine screening of all patients with cancer for psychological distress.[88] The American Society of Clinical Oncology also recommends screening for depression and anxiety in all patients with cancer so treatment can be offered because it correlates with the quality of life as well as morbidity and mortality.[89]

Adjustment disorder and major depressive disorder are the most prevalent psychiatric conditions associated with cancer.[90,91] A Swedish cohort study concluded that young patients with cancer are at substantially increased risk of suicidal behavior during the first year and another, larger study found that patients recently diagnosed with cancer had higher risk of suicide and death from cardiovascular complications.[92,93]

SUMMARY

Critically ill patients can develop a host of psychiatric and behavioral problems during and after their ICU stay. These illnesses can delay recovery from medical illness and negatively affect quality of life after discharge. Common psychiatric illnesses during ICU stay include delirium, depression, anxiety and PTSD, sleep problems, and pain. Many acute medical illnesses can also give rise to psychiatric complications, including MI and coronary artery disease, cerebrovascular illnesses, TBI, and cancer. Appropriate assessment and timely treatment, both during the ICU stay and after discharge, ensures optimal recovery and a high quality of life post-ICU.

ACKNOWLEDGMENTS

Dr A.M. Hashmi would like to thank Dr. Ali Ahsan Ali, MD, Resident Psychiatrist, Icahn School of Medicine at Mount Sinai (Elmhurst), Queens, New York, for his help in preparing this article and for designing the infographic (**Fig. 1**).

REFERENCES

1. Society of Critical Care Medicine. Critical care statistics in the United States. Available at: http://sccmwww.sccm.org/Documents/WebStatisticsPamphletFinalJune06.pdf. Accessed November 9, 2016.
2. Chahraoui K, Laurent A, Bioy A, et al. Psychological experience of patients 3 months after a stay in the intensive care unit: a descriptive and qualitative study. J Crit Care 2015;30(3):599–605.
3. Denehy L, Elliott D. Strategies for post ICU rehabilitation. Curr Opin Crit Care 2012;18(5):503–8.
4. Cavallazzi R, Saad M, Marik PE. Delirium in the ICU: an overview. Ann Intensive Care 2012;2:49.
5. Barr J, Fraser GL, Puntillo K, et al. Clinical practice guidelines for the management of pain, agitation, and delirium in adult patients in the intensive care unit. Crit Care Med 2013;41(1):263–306.
6. Girard TD, Pandharipande PP, Ely EW. Delirium in the intensive care unit. Crit Care 2008;12(Suppl 3):S3.
7. Ely EW, Margolin R, Francis J, et al. Evaluation of delirium in critically ill patients: validation of the confusion assessment method for the intensive care unit (CAM-ICU). Crit Care Med 2001;29(7):1370–9.
8. Brummel NE, Vasilevskis EE, Han JH, et al. Implementing delirium screening in the intensive care unit: secrets to success. Crit Care Med 2013;41(9):2196–208.

9. Gusmao-Flores D, Salluh JI, Chalhub RA, et al. The confusion assessment method for the intensive care unit (CAM-ICU) and intensive care delirium screening checklist (ICDSC) for the diagnosis of delirium: a systematic review and meta-analysis of clinical studies. Crit Care 2012;16(4):R115.
10. Van Rompaey B, Elseviers MM, Schuurmans MJ, et al. Risk factors for delirium in intensive care patients: a prospective cohort study. Crit Care 2009;13(3):R77.
11. Shehabi Y, Bellomo R, Reade MC, et al. Early intensive care sedation predicts long-term mortality in ventilated critically ill patients. Am J Respir Crit Care Med 2012;186(8):724–31.
12. Rivosecchi RM, Kane-Gill SL, Svec S, et al. The implementation of a nonpharmacological protocol to prevent intensive care delirium. J Crit Care 2016;31(1):206–11.
13. Chan EW, Taylor DM, Knott JC, et al. Intravenous droperidol or olanzapine as an adjunct to midazolam for the acutely agitated patient: a multicenter, randomized, double-blind, placebo-controlled clinical trial. Ann Emerg Med 2013;61(1):72–81.
14. Friese RS. Sleep and recovery from critical illness and injury: a review of theory, current practice, and future directions. Crit Care Med 2008;36(3):697–705.
15. Bosma KJ, Ranieri VM. Filtering out the noise: evaluating the impact of noise and sound reduction strategies on sleep quality for ICU patients. Crit Care 2009;13(3):151.
16. Bourne RS, Mills GH. Sleep disruption in critically ill patients–pharmacological considerations. Anaesthesia 2004;59(4):374–84.
17. Drouot X, Cabello B, d'Ortho MP, et al. Sleep in the intensive care unit. Sleep Med Rev 2008;12(5):391–403.
18. Kadiev S, Ali N. Sleep in the intensive care unit. Sleep Med Clin 2008;3(4):569–80.
19. Dew MA, Hoch CC, Buysse DJ, et al. Healthy older adults' sleep predicts all-cause mortality at 4 to 19 years of follow-up. Psychosom Med 2003;65(1):63–73.
20. Eddleston JM, White P, Guthrie E. Survival, morbidity, and quality of life after discharge from intensive care. Crit Care Med 2000;28(7):2293–9.
21. Weinhouse GL, Schwab RJ. Sleep in the critically ill patient. Sleep 2006;29(5):707–16.
22. Nelson JE, Meier DE, Oei EJ, et al. Self-reported symptom experience of critically ill cancer patients receiving intensive care. Crit Care Med 2001;29(2):277–82.
23. Kelly MA, McKinley S. Patients' recovery after critical illness at early follow-up. J Clin Nurs 2010;19(5–6):691–700.
24. Angus DC, Kelley MA, Schmitz RJ, et al. Caring for the critically ill patient. Current and projected workforce requirements for care of the critically ill and patients with pulmonary disease: can we meet the requirements of an aging population? JAMA 2000;284(21):2762–70.
25. Matthews EE. Sleep disturbances and fatigue in critically ill patients. AACN Adv Crit Care 2011;22(3):204–24.
26. Chanques G, Sebbane M, Barbotte E, et al. A prospective study of pain at rest: incidence and characteristics of an unrecognized symptom in surgical and trauma versus medical intensive care unit patients. Anesthesiology 2007;107(5):858–60.
27. Dunwoody CJ, Krenzischek DA, Pasero C, et al. Assessment, physiological monitoring, and consequences of inadequately treated acute pain. J Perianesth Nurs 2008;23(1 Suppl):S15–27.
28. Reardon DP, Anger KE, Szumita PM. Pathophysiology, assessment, and management of pain in critically ill adults. Am J Health Syst Pharm 2015;72(18):1531–43.

29. Karnatovskaia LV, Johnson MM, Benzo RP, et al. The spectrum of psychocognitive morbidity in the critically ill: a review of the literature and call for improvement. J Crit Care 2015;30(1):130–7.
30. Long AC, Kross EK, Davydow DS, et al. Posttraumatic stress disorder among survivors of critical illness: creation of a conceptual model addressing identification, prevention, and management. Intensive Care Med 2014;40(6):820–9.
31. Wade DM, Hankins M, Smyth DA, et al. Detecting acute distress and risk of future psychological morbidity in critically ill patients: validation of the intensive care psychological assessment tool. Crit Care 2014;18(5):519.
32. Stevenson JE, Colantuoni E, Bienvenu OJ, et al. General anxiety symptoms after acute lung injury: predictors and correlates. J Psychosom Res 2013;75(3): 287–93.
33. Jubran A, Lawm G, Kelly J, et al. Depressive disorders during weaning from prolonged mechanical ventilation. Intensive Care Med 2010;36(5):828–35.
34. Jackson JC, Mitchell N, Hopkins RO. Cognitive functioning, mental health, and quality of life in ICU survivors: an overview. Anesthesiol Clin 2011;29(4):751–64.
35. Peris A, Bonizzoli M, Iozzelli D, et al. Early intra-intensive care unit psychological intervention promotes recovery from posttraumatic stress disorders, anxiety and depression symptoms in critically ill patients. Crit Care 2011;15(2):418.
36. Tetrault JM, O'Connor PG. Substance abuse and withdrawal in the critical care setting. Crit Care Clin 2008;24(4):767–88.
37. Center for Behavioral Health Statistics and Quality (2016). 2015 National survey on drug use and health: detailed tables. Available at: http://www.samhsa.gov/data/sites/default/files/NSDUH-DetTabs-2015/NSDUH-DetTabs-2015/NSDUH-DetTabs-2015.pdf. Accessed November 27, 2016.
38. Dixit D, Endicott J, Burry L, et al. Management of acute alcohol withdrawal syndrome in critically ill patients. Pharmacotherapy 2016;36(7):797–822.
39. Moss M, Burnham EL. Alcohol abuse in the critically ill patient. Lancet 2006; 368(9554):2231–42.
40. Jenkins DH. Substance abuse and withdrawal in the intensive care unit. Contemporary issues. Surg Clin North Am 2000;80(3):1033–53.
41. Awissi DK, Lebrun G, Fagnan M, et al. Alcohol, nicotine, and iatrogenic withdrawals in the ICU. Crit Care Med 2013;41(9 Suppl 1):S57–68.
42. Carlson RW, Kumar NN, Wong-Mckinstry E, et al. Alcohol withdrawal syndrome. Crit Care Clin 2012;28(4):549–85.
43. Selzer ML, Vinokur A, van Rooijen L. A self-administered Short Michigan Alcoholism Screening Test (SMAST). J Stud Alcohol 1975;36(1):117–26.
44. Perry EC. Inpatient management of acute alcohol withdrawal syndrome. CNS Drugs 2014;28(5):401–10.
45. Desai SV, Law TJ, Needham DM. Long-term complications of critical care. Crit Care Med 2011;39(2):371–9.
46. Bienvenu OJ, Williams JB, Yang A, et al. Posttraumatic stress disorder in survivors of acute lung injury: evaluating the impact of event scale-revised. Chest 2013;144(1):24–31.
47. Bienvenu OJ, Colantuoni E, Mendez-Tellez PA, et al. Depressive symptoms and impaired physical function after acute lung injury: a 2-year longitudinal study. Am J Respir Crit Care Med 2012;185(8):900.
48. Patel MB, Jackson JC, Morandi A, et al. Incidence and risk factors for intensive care unit-related post-traumatic stress disorder in veterans and civilians. Am J Respir Crit Care Med 2016;193(12):1373–81.

49. Yende S, Iwashyna TJ, Angus DC. Interplay between sepsis and chronic health. Trends Mol Med 2014;20(4):234–8.
50. Needham DM, Davidson J, Cohen H, et al. Improving long-term outcomes after discharge from intensive care unit: report from a stakeholders' conference. Crit Care Med 2012;40(2):502–9.
51. Pandharipande PP, Girard TD, Jackson JC, et al. Long-term cognitive impairment after critical illness. N Engl J Med 2013;369(14):1306–16.
52. Wunsch H, Christiansen CF, Johansen MB, et al. Psychiatric diagnoses and psychoactive medication use among nonsurgical critically ill patients receiving mechanical ventilation. JAMA 2014;311(11):1133–42.
53. Hopkins RO, Weaver LK, Collingridge D, et al. Two-year cognitive, emotional, and quality-of-life outcomes in acute respiratory distress syndrome. Am J Respir Crit Care Med 2005;171(4):340–7.
54. Mikkelsen ME, Shull WH, Biester RC, et al. Cognitive, mood and quality of life impairments in a select population of ARDS survivors. Respirology 2009;14(1): 76–82.
55. Yaffe K, Weston A, Graff-Radford NR, et al. Association of plasma beta-amyloid level and cognitive reserve with subsequent cognitive decline. JAMA 2011; 305(3):261–6.
56. Iwashyna TJ, Ely EW, Smith DM, et al. Long-term cognitive impairment and functional disability among survivors of severe sepsis. JAMA 2010;304(16):1787–94.
57. Girard TD, Jackson JC, Pandharipande PP, et al. Delirium as a predictor of long-term cognitive impairment in survivors of critical illness. Crit Care Med 2010; 38(7):1513–20.
58. Bienvenu OJ, Gellar J, Althouse BM, et al. Post-traumatic stress disorder symptoms after acute lung injury: a 2-year prospective longitudinal study. Psychol Med 2013;43(12):2657–71.
59. Davydow DS, Desai SV, Needham DM, et al. Psychiatric morbidity in survivors of the acute respiratory distress syndrome: a systematic review. Psychosom Med 2008;70(4):512–9.
60. Jackson JC, Ely EW, Morey MC, et al. Cognitive and physical rehabilitation of intensive care unit survivors: results of the RETURN randomized controlled pilot investigation. Crit Care Med 2012;40(4):1088–97.
61. Nasreddine ZS, Phillips NA, Bédirian V, et al. The Montreal Cognitive Assessment, MoCA: a brief screening tool for mild cognitive impairment. J Am Geriatr Soc 2005;53(4):695–9.
62. Jackson JC, Pandharipande PP, Girard TD, et al. Depression, post-traumatic stress disorder, and functional disability in survivors of critical illness in the BRAIN-ICU study: a longitudinal cohort study. Lancet Respir Med 2014;2(5): 369–79.
63. Morandi A, Brummel NE, Ely EW. Sedation, delirium and mechanical ventilation: the 'ABCDE' approach. Curr Opin Crit Care 2011;17(1):43–9.
64. Girard TD, Kress JP, Fuchs BD, et al. Efficacy and safety of a paired sedation and ventilator weaning protocol for mechanically ventilated patients in intensive care (Awakening and Breathing Controlled trial): a randomized controlled trial. Lancet 2008;371(9607):126–34.
65. Mehlhorn J, Freytag A, Schmidt K, et al. Rehabilitation interventions for postintensive care syndrome: a systematic review. Crit Care Med 2014;42(5):1263–71.
66. Hopkins RO, Suchyta MR, Farrer TJ, et al. Improving post-intensive care unit neuropsychiatric outcomes: understanding cognitive effects of physical activity. Am J Respir Crit Care Med 2012;186(12):1220–8.

67. Jones C, Skirrow P, Griffiths RD, et al. Rehabilitation after critical illness: a randomized, controlled trial. Crit Care Med 2003;31(10):2456–61.
68. Jensen JF, Thomsen T, Overgaard D, et al. Impact of follow-up consultations for ICU survivors on post-ICU syndrome: a systematic review and meta-analysis. Intensive Care Med 2015;41(5):763–75.
69. Hoge CW, McGurk D, Thomas JL, et al. Mild traumatic brain injury in U.S. soldiers returning from Iraq. N Engl J Med 2008;358(5):453–63.
70. Van Veldhoven LM, Sander AM, Struchen MA, et al. Predictive ability of preinjury stressful life events and post-traumatic stress symptoms for outcomes following mild traumatic brain injury: analysis in a prospective emergency room sample. J Neurol Neurosurg Psychiatry 2011;82(7):782–7.
71. Fann JR, Uomoto JM, Katon WJ. Cognitive improvement with treatment of depression following mild traumatic brain injury. Psychosomatics 2001;42(1): 48–54.
72. Ayerbe L, Ayis S, Wolfe CD, et al. Natural history, predictors and outcomes of depression after stroke: systematic review and meta-analysis. Br J Psychiatry 2013;202(1):14–21.
73. Jørgensen TS, Wium-Andersen IK, Wium-Andersen MK, et al. Incidence of depression after stroke, and associated risk factors and mortality outcomes, in a large cohort of Danish patients. JAMA Psychiatry 2016;73(10):1032–40.
74. Hackett ML, Anderson CS, House A, et al. Interventions for treating depression after stroke. Cochrane Database Syst Rev 2008;(4):CD003437.
75. Williams LS, Kroenke K, Bakas T, et al. Care management of poststroke depression: a randomized, controlled trial. Stroke 2007;38(3):998–1003.
76. Mitchell PH, Veith RC, Becker KJ, et al. Brief psychosocial-behavioral intervention with antidepressant reduces poststroke depression significantly more than usual care with antidepressant: living well with stroke: randomized, controlled trial. Stroke 2009;40(9):3073–8.
77. Ziegelstein RC. Depression in patients recovering from a myocardial infarction. JAMA 2001;286(13):1621–7.
78. Jiang W, Davidson JR. Antidepressant therapy in patients with ischemic heart disease. Am Heart J 2005;150(5):871–81.
79. Colquhoun DM, Bunker SJ, Clarke DM, et al. Screening, referral and treatment for depression in patients with coronary heart disease. Med J Aust 2013;198(9): 483–4.
80. Lichtman JH, Bigger JT Jr, Blumenthal JA, et al. Depression and coronary heart disease: recommendations for screening, referral, and treatment: a science advisory from the American Heart Association Prevention Committee of the Council on Cardiovascular Nursing, Council on Clinical Cardiology, Council on Epidemiology and Prevention, and Interdisciplinary Council on Quality Of Care and Outcomes Research: endorsed by the American Psychiatric Association. Circulation 2008;118(17):1768–75.
81. Larsen KK, Agerbo E, Christensen B, et al. Myocardial infarction and risk of suicide: a population-based case-control study. Circulation 2010;122(23):2388–93.
82. US Food and Drug Administration. FDA drug safety communication: revised recommendations for Celexa (citalopram hydrobromide) related to a potential risk of abnormal heart rhythms with high doses. Available at: http://www.fda.gov/Drugs/DrugSafety/ucm297391.htm. Accessed November 29, 2016.
83. Glassman AH, O'Connor CM, Califf RM, et al. Sertraline treatment of major depression in patients with acute MI or unstable angina. JAMA 2002;288(14):1720.

84. Huffman JC, Mastromauro CA, Beach SR, et al. Collaborative care for depression and anxiety disorders in patients with recent cardiac events: the Management of Sadness and Anxiety in Cardiology (MOSAIC) randomized clinical trial. JAMA Intern Med 2014;174(8):1419.
85. Dobbels F, Skeans MA, Snyder JJ, et al. Depressive disorder in renal transplantation: an analysis of Medicare claims. Am J Kidney Dis 2008;51(5):819–28.
86. Kurella M, Kimmel PL, Young BS, et al. Suicide in the United States end-stage renal disease program. J Am Soc Nephrol 2005;16(3):774–81.
87. Burgess C, Cornelius V, Love S, et al. Depression and anxiety in women with early breast cancer: five year observational cohort study. BMJ 2005;330(7493):702.
88. National Comprehensive Cancer Network. Distress management. Clinical practice guidelines. J Natl Compr Canc Netw 2003;1(3):344–74.
89. Andersen BL, DeRubeis RJ, Berman BS, et al. American Society of Clinical Oncology. Screening, assessment, and care of anxiety and depressive symptoms in adults with cancer: an American Society of Clinical Oncology guideline adaptation. J Clin Oncol 2014;32(15):1605–19.
90. Akechi T, Okuyama T, Sugawara Y, et al. Major depression, adjustment disorders, and post-traumatic stress disorder in terminally ill cancer patients: associated and predictive factors. J Clin Oncol 2004;22(10):1957–65.
91. Walker J, Hansen CH, Martin P, et al. Prevalence, associations, and adequacy of treatment of major depression inpatients with cancer: a cross-sectional analysis of routinely collected clinical data. Lancet Psychiatry 2014;1(5):343–50.
92. Lu D, Fall K, Sparén P, et al. Suicide and suicide attempt after a cancer diagnosis among young individuals. Ann Oncol 2013;24(12):3112–7.
93. Fang F, Fall K, Mittleman MA, et al. Suicide and cardiovascular death after a cancer diagnosis. N Engl J Med 2012;366(14):1310–8.

Drugs of Abuse

Evaristo Akerele, MD, MPH, DFAPA*, Tolu Olupona, MD

KEYWORDS

• Heroin • Opioids • Cocaine • Designer drugs • Marijuana • Intoxication • Overdose

KEY POINTS

- The risk of death from opioid overdose is increasing. Timely intervention with opioid antagonists saves lives. The general public needs more education on the use of naloxone kits.
- Cocaine induced chest pain occurs more frequently than expected.
- Always consider designer drugs. Think outside the box for drug intoxication/withdrawal symptoms.
- Marijuana has significant adverse effects. However, when properly harnessed, it may be useful for medical intervention.

HEROIN AND PRESCRIPTION OPIOIDS

Heroin and prescription opioid pain relievers (fentanyl, oxycodone, acetaminophen with hydrocodone bitartrate [Vicodin], acetaminophen with oxycodone hydrochloride [Percocet], and codeine) both belong to a class of drugs known as opioids. Their effects are typically mediated by specific subtypes of opioid receptors (mu, delta, and kappa) that are activated by endogenous, opioids (endorphins, encephalin). Heroin is an opioid drug that is synthesized from morphine, a naturally occurring substance extracted from the seed pod of the Asian opium poppy plant. Heroin usually appears as a white or brown powder or as a black sticky substance, known as "black tar heroin." In 2011, 4.2 million Americans aged 12 or older (or 1.6%) had used heroin at least once in their lives. It is estimated that about 23% of individuals who use heroin become dependent on it. However, the demographics of heroin abusers are changing.

In the 1960s, heroin was used predominantly by young men from minority groups living in urban areas (82.8%; mean age at first opioid use, 16.5 years) whose first opioid of abuse was heroin (80%). The demographic of opioid users has shifted with the epidemic of prescription opioid abuse. The individuals using opioids are

Department of Psychiatry and Behavioral Health, Interfaith Medical Center, 1545 Atlantic Avenue, Brooklyn, NY 11213, USA
* Corresponding author.
E-mail address: eakerele@interfaithmedical.org

Psychiatr Clin N Am 40 (2017) 501–517
http://dx.doi.org/10.1016/j.psc.2017.05.006

0193-953X/17/© 2017 Elsevier Inc. All rights reserved.

Abbreviations	
MAT	Medication-assisted treatment
MDPV	Methylenedioxypyrovalerone
THC	Delta-9-tetrahydrocannabinol

somewhat older (mean age at first opioid use, 22.9 years), less minority, more rural/suburban, with few gender differences among those who were introduced to opioids through prescription drugs. Whites and nonwhites were equally represented in those initiating use before the 1980s, but nearly 90% of respondents who began use in the last decade were white.[1]

Racial distribution of respondents is expressed as percentage of the total sample of heroin users. Data are plotted as a function of decade in which respondents initiated their opioid abuse.[1] As a result of the data, several studies have been undertaken to clarify the path to heroin use disorder.

A recent study of heroin users in the Chicago metropolitan area identified 3 main paths to heroin addiction: prescription opioid abuse to heroin use, cocaine use to heroin use (to "come down"), and polydrug use (ie, use of multiple substances) to heroin use. Polydrug use to heroin was the most common path in this study.[2] The estimated 4% subset of people who transition from prescription opioid abuse to heroin use[3] may be predisposed to polydrug use, and the transition may represent a natural progression for them.

As the government successfully implemented initiatives to decrease availability of prescription opioid drugs, overdose deaths in states with the most aggressive policies declined, since 2010, overdose deaths related to heroin have started to increase (as detailed in the testimony from the US Centers for Disease Control and Prevention). As a result, there was some concern that the increase in heroin-related overdoses may be an unintended consequence of reducing the availability of prescription opioids. Research data suggest that prescription opioid use is a risk factor for heroin use. The incidence of heroin initiation is 19 times higher among those who report prior nonmedical pain reliever use than among those who do not (0.39% vs 0.02%).[1,3]

However, heroin use is rare in prescription drug users. According to the National Survey on Drug Use and Health, less than 4% of people who had used prescription painkillers nonmedically started using heroin within 5 years of their initiation of nonmedical use of pain medication.[4]

Because heroin is often injected, the increase in use also has implications for human immunodeficiency virus, hepatitis C virus (HCV), and other injection-related illnesses. Recent studies suggest that having used opioid pain relievers before transitioning to heroin injection is a common trajectory for young injection drug users with HCV infection.[5] A study of new HCV infections in Massachusetts found that 95% of interview respondents used prescription opioids before initiating heroin.[6]

The number of individuals being treated for prescription opioids has increased from 360,000 in 2002, representing 10.3% of the total treatment population, to 772,000 (18.6%) in 2014. Similarly for heroin treatment the number has increased from 277,000 in 2002 to 618,000 in 2014.[7] Furthermore, the number of individuals with heroin "dependence or abuse" more than doubled from 2002 to 2014, increasing from about 214,000 to 586,000.[8]

Opioid Intoxication

Signs and symptoms

Signs include small, or constricted, pupils, slowed breathing or absent breathing, extreme fatigue, changes in heart rate, and a loss of alertness. Symptoms of an opioid overdose include excessive sleepiness, not awakening when spoken to in a loud voice or when the middle of the chest is rubbed firmly, breathing either stops or is shallow, with constricted pupils.

Opioid Withdrawal

Signs and symptoms

Signs and symptoms of opioid withdrawal include lacrimation, perspiration, piloerection, restlessness, rhinorrhea, yawning, irritability, fatigue, headache, abdominal cramps, broken sleep, hot and cold flashes, mydriasis, nausea and vomiting, muscle and bone pain, muscle spasm, and low-grade fever. These symptoms eventually peak (eg, around 36–72 hours for short-acting opioids like heroin) and then patient gets better with or without treatment ("cold turkey").

Treatment

Treatment of overdose

Naloxone injection is packaged as a solution to be injected intravenously, intramuscularly, or subcutaneously. It is also packaged as a prefilled autoinjection device containing a solution to be injected intramuscularly or subcutaneously. It is usually given as needed to treat opiate overdoses.

Naloxone injection may not reverse the effects of certain opiates such as buprenorphine (Belbuca, Buprenex, Butrans) and pentazocine (Talwin) and may require additional naloxone doses. In case of emergency, even a person who has not been trained to inject naloxone should still try to inject the medication. The first dose of naloxone should be into the muscle or under the skin of the thigh. The medication may be injected through the clothing if necessary in an emergency. After injecting naloxone, should the symptoms return additional injections may be given every 2 to 3 minutes until additional medical assistance is available. Each prefilled automatic injection device (0.4 mg) should be used only once. Narcan 4 mg (naloxone HCL) nasal spray may also be used in opioid overdose.

Treatment for Chronic Use

Three types of medications are used: (1) agonists, which activate opioid receptors, (2) partial agonists, which also activate opioid receptors but produce a smaller response, and (3) antagonists, which block the receptor and interfere with the rewarding effects of opioids. The choice of medication used is based on a patient's specific medical needs and other factors. Effective medications include: methadone, buprenorphine and naltrexone.[9]

Summary

The primary solution to the opioid epidemic and its dire consequences is prevention. However, prevention is only the first step; it is imperative that we provide evidence-based treatments for these individuals. Treatment should include access to the medication-assisted treatment (MAT). Currently, far fewer people receive MAT than could potentially benefit from it. Nearly all US states have higher rates of opioid abuse and dependence than their buprenorphine treatment capacity,[10] and fewer than 1 million of the 2.5 million Americans who abused or were dependent on opioids in 2012 received MAT.[11] Removing barriers to MAT access and utilization is a top priority for the US Department of Health and Human Services and is a key objective of the Secretary's Opioid Initiative to combat opioid drug-related dependence and overdose.

COCAINE

The term "coca" may refer to any of the 4 cultivated plants that belong to the family Erythroxylaceae *Erythroxylon coca*, which is native to western South America. Raw coca leaves, chewed or consumed as tea or "mate de coca," are rich in nutritional properties. Leaves of this plant have been chewed by Amerindian peoples for thousands of years, making coca one of the most venerable of "lifestyle drugs,"[12] but aboriginal chewing or drinking of coca tea does not produce the euphoria experienced with cocaine. In the early 1900s, purified cocaine was the main active ingredient in many tonics and elixirs developed to treat a wide variety of illnesses and was even an ingredient in the early formulations of Coca-Cola. Before the development of synthetic local anesthetic, surgeons used cocaine to block pain.[13] Today cocaine is a schedule II drug.[14]

Cocaine plays a significant role in drug-related emergency room visits. Data from the 2011 Drug Abuse Warning Network report showed that cocaine was involved in 505,224 of the nearly 1.3 million visits to emergency departments for drug misuse or abuse. This translates to more than 1 in 3 drug misuse or abuse-related emergency department visits (40%) that involved cocaine.[15] Rates for cocaine were highest in individuals ages 35 to 44; rates for heroin were highest among individuals ages 21 to 24; stimulant use was highest among those 25 to 29; and marijuana use was highest for those ages 18 to 20.

Cocaine has also become one of the primary drugs involved in drug-related emergency room deaths. According to the US Centers for Disease Control and Prevention, among the deaths attributed to drug overdose, cocaine, heroin, and opioid painkillers are the most common substances involved.

There are 2 chemical forms of cocaine that are abused: the water-soluble hydrochloride salt and the water-insoluble cocaine base, or freebase. Cocaine is generally sold on the street as a fine, white, crystalline powder; it is also known as "coke," "C," "snow," "flake," or "blow." Street dealers generally dilute it with inert substances such as cornstarch, talcum powder, or sugar, or with active drugs such as procaine (a chemically related local anesthetic) or amphetamine.[16] Some users combine cocaine with heroin in what is termed a "speedball."

When abused, the water-soluble hydrochloride salt, or powdered form of cocaine, can be injected or snorted. The water-insoluble cocaine base, or freebase form of cocaine, is processed with ammonia or sodium bicarbonate and water, then heated to remove the hydrochloride to produce a smokable substance. The freebase cocaine is referred to as "crack" in the streets owing to the crackling sound heard when the mixture is smoked.

The principal routes of cocaine administration are oral, intranasal, inhalation, and intravenous. Snorting is the process of inhaling cocaine powder through the nose, where it is absorbed into the bloodstream through the nasal tissues. The drug also can be rubbed onto mucous tissues. Smoking involves inhaling cocaine vapor or smoke into the lungs, where absorption into the bloodstream is as rapid as it is by injection. Injecting the drug directly into the bloodstream, heightens the intensity of the drug's effects.

A common pharmacokinetic-based issue is the increased risk when cocaine is taken in combination with alcohol. In most users, it produces more euphoria and possesses a longer duration of action than cocaine. Data suggest that it may be more cardiotoxic than cocaine and is associated with a greater risk of sudden death than with cocaine alone.[17,18]

Intoxication

Cocaine increases alertness, feelings of well-being and euphoria, energy and motor activity, and feelings of competence and sexuality. Its effects appear almost immediately after a single dose and disappear within a few minutes or an hour. Taken in small amounts, cocaine usually makes the user feel euphoric, energetic, talkative, and mentally alert, especially to the sensations of sight, sound, and touch. It can also temporarily decrease the need for food and sleep.

The duration of cocaine's euphoric effects depends on the route of administration. The faster the drug is absorbed, the more intense the resulting high, but also the shorter the duration. The high from snorting is relatively slow to arrive, but it may last 15 to 30 minutes; in contrast, the effects from smoking are more immediate but may last only 5 to 10 minutes. The short-term physiologic effects of cocaine use include constricted blood vessels and dilated pupils, and increased body temperature, heart rate, and blood pressure. Large amounts of cocaine may intensify the user's high, but can also lead to bizarre, erratic, and violent behavior. Some cocaine users report feelings of restlessness, irritability, anxiety, panic, and paranoia. Users may also experience tremors, vertigo, and muscle twitches.[14]

Overdose

The signs and symptoms of cocaine overdose are related to the psychological and stimulant effects of the drug. The use of cocaine causes tachyarrhythmia and a marked elevation of blood pressure, which can be life threatening. This increase in blood pressure can lead to death from respiratory failure, stroke, cerebral hemorrhage, or heart failure. Cocaine is also highly pyrogenic, because the stimulation and increased muscular activity cause greater heat production. Heat loss is inhibited by the intense vasoconstriction. Cocaine-induced hyperthermia may cause muscle cell destruction and myoglobinuria, resulting in renal failure. The classic signs are hypertension, tachycardia, and tachypnea. This occurs with agitation, confusion, irritability, sweating, and hyperthermia. Sometimes seizures may occur.

Cocaine overdose can also present as a myocardial infarction with chest pain. This is thought to result from "spasm" of the coronary arteries that feed the heart muscle or from insufficient supply of blood flow to meet the needs of the stimulated heart muscle. Unfortunately, sudden death may also be the initial presentation to the emergency department; this is due to a lethal heart rhythm precipitated by cocaine consumption. It is important to avoid beta blockers.

Stroke, seizures, fever, infection, kidney failure, liver hepatitis, pneumonia, thrombophlebitis, and human immunodeficiency virus are other potential complications of cocaine use and cocaine overdose. According to the US Centers for Disease Control and Prevention, 33,000 people died from cocaine overdose in 2005, which is a 60% increase since 1990. It is estimated that 70% to 80% of these were accidental deaths owing to heart failure.

Acute cocaine-related toxicity is a common cause of presentation to accident and emergency departments. The clinical features of acute toxicity include tachycardia, dysrhythmias, agitation and aggressive behavior, hallucinations, dilated pupils, hypertonia, hyperreflexia, hyperpyrexia, acid–base disturbance, and arterial dissection.

Hoffman in 2010[19] suggested dysrhythmias in the setting of slow-on slow-off (Vaughan Williams class IC) sodium channel blockade (with prolonged depolarization, characterized by prolongation of the QRS complex as the precursor to ventricular tachycardia, and on occasion a Brugada-like pattern on the electrocardiogram), potassium channel blockade (QT prolongation, Torsade de pointes) primarily of the inward potassium rectifier current, and catecholamine excess.

Withdrawal

Withdrawal symptoms are characterized by symptoms and signs that appear over a period of a few hours to several days after the cessation or reduction in heavy or prolonged use of cocaine. It consists of dysphoric mood and 2 or more of the following: fatigue, vivid and unpleasant dreams, insomnia or hypersomnia, increased appetite, and either psychomotor agitation or retardation. Cocaine craving and anhedonia are also present. Cocaine withdrawal peaks in 2 to 4 days with symptoms such as lowering of mood, fatigue, and general malaise lasting for several weeks.

Effects of Cocaine

Psychiatric comorbidity and sequelae

Treatment of cocaine use disorder in comorbid populations is even more challenging. One potential solution might be to target such medication development toward specific subpopulations. Some data suggest that antipsychotics may be useful in the treatment of cocaine use disorder in individuals with schizophrenia.[20]

Injecting cocaine can bring about severe allergic reactions and increased risk for contracting human immunodeficiency virus/AIDS, HCV, and other blood-borne diseases. Risk begins with the first injection, and within 2 years, nearly 40% of injecting drug users are exposed to HCV. By the time injecting drug users have been injecting for 5 years, their chances of being infected with HCV are between 50% and 80%.[21] Cocaine-related deaths are often a result of cardiac arrest or seizure, followed by respiratory arrest.

Lamy and Thibaut[22] in 2010 indicated that babies born to mothers who abuse cocaine during pregnancy are more likely to be premature, have low birth weights, have smaller head circumferences, and to be shorter than babies born to mothers who do not abuse cocaine. Multiple factors influence the effect of mothers' drug abuse on their babies. These factors include but are not limited to the amount and number of drugs abused, including nicotine, extent of prenatal care, possible neglect or abuse of the child, exposure to violence in the environment, socioeconomic conditions, maternal nutrition, other health conditions, and exposure to sexually transmitted diseases. Exposure to cocaine during fetal development may also lead to later subtle, yet significant, deficits in some children, including deficits in some aspects of cognitive performance, information processing, and attention to tasks and abilities that are important for the realization of a child's full potential.

Treatment

Cocaine intoxication or overdose

Cocaine overdose is treated as a medical emergency owing to the risk of cardiac toxicity. Physical cooling (ice, cold blankets, etc) and acetaminophen may be used to treat hyperthermia, while specific treatments are then developed for any further complications. Sedation with agents such as diazepam (Valium) is recommended for the agitation, irritability, seizures, and hyperexcitable state. This measure also helps to control the rapid heart rate and elevated blood pressure. If the body temperature is elevated, this is brought down with cold water, fans, cooling blankets, and acetaminophen. Specific therapies are geared to the specific complaint or system involved. For example, if the cocaine overdose has led to a heart attack, thrombolytic drugs may be used. Further testing with cardiac catheterization may be done. If this test shows a blocked vessel, a balloon angioplasty may also be done. Treatment depends on the presenting complaint and organ system involved. In addition, a history of high blood pressure or cardiac problems puts the patient at high risk of cardiac arrest or stroke, and requires immediate medical treatment.

Cocaine withdrawal

Withdrawal from cocaine may not be as unstable as withdrawal from alcohol. However, withdrawal from any chronic substance abuse is very serious. There is a risk of suicide or overdose. Symptoms usually disappear over time. Individuals may benefit from anxiolytics and antidepressants. Almost one-half of all people who are addicted to cocaine also have a mental disorder.[23] These conditions should be suspected and treated. When cocaine use disorder is diagnosed and treated, relapse rates are reduced dramatically.

Chronic cocaine use disorder

Currently, there are no US Food and Drug Administration–approved medications for treating cocaine use disorder. Behavioral interventions—particularly cognitive–behavioral therapy—have been shown to effectively decrease cocaine use and prevent relapse.

A significant number of medications have been evaluated for the treatment of cocaine use disorder. Randomized controlled trials focusing on the use of antidepressants, carbamazepine, dopamine agonists, and other drugs used in the treatment of cocaine dependence showed mixed results.[24] Several medications marketed for other diseases (eg, vigabatrin, modafinil, tiagabine, disulfiram, and topiramate) show promise and have been reported to reduce cocaine use in controlled clinical trials. Among these, disulfiram (used to treat alcoholism) has produced the most consistent reductions in cocaine abuse. In contrast, new knowledge of how the brain is changed by cocaine is directing attention to novel targets for medications development. Compounds that are currently being tested for addiction treatment take advantage of underlying cocaine-induced adaptations in the brain that disturb the balance between excitatory (glutamate) and inhibitory (gamma-aminobutyric acid) neurotransmission.[25] Finally, a cocaine vaccine that prevents entry of cocaine into the brain holds great promise for reducing the risk of relapse.

In addition to treatments for addiction, medical treatments are being developed to address the acute emergencies that result from cocaine overdose each year. Modafinil, a medication used to treat narcolepsy and related disorders, dramatically improves sleep among recently abstinent cocaine abusers. Cocaine abusers treated with modafinil for 16 days demonstrated improvements in several characteristics of sleep, including total sleep time.[26] Better sleep may boost patients' attention, memory, and mood—helping them to benefit from behavioral therapy for addiction.

The cocaine vaccine consists of a small amount of the drug chemically bonded to a protein, derived from cholera toxin that stimulates the immune system to produce antibodies. Anticocaine antibodies latch onto cocaine molecules in the bloodstream, forming drug–antibody complexes that are too large to pass through the fine-grained tissue filter that enwraps and protects the brain.[27] If the vaccinated person develops enough antibodies to capture and hold onto most of the cocaine molecules circulating in the blood, the drug will not produce the euphoria or other psychoactive effects that reinforce drug taking and addiction. A subgroup of vaccinated patients generated levels of antibodies that were sufficient to block cocaine's effects, and during the period of peak antibody production, they submitted more drug-free urine samples than participants in the placebo group or those who did not respond strongly to the vaccine.[28] With further refinement to increase response, a vaccine might someday be available as a therapy for cocaine abuse.

Behavioral and psychosocial treatments

These treatments are similar to modalities used for other substance use disorders. They include but are not limited to cognitive–behavioral therapy and contingency management and motivational incentives. Motivational incentives may be particularly useful for helping patients achieve initial abstinence from cocaine and stay in treatment.[29]

Summary

Cocaine still accounts for 25% of emergency department presentations for drug-related visits. Pharmacologic treatment remains elusive despite multiple promising agents. The primary modality of treatment is currently psychosocial. One modality for developing treatment is to target patients before the development of a cocaine use disorder.

DESIGNER DRUGS

Synthetic drugs, also known as designer drugs, are man-made recreational psychotropic chemical compounds with substantial variability in product structure, composition, and concentration. These include but are not limited to synthetic cannabinoids and cathinones.

Synthetic cannabinoids refer to a growing number of man-made, mind-altering chemicals that are either sprayed on dried, shredded plant material so they can be smoked (herbal incense) or sold as liquids to be vaporized and inhaled in e-cigarettes and other devices (liquid incense). Users usually smoke the dried plant material sprayed with synthetic cannabinoids. Sometimes they mix the sprayed plant material with marijuana, or they brew it as tea. Other users buy synthetic cannabinoid products as liquids to vaporize them in e-cigarettes.

The synthetic cannabinoids, which are also known as synthetic marijuana, K2, and spice, are the most prevalent and are widely available in head shops, convenience stores, gas stations, and on the Internet despite governmental efforts to regulate them. Synthetic cannabinoids are produced in clandestine laboratories; they often contain more than 10 additives and these chemicals are sprayed onto plant materials and advertised as giving "legal" highs.

These chemicals are called *cannabinoids* because they are related to chemicals found in the marijuana plant. Because of this similarity, synthetic cannabinoids are sometimes misleadingly called "synthetic marijuana" (or "fake weed"), and they are often marketed as "safe," legal alternatives to marijuana. In fact, they may affect the brain much more powerfully than marijuana; their actual effects can be unpredictable and, in some cases, severe or even life threatening.

Manufacturers sell these herbal incense products in colorful foil packages and sell similar liquid incense products, like other e-cigarette fluids, in plastic bottles. They market these products under a wide variety of specific brand names such as K2, spice, Joker, Black Mamba, Kush, and Kronic.

The use of synthetic cathinones such as mephedrone, methylone, and methylenedioxypyrovalerone (MDPV), which are often referred to as "bath salts," "Khat," or "jewelry cleaner," is comparably lower than synthetic cannabinoids, but rapidly growing. Cathinone and its metabolite cathine, which are known to give euphoric effects, are derived from chewing the leaves and twigs of the khat plant, *Catha edulis*. Lesser known synthetic drugs include synthetic hallucinogens such as 25I-NBOMe and N-bomb.

Synthetic drugs are disguised with the label, "not for human consumption," and they are able to evade the regulatory process and the Controlled Substances Analogues Enforcement Act of the United States. The popularity of synthetic drugs is attributed to easy accessibility, novelty, attractive packaging and enticing names, low cost, intense psychoactive effects, lack of detection in routine drug screen tests, and perceived harmlessness.

Synthetic drugs, in the absence of dose control and strict regulation, are serious public health threats because of their frequent alterations in chemical structures and combination of ingredients with unknown and unpredictable risk profiles. According to the report produced by White House Office of National Drug Control Policy,[30] 51 new synthetic cannabinoids were identified in 2012, which is a significant increase from 2 synthetic cannabinoids in 2009. Similarly, during this time period, the number of synthetic cathinones increased from 4 to 31. In addition, 76 other synthetic drugs were identified in 2012. Although many synthetic cannabinoids are schedule I drugs under the US controlled substance act, structurally altered compounds continue to emerge and evade government bans. Although data are not as well-established, other synthetic drugs present similar threats to the public.

Effects on the Central Nervous System

Synthetic cannabinoids act on the same brain cell receptors as delta-9-tetrahydrocannabinol (THC), the mind-altering ingredient in marijuana. So far, there have been few scientific studies of the effects of synthetic cannabinoids on the human brain, but researchers do know that some of them bind more strongly than marijuana to the cell receptors affected by THC, and may produce much stronger effects. The resulting health effects can be unpredictable.

Synthetic cannabinoid users report some effects similar to those produced by marijuana: elevated mood, relaxation, altered perception (awareness of surrounding objects and conditions), and symptoms of psychosis (delusional or disordered thinking detached from reality). Psychotic effects include extreme anxiety, confusion, paranoia (extreme and unreasonable distrust of others), and hallucinations (sensations and images that seem real although they are not).

Other Health Effects of Synthetic Cannabinoids

People who have used synthetic cannabinoids and have been taken to emergency rooms have shown severe effects including rapid heart rate, vomiting, violent behavior, and suicidal thoughts. Synthetic cannabinoids can also raise blood pressure and cause reduced blood supply to the heart, as well as kidney damage and seizures. Use of these drugs is associated with a rising number of deaths.

Synthetic cannabinoids can be addictive. Withdrawal symptoms include headaches, anxiety, depression and irritability. Synthetic cannabinoids are defined as any chemical compound that is a cannabinoid receptor agonist. In-vitro and in-vivo animal studies suggest synthetic cannabinoids are 2 to 100 times more potent than THC.[31] Furthermore, synthetic cannabinoids does not contain cannabidiols, which are found in cannabis and have potentially antipsychotic effects. However, it is important to note that synthetic cannabinoids binding affinities to CB1 and CB2 receptors vary depending on the ingredient compositions, which are frequently altered. Some synthetic cannabinoids metabolites may be active and prolong psychoactive and physiologic effects of intoxication. No human evidence describing absorption, distribution, metabolism, or elimination exists. Effects start to manifest within 10 minutes after inhalation, and may disappear 2 to 6 hours after use.

Young adults, primarily males in their mid to late 20s, account for the majority of synthetic drug use. Synthetic cannabinoids are popular among young cannabis and polydrug users because their perceived safety relative to other substances. Their prevalence is greater among regular cannabis users, university students, and dance club attendees. The 2012 Monitoring the Future survey of youth drug use trends reported 11% of 12th graders in the United States as having used synthetic cannabinoids in the past year.[31] After marijuana, synthetic cannabinoids is the most commonly used illegal drug among high school seniors. Risk factors for adolescent synthetic drugs use include parents with substance use disorders, poor family relationships, poor discipline, high family conflict, and adolescents involved in the foster care or the criminal justice systems.

Data from the American Association of Poison Control Centers suggest, synthetic cannabinoids–related calls have steadily increased from 2668 in 2013 to 3682 in 2014, and more than doubling to 7779 in 2015. In addition, national estimates on synthetic cannabinoids related emergency department visits obtained from the Drug Abuse Warning Network, managed by the Substance Abuse and Mental Health Services Administration, revealed there were 28,531 synthetic cannabinoid–related emergency department visits in 2011, which is more than a 2-fold increase from 2010. Males accounted for 79% of those visits. Approximately one-quarter of all visits were made by patients aged 12 to 17 years, and 29% of visits were made by patients aged 18 to 20 years. In sum, 12- to 20-year-olds accounted for 55% of all synthetic cannabinoids related emergency department visits in 2011, whereas 41% visits were made by 21- to 44-year-olds; with the remaining 4% by those aged 45 or older.[32]

A worldwide survey from Internet drug forum participants (n = 168, representing 13 countries and 42 states) revealed that the majority were Caucasian (90%), single (67%), men (83%), with at least a high school education (96%). Smoking was the most common route, although oral, rectal, and vaporized administrations were mentioned. Curiosity was the primary reason (78%) for synthetic cannabinoids use, and 58% favored the drugs' effects. Among synthetic cannabinoids users, abuse was reported by 37%, 15% reported dependence, and 15% withdrawal.[33]

An anonymous email survey (n = 852) at the University of Florida in September 2010 found that of 8.1% of those surveyed reported lifetime synthetic cannabinoids use, and among them 68% were male and 32% female. Smoking was the most popular route (88%), and 25% consumed with a hookah or joint. The majority of synthetic cannabinoids users (91.3%) also smoked cannabis.[34]

The prevalence of synthetic cathinones is rapidly increasing. According to the American Association of Poison Control Centers data from 2010 to 2011, calls pertaining to synthetic cannabinoids increased more than almost 20-fold from 304 to 6138. According to National Forensic Laboratory Information System data, 628 cases from 27 states were reported in 2010, which is a significant increase from 34 cases from 8 states in 2009. Among those reports in 2010, 48% was mephedrone, 40% MDPV, and 10% methylone. The majority of cases were reported in the South (57%), with 25% in the Midwest and 16% in the Northeast.[35]

Synthetic cathinones

Synthetic cathinones are β-ketophenethylamines that are similar structurally to amphetamines and MDMA. Cathinone derivatives are more hydrophilic, which decreases their ability to cross the blood–brain barrier, resulting in less potency as compared with amphetamines.

It has been speculated that the presence of carbonyl groups makes the molecule more planar, in turn facilitating its insertion into the DNA and producing cellular toxicity. They strongly inhibit reuptake of dopamine, serotonin, and norepinephrine, while simultaneously increasing presynaptic release of those neurotransmitters to a small extent.[36] Overall, it increases the extracellular levels of neurotransmitters, which is similar to how other stimulants like amphetamines and cocaine produce their effects. Commonly reported effects are increased energy, alertness, mood enhancement, euphoria, and decreased appetite. Also, they are often contaminated with benzocaine, lidocaine, procaine, caffeine, or even controlled drugs.

The most popular route of administration is through nasal insufflation followed by other routes such as oral ingestion, rectal insertion, and intravenous or intramuscular injection. A typical dose is 100 to 200 mg orally, and the onset of effect takes 30 to 45 minutes with the duration of action lasting 2 to 5 hours. MDPV is the more potent type, and a dose of 10 to 15 mg causes effects within 15 to 30 minutes of intake with duration of action la (<3.5 mEq/L), or hyperglycemia are occasionally observed sting 2 to 7 hours.

Clinical Manifestations and Diagnosis

Synthetic cannabinoids

Synthetic cannabinoids result in physiologic and psychoactive effects similar to THC, but with greater intensity and duration, which often requires medical and psychiatric emergency department visits. Acute synthetic cannabinoids intoxication psychoactive symptoms include anxiety, paranoia, agitation, delusions, and hallucinations. Physical signs include tachycardia, diaphoresis, xerostomia, conjunctival injection, and seizures in severe cases. Other reported manifestations are dilated pupils, decreased reflexes, nausea, vomiting, slurred speech, shortness of breath, hypertension, chest pain, muscle twitches, and skin pallor. In laboratory tests, mild leukocytosis (white blood cell count, 12,000–14,000), hypokalemia (<3.5 mEq/L), or hyperglycemia are occasionally observed.[31]

Some report the effect of onset to take place within minutes of smoking and intoxication lasting 2 to 5 hours, with most recovering in less than 24 hours. Adverse effects from acute intoxication generally subside within 24 to 48 hours after treatment with benzodiazepines and supportive care. Withdrawal symptoms were observed in chronic synthetic cannabinoids smokers after at least 1 week of abstinence.

Synthetic cannabinoids do not cross-react with routine laboratory cannabis tests. Instead, they can be detected by gas chromatography-mass spectrophotometry testing and also matrix-assisted laser desorption/ionization time of flight mass spectrometry. Blood tests are also available for some metabolites of various compounds. Detection time is not known, but may range from 48 to 72 hours.

Synthetic cathinones

Signs of acute intoxication overlap with central nervous system stimulation caused by cocaine and amphetamines. They include euphoria, heightened alertness, increased energy, talkativeness, increased sexual arousal, aggression, psychosis, self-mutilation, and suicide attempts. They also result in various physical symptoms involving different organ systems in serious cases involving renal and liver dysfunction.

Adverse reactions are mainly from sympathomimetic toxicity leading to hypertension, tachycardia, hyperthermia, dehydration, and psychomotor agitation. Cases of myocardial infarction and mephedrone-related myocarditis have been reported. Other common adverse reactions include palpitations, headache, chest pain, trismus, bruxism, tremors, insomnia, and paranoia. Significant hyponatremia has been related to mephedrone use, similar to hyponatremia seen with 3,4 Methylenedioxmethamphetamine MDMA (ecstasy), and may be caused by sweating, electrolyte loss, and antidiuretic hormone secretion. Even death was reported with mephedrone and MDPV (methylenedioxypyrovalerone).[36]

Users report persistent symptoms of paresthesia and mood changes for days to weeks after using both mephedrone and MDPV. Thirty percent of mephedrone users reported symptoms of dependence, such as tolerance, impaired control, and craving. Withdrawal effects of chronic users include tiredness, insomnia, difficulty concentrating, irritability, depression, and nasal congestion.

Synthetic cathinone derivatives are not detected on routine urine enzyme-linked immunosorbent assay–based drug screening for amphetamines. Comprehensive analysis of serum and urine using gas chromatography-mass spectrophotometry for synthetic cathinones has been described. In addition, testing kits are available commercially for mephedrone, MDPV, and methylone.

Treatment

Synthetic cannabinoids

The treatment of choice for synthetic cannabinoids is supportive care. Most physical symptoms are self-limited and tend to resolve within 1 to several days. However, for psychiatric manifestations, benzodiazepines such as lorazepam are used for agitation, and verbal reassurance or a "talk down" is effective. In some cases, psychotic symptoms persist from 1 week to 5 months. Seclusion and restraint are recommended only in patients with serious danger. Ongoing psychiatric care might be necessary. For neurologic symptoms, the presence of seizure should be monitored, which might require intubation. In addition, muscle injury can be suspected by muscle pain/weakness and decreased kidney function detectible in laboratory testing. For cardiovascular symptoms, blood pressure and heart rate must be monitored as well as electrocardiography and laboratory tests that can detect enzymes such as troponin and creatine kinase myocardial band. For gastrointestinal symptoms, medication for nausea can be given in addition to intravenous fluids. Laboratory tests must be monitored for low potassium levels. Some of the lasting, potentially lethal consequences include heart attacks, psychosis, self-harm, and suicidal thoughts while intoxicated. Intravenous fluid and benzodiazepine administration, and possibly antipsychotic medications in severe situations are helpful.

Synthetic cathinones

The mainstream management and treatment of synthetic cathinones users include supportive care and symptom targeted treatment such as use of benzodiazepines and vasodilators in case of persistent hypertension. Beta blockers should be avoided. Routine monitoring should follow temperature, electrolytes, creatine phosphokinase for muscle damage, renal/hepatic function, and cardiac function including electrocardiography.

Summary

The primary modality for the prevention of synthetic drug use needs to be the enactment of enforceable legislation. The tracking and reclassification of food supplements and drugs distributed through the Internet and gas stations is imperative. In March 2011, the Administrator of the drug enforcement agency issued an order to temporarily place 2 synthetic cannabinoids under the Controlled Substances Act.[37]

MARIJUANA

Epidemiology

Cannabis use remains prevalent world wide. Recent data from the United Nations show that 182 million people, approximately 3.8% of the world's population of people ages 15 to 64 years, use cannabis.[38] Cannabis remains one of the most widely used substances in the United States. Cannabis is the most prevalent illicit drug in the United States.[39] A recent prevalence study by National Survey on Drug Use and Health shows a lifetime prevalence of 46% among adults ages 26 or older, a 52.7% lifetime prevalence rate among adults age 18 to 25, and a 15.7% lifetime prevalence among adolescents ages 12 to 17. Among adolescents, 21.3% of 12th graders report use in the past month, 14.8% of 10th graders report use in the past month, and 6.5% of 8th graders report use in the past month.[40]

Cannabis is consumed by different methods, including inhaled after being hand-rolled into joints or blunts (empty cigar filled with cannabis). It is also smoked via bongs or vaporizers. Some individual also enjoy eating cannabis in the form of cannabis brownies, cookies, or candy. Cannabis resin are also increasingly being extracted and made into various products that are now consumed by users including products such as hash oil (liquid format), wax (softer liquid), or harder solids called Shatter.[41] Cannabis is considered a gateway drug in use among adolescents with adolescent often progressing from alcohol, cigarettes to cannabis, and eventually experimenting with hard drugs such as stimulants, opiates, and hallucinogens.[42]

Clinical Manifestations

The physiologic effects of cannabinoid ingestion include dry mouth, red eyes, lowering of blood pressure, fine shakes or tremors, decreased body temperature, and decreases in muscle strength and balance. Respiratory effects include acute dilation of the bronchial tubes, decreased bronchial diameter, and worsening of breathing problems. Cardiac effects include increased heart rate and an increased cardiac workload, which may be associated with heart attacks. Urinary effects include increased urinary frequency. Gastrointestinal effects include decreased nausea/vomiting.

The effects of cannabis on mood are variable. Mood effects include altered consciousness, mild euphoria, increased giddiness, increased and then decreased social interaction, and a decrease in feeling of anxiety or stress. However, some people report increased feeling of anxiety, depression, and panic symptoms with use of cannabis. Animal studies have shown that cannabis has a double edge effect on mood, improving depressive symptoms at lower dosages and increasing depressive symptoms at higher dosages.[43] A metaanalysis reviewing effects of cannabis and depression showed that heavy cannabis use increases the risk of patients developing depressive symptoms.[44]

A metaanalysis of 267 studies showed that cannabis use is associated with increased anxiety.[45] Some patients also experience increased sexual arousal, feeling of decreased slowing of time, and increased feeling of hunger (munchies). Some patients also experienced impaired short-term memory, reduced distance perception, and also increased sleepiness. Cannabis-induced psychotic symptoms are of concern in the emergency room setting. Acute intoxication has been associated with increased suspiciousness, paranoia, derealization, lack of insight, and also increased anxiety. At very high doses, cannabis has been known to cause increased hallucinations and paranoid delusions. Some patients have also reported increased severe anxiety including increased panic symptoms during acute intoxication. Some patients experience increased aggressiveness with cannabis intoxication, although there are patients who report reduced aggression. During acute intoxication, the main concerns include cardiac risk factors associated with intoxication including arrhythmia. Cannabis is often mixed with other serious substances that may cause other side effects, including chest pain, heart attacks, strokes, seizures, and so on.

Cannabis also has cognitive effects, including slowed reaction time, decreased short*term memory, decreased concentration, and attention, and also causes slower processing speed for information. Early onset cannabis users (use before age 17) have been shown to have lower performance on cognitive test than late onset or control group users, even after 1 month of abstinence.[46]

The role of cannabis use and increased in psychotic symptoms have been subject of much debate. A review of 6 longitudinal studies suggest that regular use of cannabis predicted increased risk of a schizophrenia diagnosis or reporting of psychotics symptoms.[46] Some studies have also shown that cannabis use aggravates symptoms and worsens the clinical course in patients with schizophrenia. Cannabis use has also been associated with increased risk of first break psychotic symptoms compared with patients who did not abuse cannabis. A case control study of 410 patients with first-episode psychosis versus 370 controls showed risk of psychosis was 3 times in users who used skunk cannabis versus individuals who do not use cannabis.[47]

Diagnosis

Diagnostic workup including urine toxicology or blood test should be done. Testing should also be done to rule out use of other substances that could be affecting the presentation. Electrolyte levels should be obtained. Electrocardiography should also be obtained to rule out cardiac-related issues. Patients should be evaluated for respiratory distress, particularly if cannabis has been mixed with other substances before being smoked.

Treatment

Treatment should focus on managing presenting symptoms. If patients are agitated, benzodiazepines should be used to manage symptoms. If there are psychotic symptoms present, antipsychotics should be used to treat presenting symptoms. Charcoal may be needed depending on the amount ingested. Intravenous fluid supplementation may also be needed. There is no agent that has been shown to have superior efficacy in managing cannabis dependence. Dronabinol is a drug that contains active ingredients similar to marijuana and is used for treatment of cannabis use disorder.

Summary

Marijuana use remains a significant public health issue. There are significant medical and psychiatric issues associated with the use of marijuana. Similarly, there are potential health benefits from the use of marijuana.

REFERENCES

1. Cicero TJ, Ellis MS, Surratt HL, et al. The changing face of heroin use in the United States: a retrospective analysis of the past 50 years. JAMA Psychiatry 2014;71(7):821–6.
2. Kane-Willis K, Schmitz S, Bazan M, et al. Understanding suburban heroin use. Roosevelt University; 2015.
3. Muhuri PK, Gfroerer JC, Davies MC. Associations of nonmedical pain reliever use and initiation of heroin use in the United States. CBHSQ Data Rev 2013;17.
4. Franklin G, Sabel J, Jones CM, et al. A comprehensive approach to address the prescription opioid epidemic in Washington State: milestones and lessons learned. Am J Public Health 2015;105(3):463–9.

5. Klevens RM, Hu DJ, Jiles R, et al. Evolving epidemiology of hepatitis C virus in the United States. Clin Infect Dis 2012;55(Suppl 1):S3–9.
6. Church DBK, Elson F, DeMaria A, et al. Notes from the field: risk factors for hepatitis C virus infections among young adults–Massachusetts, 2010. MMWR Morb Mortal Wkly Rep 2011;60(42):1457–8.
7. Center for Behavioral Health Statistics and Quality (CBHSQ). 2014 National survey on drug use and health: detailed tables. Substance Abuse and Mental Health Services Administration. (Table 7.62A).
8. Center for Behavioral Health Statistics and Quality (CBHSQ). 2014 National survey on drug use and health: detailed tables. Substance Abuse and Mental Health Services Administration. (Table 7.50A).
9. National Institute on Drug Abuse. Heroin; 2014. Available at: https://www.drugabuse.gov/publications/research-reports/heroin. Accessed June 28, 2017.
10. Jones CM, Campopiano M, Baldwin G, et al. National and state treatment need and capacity for opioid agonist medication-assisted treatment. Am J Public Health 2015;105(8):e55–63.
11. Volkow ND, Frieden TR, Hyde PS, et al. Medication-assisted therapies—tackling the opioid-overdose epidemic. N Engl J Med 2014;370(22):2063–6.
12. Flower R. Lifestyle drugs: pharmacology and the social agenda. Trends Pharmacol Sci 2004;25(4):182–5.
13. Calatayud J, Gonzalez A. History of the development and evolution of local anesthesia since the coca leaf. Anesthesiology 2003;98(6):1503–8.
14. Akerele E, Nahar N. Part III, Chapter 12. Substance abuse: cocaine. In: Mack AH, Brady KT, Frances RJ, et al, editors. Clinical textbook of addictive disorders. New York: Guilford Publications; 2016. p. 220–38.
15. National Institute on Drug Abuse (NIDA). Cocaine. 2016. Available at: https://www.drugabuse.gov/publications/research-reports/cocaine. Accessed June 28, 2017.
16. National Institute on Drug Abuse (NIDA). Research Report Series. 2010. Cocaine abuse and addiction. Available at: www.drugabuse.gov/sites/default/files/rrcocaine.pdf. Accessed March 5, 2012.
17. Bradberry CW, Nobiletti J, Elsworth J, et al. Cocaine and cocaethylene: microdialysis comparison of brain drug levels and effects on dopamine and serotonin. J Neurochem 1993;60(4):1429–35.
18. Jatlow P, McCance EF, Bradberry CW, et al. Alcohol plus cocaine: the whole is more than the sum of its parts. Ther Drug Monit 1996;18(4):460–4.
19. Hoffman RS. Treatment of patients with cocaine-induced arrhythmias: bringing the bench to the bedside. Br J Clin Pharmacol 2010;69(5):448–57.
20. Akerele E, Levin FR. Comparison of olanzapine to risperidone in substance-abusing individuals with schizophrenia. Am J Addict 2007;16(4):260–8.
21. Academy for Educational Development. Hepatitis C virus and HIV coinfection; 2002. Available at: www.cdc.gov/idu/hepatitis/hepc_and_hiv_co.pdf. Accessed May 21, 2012.
22. Lamy S, Thibaut F. Psychoactive substance use during pregnancy: a review. Encephale 2010;36(1):33–8 [in French].
23. Falck RS, Wang J, Siegal HA, et al. The prevalence of psychiatric disorder among a community sample of crack cocaine users: an exploratory study with practical implications. J Nerv Ment Dis 2004;192(7):503–7.
24. Lima MS, Soares BG, Reisser AAP, et al. Pharmacological treatment of cocaine dependence: a systematic review. Addiction 2002;97(8):931–49.
25. Schmidt HD, Pierce RC. Cocaine-induced neuroadaptations in glutamate transmission. Ann N Y Acad Sci 2010;1187(1):35–75.

26. Morgan PT, Pace-Schott E, Pittman B, et al. Normalizing effects of modafinil on sleep in chronic cocaine users. Am J Psychiatry 2010;167(3):331–40.
27. Orson FM, Kinsey BM, Singh RA, et al. Vaccines for cocaine abuse. Hum Vaccin 2009;5(4):194–9.
28. Martell BA, Orson FM, Poling J, et al. Cocaine vaccine for the treatment of cocaine dependence in methadone-maintained patients: a randomized, double-blind, placebo-controlled efficacy trial. Arch Gen Psychiatry 2009; 66(10):1116–23.
29. National Institute on Drug Abuse. Incentives Promote Abstinence; 2010. Available at: https://www.drugabuse.gov/news-events/nida-notes/2010/12/incentives-promote-abstinence. Accessed June 28, 2017.
30. Washington DC. The White House; c2015. The White House [Internet] Office of National Drug Control Policy: Synthetic Drugs (a.k.a. K2, Spice, Bath Salts, etc.); 2015.
31. Castaneto MS, Gorelick DA, Desrosiers NA, et al. Synthetic cannabinoids: epidemiology, pharmacodynamics, and clinical implications. Drug Alcohol Depend 2014;144:12–41.
32. Bush DM, Woodwell DA. Update: drug-related emergency department visits involving synthetic cannabinoids. The CBHSQ report. Rockville (MD): Substance Abuse and Mental Health Services Administration; 2013.
33. Vandrey R, Dunn KE, Fry JA, et al. A survey study to characterize use of Spice products (synthetic cannabinoids). Drug Alcohol Depend 2012;120(1):238–41.
34. Hu X, Primack BA, Barnett TE, et al. College students and use of K2: an emerging drug of abuse in young persons. Substance Abuse Treat Prev Pol 2011;6(1):1.
35. US Drug Enforcement Administration. Special report: synthetic cannabinoids and synthetic cathinones reported in and synthetic cathinones reported in NFLIS, 2009-2010.
36. Weaver MF, Hopper JA, Gunderson EW. Designer drugs 2015: assessment and management. Addict Sci Clin Pract 2015;10(1):1.
37. Sacco LN, Finklea KM. Synthetic drugs: overview and issues for congress. J Drug Addict Educ Eradication 2012;8(4):197.
38. Drugs UNO, Crime. World drug report 2010. United Nations Publications; 2010.
39. Hedden SL. Behavioral health trends in the United States: results from the 2014 National Survey on Drug Use and Health. Rockville (MD): Substance Abuse and Mental Health Services Administration, Department of Heath & Human Services; 2015.
40. National Institute on Drug Abuse. Marijuana. Available at: https://www.drugabuse.gov/drugs-abuse/marijuana. Accessed December 13.
41. Medical Jane. Cannabis extraction: learn about the various methods in which cannabis is extracted. Available at: https://www.medicaljane.com/category/cannabis-classroom/extractions-methods/#what-are-cannabis-extracts. Accessed June 28, 2017.
42. Fiellin LE, Tetrault JM, Becker WC, et al. Previous use of alcohol, cigarettes, and marijuana and subsequent abuse of prescription opioids in young adults. J Adolesc Health 2013;52(2):158–63.
43. Bambico FR, Katz N, Debonnel G, et al. Cannabinoids elicit antidepressant-like behavior and activate serotonergic neurons through the medial prefrontal cortex. J Neurosci 2007;27(43):11700–11.
44. Lev-Ran S, Roerecke M, Le Foll B, et al. 892–The association between cannabis use and depression: a systematic review and meta-analysis of longitudinal studies. Eur Psychiatry 2013;28:1.

45. Kedzior KK, Laeber LT. A positive association between anxiety disorders and cannabis use or cannabis use disorders in the general population-a meta-analysis of 31 studies. BMC Psychiatry 2014;14(1):1.
46. Pope HG, Gruber AJ, Hudson JI, et al. Early-onset cannabis use and cognitive deficits: what is the nature of the association? Drug Alcohol Depend 2003; 69(3):303–10.
47. Di Forti M, Marconi A, Carra E, et al. Proportion of patients in south London with first-episode psychosis attributable to use of high potency cannabis: a case-control study. Lancet Psychiatry 2015;2(3):233–8.

Toxicologic Emergencies in Patients with Mental Illness

When Medications Are No Longer Your Friends

Spencer Greene, MD, MS*, Erin AufderHeide, MD,
Lindsay French-Rosas, MD

KEYWORDS

• Psychiatric disorders • Toxicologic emergencies • Psychotropic medications
• Overdose

KEY POINTS

- Patients with psychiatric disorders are at risk for toxicologic emergencies.
- Psychotropic medications have numerous effects on the neurologic, cardiac, and other organ systems and interact with other medications, potentially leading to further side effects.
- It is important to become familiar with accepted psychiatric practice guidelines, common toxidromes, medical sequelae associated with prescribed medications, and the specific work-up and treatment of overdoses of frequently prescribed psychotropics.

INTRODUCTION

Patients with psychiatric disorders are at risk for toxicologic emergencies. Psychotropic medications have numerous effects on the neurologic, cardiac, and numerous other organ systems and interact with other medications that can lead to further side effects. According to the American Association of Poison Control Center's National Poison Data System, sedatives, hypnotics, and antipsychotics were implicated in 117,682 adult exposures in 2014, second only to analgesics. Antidepressants were third, with 75,662 exposures reported.[1] It is important to become familiar with accepted psychiatric practice guidelines, common toxidromes, medical sequelae associated with prescribed medications, and the specific work-up and treatment of overdoses of frequently prescribed psychotropics.

Ben Taub General Hospital, Houston, TX 77030, USA
* Corresponding author.
E-mail address: spencer.greene@bcm.edu

Psychiatr Clin N Am 40 (2017) 519–532
http://dx.doi.org/10.1016/j.psc.2017.05.007
0193-953X/17/© 2017 Elsevier Inc. All rights reserved.

The number of safe and effective medication treatments for mental illnesses has significantly increased over the past several years. As a broad principle, pharmacologic management depends on accurate diagnosis, whereas the optimal care of patients with acute or chronic psychiatric illness involves consideration of nonmedication treatments, such as therapies or lifestyle modification, in addition to, or instead of, pharmacologic approaches.[2] Besides clarifying diagnosis, key target symptoms and goals of treatment must be identified. Once a choice is made to pursue pharmacologic treatment, a specific treatment must be selected. Clinically useful biological predictors are commonly lacking, so an individual agent is usually chosen based on prior treatment response, ease of dosing and monitoring, drug interactions, side effects, comorbid conditions that could be affected, and cost.[2]

PSYCHOTROPIC CLASSIFICATION

Depressive disorders are prevalent, potentially disabling, and associated with increased suicide risk.[3] For most patients, including those with anxiety disorders, selective serotonin reuptake inhibitors (SSRIs) are the first-line choice.[2] SSRIs are effective for major depressive disorder, persistent depressive disorder, posttraumatic stress disorder, obsessive-compulsive disorder, and anxiety disorders. SSRIs inhibit the reuptake of serotonin and have minimal antimuscarinic, antihistaminic, and peripheral α_1-adrenergic antagonistic effects. In general, they are well tolerated and not as dangerous in overdose as older agents such as tricyclic antidepressants (TCAs) and monoamine oxidase inhibitors (MAOIs).[2] The lowest therapeutic dose is ideal but should be increased if there is less than 20% to 30% improvement 2 to 4 weeks after treatment is initiated. If symptoms persist despite appropriate dosing, another SSRI or a drug from a different class may be tried.[2]

Other commonly used classes of antidepressants include selective norepinephrine reuptake inhibitors (SNRIs), trazodone, atypical antidepressants such as bupropion and mirtazapine, TCAs, and MAOIs. SNRIs are effective for depression and some anxiety disorders and work by blocking the reuptake of both serotonin and norepinephrine. Similar to SSRIs, they are generally well tolerated and safer in overdose compared with older agents.[2] Trazodone works by inhibiting serotonin reuptake and agonizing serotonin receptors. Mirtazapine's mechanism of action has been debated but it seems to work by antagonizing α_2-adrenergic receptors and inhibiting the reuptake of serotonin. Bupropion works by inhibiting the reuptake of norepinephrine and dopamine. TCAs exert their antidepressant effect by inhibiting the reuptake of both serotonin and norepinephrine but have greater toxicity in overdose because of their effects at other sites. MAOIs increase catecholamine concentrations by preventing their degradation but their use is limited by severe toxicity caused by excessive catecholamine activity and multiple dietary and drug interactions.

Anxiety disorders are the most frequent psychiatric illness, with specific phobia being the most common type with a lifetime prevalence of 15.6%, followed by social anxiety disorder (10.7%), generalized anxiety disorder (4.3%), and panic disorder (3.8%)[4] The most commonly used anxiolytics are benzodiazepines (BZD), which act as agonists at the chief inhibitory neurotransmitter in the central nervous system (CNS), gamma-aminobutyric acid (GABA). Benzodiazepines specifically act on $GABA_A$ receptors and are rapidly effective but increase the risk of falls, delirium, and other cognitive concerns and can cause respiratory depression in overdose.[2] Current practice guidelines suggest caution in the long-term use of BZD because of their potential for misuse, physical dependency, and side effects.[4]

Agitation is defined as excessive motor activation with concurrent inner tension. If untreated, agitation can escalate to behavioral dyscontrol, and aggression toward others, self, or environment. Both benzodiazepines and various antipsychotics are frequently used to treat agitation, often in combination. Antipsychotics, often referred to as neuroleptics, are divided into typical and atypical types, and each group can be further divided into various categories. Typical antipsychotics antagonize dopaminergic D_2receptors and are used primarily for schizophrenia spectrum disorders but also for psychosis associated with other illnesses such as major depressive disorder, bipolar disorder, and delirium. These medications are very effective and studies have found they may be as effective as the atypical antipsychotics in the treatment of schizophrenia.[2] Atypical antipsychotics differ from their predecessors by their blockade of serotonergic $5HT_{2A}$ receptors and variable blockade of D_2 receptors. Atypical antipsychotics are effective for all conditions treated by typical antipsychotics and may be effective in patients with bipolar disorder for acute mania and as maintenance mood stabilizers.

Nearly all neuroleptics, but particularly high-potency typical antipsychotics, can cause various extrapyramidal side effects (EPS), including dystonia, akathisia, parkinsonism, bradykinesia, and tardive dyskinesia. Weight gain and poor glycemic control may result from chronic use of various antipsychotics, including clozapine and olanzapine. Clozapine is also associated with agranulocytosis and cardiomyopathy, and in many settings its use is restricted to psychiatrists when other neuroleptics have failed.

Lithium is the classic pharmacologic treatment choice for bipolar disorder characterized by full mania and depression. Lithium is used to treat both manic and depressive illness phases as well as bipolar maintenance and can reduce suicide risk. Caution must be practiced because of its multiple drug interactions, narrow therapeutic index, and potential teratogenicity leading to Ebstein anomaly. Chronic use may also result in multiple organ dysfunction, primarily the CNS and thyroid, although nephrogenic diabetes insipidus is also sometimes observed.[2]

Valproic acid (VPA) is indicated for acute manic episodes, bipolar maintenance, and for aggression or impulsivity. VPA can be titrated more aggressively than lithium and has a wider therapeutic index but still commonly causes sedation, weight gain, and gastrointestinal (GI) upset. It is also a teratogen that causes neural tube defects and is associated with significant drug interactions. Idiosyncratic effects of VPA may include increased transaminase levels, pancreatitis, and thrombocytopenia.[2]

ADVERSE DRUG REACTIONS

In light of the vast amount of psychotropic medication available, clinicians must watch for various adverse drug reactions, defined as responses to a medication that are noxious, unintended, and may occur at therapeutic doses. Adverse events from medications are now the fourth leading cause of death in the United States.[5] Particularly dangerous adverse drug reactions include EPS and the related but different neuroleptic malignant syndrome (NMS), serotonin syndrome (SS), dysrhythmias, and antimuscarinic toxicity, which are all described in greater detail later.

Extrapyramidal Side Effects

EPS can occur with therapeutic use of neuroleptics or following overdose. They are thought to result from excessive blockade of dopamine receptors in the basal ganglia or secondary to an altered ratio of cholinergic and dopaminergic activity.[6] Manifestations include acute dystonia, akathisia, parkinsonism, and tardive dyskinesia. Acute dystonia occurs within hours of starting antipsychotic treatment and is characterized by intermittent, involuntary motor tics and spasms of the face, neck, back, and extremities. Akathisia occurs within days of starting treatment and is characterized by a sensation of restlessness associated with objective motor hyperactivity. Parkinsonism develops within months of starting neuroleptics and is characterized by bradykinesia, masked faces, muscular rigidity, and resting tremor. Tardive dyskinesia occurs after years of antipsychotic treatment and is a chronic movement disorder, characterized by involuntary tics of the face, extremities, or trunk.

Neuroleptic Malignant Syndrome

A similar condition, NMS is a potentially lethal drug reaction characterized by some combination of hyperthermia, muscle rigidity, altered mental status (AMS), diaphoresis, labile blood pressure, tachycardia, and bradykinesia. The exact mechanism of NMS is unknown, but it is thought to be secondary to dopamine receptor blockade in the hypothalamus leading to hyperthermia and dysautonomia, as well as dopamine receptor blockade in the nigrostriatal pathway, leading to rigidity, tremor, and parkinsonism.[7,8] Although NMS is most often seen with the typical high-potency neuroleptic agents (eg, haloperidol, droperidol), it can develop after exposure to any antipsychotic.[9]

NMS typically presents within 2 weeks of starting an antipsychotic but has been known to occur months and even years later.[10] Mortality exceeded 70% when NMS was first described in the 1960s, but earlier recognition and better intensive care has reduced mortality to less than 20%.[11] Diagnostic criteria were developed by a multispecialty physician panel in 2011 to better characterize NMS and consequently improve clinical management of patients receiving antipsychotic medications.[12] In order to make the diagnosis of NMS, certain criteria must be met (**Box 1**).

Serotonin Toxicity

Serotonin toxicity results from excessive activity at the 5-HT_{1A} and 5-HT_{2A} receptors, which may follow a dose increase (including overdose) of a serotonergic agent or when 2 or more serotonergic agents are used simultaneously.[13] It is especially common when drugs with different mechanisms of action are combined; for example, a serotonin reuptake inhibitor combined with a drug that enhances serotonin release. Commonly implicated medications include antidepressants (eg, SSRIs, SNRIs, TCAs, MAOIs), drugs of abuse (eg, cocaine, lysergic acid diethylamide [LSD]), analgesics (eg, tramadol, meperidine), dextromethorphan, lithium, and St John's Wort.[14]

Box 1
Diagnosis of neuroleptic malignant syndrome

1. Recent dopamine antagonist exposure or dopamine agonist withdrawal
2. Hyperthermia (≥38.0°C)
3. Rigidity
4. Mental status alteration
5. Creatine kinase level increased to more than 4 times normal
6. Sympathetic nervous system lability (blood pressure increased 25% above baseline, blood pressure fluctuation ≥20 mm Hg diastolic or ≥25 mm Hg systolic within 24 hours)
7. Tachycardia greater than 25% increase from baseline plus tachypnea greater than 50% increase from baseline

When certain conditions are satisfied, the diagnosis of SS can be made. However, toxicity can be diagnosed even if all the criteria are not satisfied. One approach to diagnosing SS is to use the Hunter criteria.[15] To make the diagnosis using Hunter criteria, the patient must have history of serotonergic agent use and must have certain features (**Box 2**).

Several conditions resemble NMS and SS, including sympathomimetic toxicity, salicylate toxicity, thyrotoxicosis, malignant hyperthermia, sepsis, and *N*-methyl-D-aspartate receptor antibody encephalitis. A thorough evaluation is often needed to arrive at the correct diagnosis. However, there are certain historical and clinical features that can help distinguish NMS from SS, the 2 toxidromes that are most commonly confused (**Table 1**).

The antimuscarinic (anticholinergic) toxidrome results from antagonism at peripheral and central muscarinic acetylcholine receptors. It is characterized by AMS ranging from lethargy to delirium; hot, dry, flushed skin; mydriasis; hyperthermia; tachycardia; hypertension; decreased bowel sounds; and urinary retention. Both nonpsychiatric medications (eg, diphenhydramine, tolterodine) and psychotropics (eg, TCAs, carbamazepine, and multiple antipsychotics) can cause antimuscarinic effects in therapeutic use and overdose. Several plants (eg, *Datura* spp), some of which are occasionally abused for their hallucinogenic effect, can also cause antimuscarinic effects.

PSYCHOTROPIC OVERDOSE

In addition to the important but rare idiosyncratic reactions described earlier, all psychotropic medications have the potential to cause serious toxicity in acute overdose and/or when used chronically. The clinical features of acute intoxications of various psychiatric medications are described here, as well as some of the more significant toxicities associated with chronic use.

Antipsychotics

Both NMS and EPS may develop after antipsychotic ingestions. More commonly, CNS depression is observed in overdose. Low-potency antipsychotics of the aliphatic phenothiazine class antagonize muscarinic receptors, and an antimuscarinic toxidrome may be observed in overdose.[16] However, a notable exception to the classic toxidrome is the absence of mydriasis. Pupils are miotic in overdose because phenothiazines such as chlorpromazine also antagonize peripheral α_1-adrenergic receptors, which results in constricted pupils. Orthostatic hypotension associated with a reflex tachycardia secondary to vasodilation is also observed. Electrocardiographic abnormalities such as QRS widening and QT prolongation are also observed in some

Box 2
Hunter criteria for the diagnosis of serotonin syndrome

Patients must have at least 1 of the following:

1. Spontaneous clonus
2. Inducible clonus plus agitation or diaphoresis
3. Ocular clonus plus agitation or diaphoresis
4. Tremor plus tachycardia
5. Hypertonia plus temperature more than 38° C plus ocular clonus or inducible clonus

Table 1
Distinguishing neuroleptic malignant syndrome from serotonin syndrome

	Serotonin Syndrome	Neuroleptic Malignant Syndrome
Inciting drug	Serotonin agent	Dopamine antagonist
Onset	Hours	Days to weeks
Duration	≤24 h	Days to weeks
Clonus	Common	Uncommon
Shivering	Common	Not observed
Lead pipe rigidity	Uncommon	Common
Bradykinesia	Not observed	Common

overdoses of low-potency antipsychotics. Thioridazine, a piperidine phenothiazine that was removed from the market recently, was commonly associated with significant cardiotoxicity in large ingestions.[17]

Atypical antipsychotics of the benzepine class include quetiapine, olanzapine, and clozapine, and acute overdoses resemble those of the low-potency typicals, although cardiotoxicity is less prominent.[18] Antimuscarinic toxicity associated with miosis, as well as orthostatic hypotension, is observed. Although xerostomia is common in antimuscarinic toxicity, clozapine is associated with sialorrhea in overdose because it acts as an agonist at the M4 receptor.[19]

Indole antipsychotics such as risperidone, paliperidone, ziprasidone, and lurasidone have the same peripheral α_1-adrenergic antagonism as described earlier, but they do not affect muscarinic receptors. Acute poisoning is characterized by CNS depression, orthostatic hypotension, tachycardia, and profound miosis.[18] QT prolongation may also be observed, particularly in ziprasidone ingestions.[20] Toxicity typically presents early, except for paliperidone, which is formulated in such a way that peak effects may not be observed for more than 24 hours.[21]

Antimuscarinic toxicity is not observed in overdoses of high-potency butyrophenone antipsychotics such as haloperidol and droperidol. CNS depression is common, and seizures and QT prolongation have been reported.[22]

Aripiprazole, a commonly prescribed atypical antipsychotic of the quinolinone class, causes sedation in overdose.[23] Electrocardiographic abnormalities are not typically observed, although hypotension secondary to α_1-adrenergic antagonism may be present. Rarely priapism develops after overdose.[24]

Antidepressants

Although SSRIs are often treated as a single class of drugs, it may be more practical to separate them by their potential toxicities. All SSRIs can cause CNS depression, tachycardia, and GI signs and symptoms in overdose. Serotonin toxicity may also be observed in large ingestions. Seizures and electrocardiographic changes are almost always caused by citalopram and, to a lesser extent, escitalopram.[25,26]

SNRIs cause similar toxicity in overdose. Hypertension is more common because of the impaired norepinephrine reuptake, but severe cases can cause significant hypotension.[27] Trazodone typically causes little more than sedation in overdose, although orthostatic hypotension and dysrhythmias are possible. Seizures, syndrome of inappropriate antidiuretic hormone secretion, and priapism are reported rarely in overdose.[28] Bupropion toxicity is characterized by seizures, tachycardia, hypertension, and occasionally electrocardiographic abnormalities.[29,30] Mirtazapine overdoses produce primarily CNS depression. Whether or not serotonin toxicity results from these ingestions has been debated in the literature.[31,32]

Toxicity from TCAs may manifest in a variety of ways, including AMS, seizures, hypotension, and dysrhythmias.[33,34] Antimuscarinic and/or serotonin toxicity may be observed. Signs appear early, and typically, if no life-threatening toxicity occurs in the first 2 hours, it is unlikely to develop later.

MAOI toxicity is characterized by tachycardia, labile blood pressure, seizures, AMS, and GI symptoms. Toxicity may result from acute overdoses, in the setting of SS, or secondary to hyperadrenergic crisis precipitated by exposure to tyramine-containing foods.[35,36]

Mood Stabilizers

Lithium poisoning can present in 3 different ways: acute, acute on chronic, and chronic. Acute toxicity results from an overdose by someone who is not taking lithium regularly. Clinical features may include nausea, vomiting, and diarrhea.[37,38] Neurologic toxicity is typically absent early on unless a coingestant is present, but, if the patient goes untreated, encephalopathy and other neurologic findings may develop as the drug crosses the blood-brain barrier. Serum lithium levels may be extremely increased in acute overdose, but the magnitude does not correlate with the degree of neurotoxicity.[39]

Chronic toxicity may develop when a patient is using an excessive dose for a prolonged period. More commonly, it results from impaired lithium excretion, typically in the setting of volume depletion or salt restriction. Risk factors for chronic lithium toxicity include advanced age, low-output heart failure, decreased sodium intake, and concomitant use of thiazide diuretics, nonsteroidal antiinflammatory drugs, and/or angiotensin-converting enzyme inhibitors.[40] Neurologic dysfunction is the primary manifestation of chronic toxicity. Signs may range from tremor to encephalopathy to seizure. On occasion, the syndrome of irreversible lithium-effectuated neurotoxicity (SILENT) may develop. This syndrome is characterized by persistent (ie, at least 2 months) neurologic dysfunction (particularly cerebellar findings) in someone with no prior neurologic illness who uses lithium chronically.[41]

Other organs may be affected in chronic lithium toxicity. Nephrogenic diabetes insipidus is among the most common adverse effects noted in patients using lithium toxicity.[42] Less often, patients develop a tubulointerstitial nephropathy resulting in renal insufficiency. However, the renal injury in patients with chronic lithium poisoning more often causes the lithium toxicity than results from it.

Other manifestations of chronic lithium toxicity include thyroid dysfunction, hyperparathyroidism, and leukocytosis.[43] Hypothyroidism is most common, but hyperthyroidism, and even thyrotoxicosis, have been reported. Cardiotoxicity may be observed, particularly in patients with underlying cardiac disease.[44]

Acute-on-chronic toxicity occurs when a patient who is on lithium therapeutically acutely overdoses on lithium. GI signs and symptoms may be present but are often less profound. Neurologic signs appear much sooner than in acute toxicity.

Although used initially as an anticonvulsant, valproic acid and its derivatives are now used extensively for mood stabilization. Acute overdoses of valproic acid and divalproex sodium manifest primarily as CNS depression, although seizures, transient myelosuppression, and a variety of laboratory abnormalities may be observed.[45] Hyperammonemia frequently accompanies acute toxicity and may also be observed in therapeutic use.[46] Valproic acid has many metabolic fates. Normally it undergoes beta oxidation in the mitochondrion, producing a nontoxic metabolite. This pathway requires carnitine. When carnitine gets depleted, VPA undergoes omega oxidation in the endoplasmic reticulum. A toxic metabolite inhibits the enzyme carbamoyl phosphate synthase I (CPSI), which normally converts ammonia to urea. Because of the CPSI inhibition, patients develop hyperammonemia. Other laboratory abnormalities that may accompany valproic toxicity include both hypernatremia and hyponatremia, metabolic acidosis, and hypocalcemia, which may manifest clinically as tetany and carpopedal spasm and electrocardiographically as a prolonged corrected QT. Because many of the products are delayed or sustained release, toxicity may not be readily apparent.

Attention-deficit/Hyperactivity Disorder Medications

There are two broad classes of medications prescribed to treat attention-deficit/hyperactivity disorder (ADHD). Amphetamines and atomoxetine can cause sympathomimetic toxicity in overdose. Features include tachycardia, mydriasis, diaphoresis, paranoia, and psychomotor agitation.[47,48] Hypertension is typically observed, but hypotension may result from volume depletion or decreased stroke volume secondary to severe tachycardia. Seizures may also occur, and signs of serotonin excess, such as clonus, tremor, hyperreflexia, and rigidity, may be present. Common laboratory abnormalities include a wide-gap metabolic acidosis, lactic acidosis, hypokalemia, hyperglycemia, and rhabdomyolysis.

Central sympatholytics such as clonidine and guanfacine are also frequently used in the treatment of ADHD. Toxicity is characterized primarily by CNS depression, but bradycardia and hypotension are also frequently observed.[49] Profound miosis is typically present, and sympatholytic toxicity may be mistaken for opioid toxicity.

Sedative-Hypnotics and Anxiolytics

Commonly prescribed medications in this group include buspirone, various benzodiazepines, and the so-called Z drugs (zolpidem, zopiclone, eszopiclone, and zaleplon). Antihistamines and antidepressants are also often used in this capacity but are not discussed here. Barbiturates are less commonly prescribed but may produce significant toxicity in overdose. Toxicity from these medications is primarily limited to CNS depression, although respiratory depression and hypotension may result from large overdoses, particularly from barbiturates.[50,51]

TREATMENT OF PSYCHIATRIC MEDICATION TOXICITY

The initial steps in the management of psychotropic medication toxicity focuses on identifying and correcting life-threatening conditions. Endotracheal intubation should be performed in any patient with significant CNS depression resulting in the loss of airway reflexes. Supplemental oxygen should be provided to hypoxic patients, and end-tidal CO_2 monitoring should be considered for patients with impaired ventilation. It is reasonable to treat bradypneic patients with naloxone. In addition to its benefits in opioid toxicity, there are numerous case reports of medications such as clonidine, guanfacine, and valproic acid responding to naloxone.[52–55] The optimal dose has not been determined and many algorithms exist.[56,57] Flumazenil, the reversal agent for benzodiazepines, has fallen out of favor because of a perceived risk of seizures in benzodiazepine-dependent patients. However, it has proved to be safe and effective in a variety of settings, including following unknown ingestions and in benzodiazepine overdoses in chronic benzodiazepine users.[58,59]

Hypotension following psychotropic overdose may be multifactorial. Impaired inotropy, insufficient stroke volume, vasodilation, and volume depletion may all result in impaired tissue perfusion. Fluid resuscitation is the initial treatment regardless of the cause. If hypotension persists, direct-acting vasopressors are recommended. However, if the hypotension is secondary to sodium channel poisoning (eg, TCA toxicity), boluses of sodium bicarbonate 1 to 2 mEq/kg every 5 to 10 minutes should be considered.[60] Sodium bicarbonate is also recommended for QRS widening, typically if the QRS duration exceeds 120 milliseconds.[60,61]

Magnesium sulfate should be administered empirically in cases of prolonged QT interval. Any hypocalcemia and/or hypokalemia should also be corrected.

All patients with CNS depression should also have their blood glucose levels measured. If hypoglycemia is present, adults should be treated with 25 to 50 g of 50% dextrose intravenously. Hyperthermia and hypothermia should also be corrected as part of the initial resuscitation.

Once the patient is stabilized, a thorough assessment is required. A complete history should be obtained (**Box 3**). Physical examination should be performed to identify particular toxidromes that may suggest a specific drug or class of drugs.

An electrocardiogram is recommended because abnormalities such as QRS widening and QT prolongation may suggest certain types of poisoning. Furthermore, the choice of pharmacotherapy may be influenced by the electrocardiogram findings.

Laboratory tests are an essential component of evaluating patients with suspected ingestions. In addition to standard tests that most psychiatric facilities require (eg, complete blood count, basic metabolic profile, pregnancy test in women of childbearing age), serum acetaminophen and salicylate levels are recommended. Serum levels of specific drugs, such as lithium, valproic acid, carbamazepine, phenytoin, phenobarbital, and digoxin, are recommended in patients known to have access to these medications or if the history or physical examination suggest toxicity from 1 or more of these agents.

Arguably the most controversial laboratory test obtained in patients with overdose is the urine drug screen (UDS). Although many psychiatric facilities require a UDS before accepting a patient, the usefulness of a UDS is limited by its limited scope and frequent false-positive and false-negative results. Some toxicologists have argued that there is no benefit from this test.[62]

Radiographic studies are rarely necessary following psychotropic overdose but are recommended if concomitant injury or illness is suspected (**Table 2**). Because most pills are radiolucent, abdominal radiographs should not be performed routinely.

Although once considered a mainstay of poisoning treatment, GI decontamination (GID) has fallen out of favor because evidence suggests it is rarely helpful and may be harmful. However, if certain criteria are satisfied, single-dose activated charcoal (SDAC) should be administered at a dose of 1 g/kg by mouth up to 100 g (**Box 4**). Whole-bowel irrigation using polyethylene glycol electrolyte solution should be

Box 3
Important information to be obtained when taking a history

1. What substances did the patient ingest?
2. To what substances did the patient potentially have access?
3. When did the ingestion occur?
4. What treatments were attempted before arrival in the emergency department?
5. What signs and symptoms has the patient had so far?
6. What is the past medical, surgical, social, and psychiatric history?

Table 2
Indications for radiographic studies in the overdose patient

Head CT	Chest Radiograph
Unexplained AMS (ie, signs not consistent with known ingestants)	Respiratory signs or symptoms
Concomitant trauma	Patient at risk for aspiration or other pulmonary toxicity
Patient at high risk for intracranial catastrophe	Unexplained fever
Focal neurologic deficit	Confirmation of central venous line or endotracheal tube placement
Examination findings suggestive of increased intracranial hypertension	

considered in situations in which GID may be helpful but SDAC is not advised; for example, acute lithium overdoses or ingestions of transdermal patches.[63,64]

Benzodiazepines are considered the first-line treatment of patients with seizures, SS, NMS, or agitation following overdose. These patients may also relieve neuroleptic-induced akathisia. Benzodiazepines raise the seizure threshold, provide sedation, reduce anxiety, and have minimal cardiovascular effects. The choice of benzodiazepine depends on availability, route, urgency, and desired duration of effect.[14]

Some psychotropic medications can be treated with specific antidotes. Physostigmine salicylate is a cholinesterase inhibitor that effectively reverses antimuscarinic toxicity. It has proved to be superior to benzodiazepines in reversing both agitation and delirium.[65] It is contraindicated in patients with an allergy to any of its components. It should also be withheld in patients with atrioventricular block, severe asthma, and relative or absolute bradycardia. Although older references list TCA toxicity as a contraindication, multiple recent studies suggest that physostigmine is safe and effective in TCA overdose.[65,66]

Other antidotes that may be indicated in psychotropic overdoses include levocarnitine for VPA toxicity, cyproheptadine for patients with serotonin toxicity refractory to benzodiazepines, and bromocriptine for patients with refractory NMS.[14,67] Dantrolene,

Box 4
Indications for single-dose activated charcoal

Potentially toxic ingestion

Protected airway (ie, patient is awake and alert or is intubated)

Patient is cooperative

GI tract is functioning normally (eg, no vomiting and no evidence of perforation or obstruction)

The suspected toxicant is adsorbable by SDAC (eg, not a hydrocarbon, elemental metal, or caustic agent)

There is no anticipated need for endoscopy

The xenobiotic has not yet been absorbed from the GI tract (ie, patient does not yet show signs of toxicity)

the antidote for malignant hyperthermia, should not be used as monotherapy for either SS or NMS because it has no CNS effects, but it may be used as adjunctive therapy. Antimuscarinic agents such as benztropine and diphenhydramine may correct dystonia. Additional antidotes may be needed if there is evidence of a nonpsychotropic coingestion; for example, *N*-acetylcysteine for acetaminophen toxicity.

Because patients who overdose on psychotropic medications may be indigent or otherwise unable to care for themselves, ensuring proper nutrition is an important aspect of treatment. Thiamine and folate supplementation should be considered along with electrolyte replacement. Pyridoxine and vitamin B_{12} may also be required.

One other intervention to consider in selected psychotropic overdoses is enhancing elimination via urinary alkalinization and/or hemodialysis. Most medications are not amenable to either treatment, but there are xenobiotics for which these are options. Lithium is readily dialyzable.[68] Phenobarbital can be eliminated through both alkalinization and dialysis.[69,70] Although valproic acid is not dialyzable in therapeutic use or mild overdose because it is so highly protein bound, in overdose the free concentration increases enough to make this a potentially useful treatment.[71]

SUMMARY

New psychotropic medications are constantly being developed, and the spectrum of toxicity they may manifest idiosyncratically or in overdose continues to grow. Clinicians should have at least a rudimentary understanding of adverse drug effects, but they should also know when to seek assistance. Many facilities have a staff medical toxicologist but, for those that do not, help is available at all hours by calling a regional poison center at 1-800-222-1222.

REFERENCES

1. Mowry JB. 32nd annual report of the American Association of Poison Control Center's National Poison Data System. Clin Toxicol 2016;53(1):962–1146.
2. Huffman JC, Alpert JE. An approach to the psychopharmacologic care of patients: antidepressants, antipsychotics, anxiolytics, mood stabilizers, and natural remedies. Med Clin North Am 2010;94:1141–60.
3. Dunlop BW. Evidence-based applications of combination psychotherapy and pharmacotherapy for depression. Focus 2016;14(2):156–73.
4. Perna G, Alciati A, Riva A, et al. Long-term pharmacological treatments of anxiety disorders: an updated systematic review. Curr Psychiatry Rep 2016;18(23):1–16.
5. Jones PB, Barnes TR, Davies L, et al. Randomized controlled trial of the effect on quality of life of second- vs first-generation antipsychotic drugs in schizophrenia: Cost Utility of the Latest Antipsychotic Drugs in Schizophrenia Study (CUtLASS 1). Arch Gen Psychiatry 2006;63:1079–87.
6. Tarsy D, Baldessarini RJ. Tardive dyskinesia. Ann Rev Med 1984;35:605–23.
7. Henderson VW, Wooten GF. Neuroleptic malignant syndrome: a pathogenetic role for dopamine receptor blockade? Neurology 1981;31(2):132–7.
8. Andreassen MD, Pedersen S. Malignant neuroleptic syndrome. A review of epidemiology, risk factors, diagnosis, differential diagnosis and pathogenesis of MNS. Ugeskr Laeger 2000;162(10):1366–70 [in Danish].
9. Caroff SN, Mann SC. Neuroleptic malignant syndrome. Med Clin North Am 1993; 77(1):185–202.
10. Pope HG Jr, Aizley HG, Keck PE, et al. Neuroleptic malignant syndrome: long-term follow-up of 20 cases. J Clin Psychiatry 1991;52(5):208–12.

11. Shalev A, Hermesh H, Munitz H. Mortality from neuroleptic malignant syndrome. J Clin Psychiatry 1989;50(1):18–25.
12. Gurrera RJ, Caroff SN, Cohen A, et al. An international consensus study of neuroleptic malignant syndrome diagnostic criteria using the Delphi method. J Clin Psychiatry 2011;72(9):1222–8.
13. Mills KC. Serotonin syndrome. A clinical update. Crit Care Clin 1997;13(4):763–83.
14. Boyer EW, Shannon M. The serotonin syndrome. N Engl J Med 2005;352(11):1112–20.
15. Dunkley EJ, Isbister GK, Sibbritt D, et al. The Hunter Serotonin Toxicity Criteria: simple and accurate diagnostic decision rules for serotonin toxicity. QJM 2003;96(9):635–42.
16. Isbister GK, Balit CR, Kilham HA. Antipsychotic poisoning in young children. Drug Saf 2005;28(11):1029–44.
17. Buckley NA, Whyte IM, Dawson AH. Cardiotoxicity more common in thioridazine overdose than with other neuroleptics. J Toxicol Clin Toxicol 1995;33(3):199–204.
18. Minns AB, Clark RF. Toxicology and overdose of atypical antipsychotics. J Emerg Med 2012;43(5):906–13.
19. Praharaj SK, Arora M, Gandotra S. Clozapine-induced sialorrhea: pathophysiology and management strategies. Psychopharmacology 2006;185(3):265–73.
20. Wenzel-Seifert K, Wittmann M, Haen E. QTc prolongation by psychotropic drugs and the risk of torsade de pointes. Dtsch Arztebl Int 2011;108(41):687–93.
21. Levine M, Lovecchio F, Tafoya P, et al. Paliperidone overdose with delayed onset of toxicity. Ann Emerg Med 2011;58(1):80–2.
22. Knight ME, Roberts RJ. Phenothiazine and butyrophenone intoxication in children. Pediatr Clin North Am 1986;33(2):299–309.
23. Carstairs SD, Williams SR. Overdose of aripiprazole, a new type of antipsychotic. J Emerg Med 2005;28(3):311–3.
24. Mago R, Anolik R, Johnson RA, et al. Recurrent priapism associated with use of aripiprazole. J Clin Psychiatry 2006;67(9):1470–1.
25. Klein-Schwartz W, Benson BE, Lee SC, et al. Comparison of citalopram and other selective serotonin reuptake inhibitor ingestions in children. Clin Toxicol 2012;50(5):418–23.
26. Engebretsen KM, Harris CR, Wood JE. Cardiotoxicity and late onset seizures with citalopram overdose. J Emerg Med 2003;25(2):163–6.
27. Mazur JE, Doty JD, Krygiel AS. Fatality Related to a 30-g venlafaxine overdose. Pharmacotherapy 2003;23(12):1668–72.
28. Ali CJ, Henry JA. Trazodone overdosage: experience over 5 years. Neuropsychobiology 1986;15(Suppl 1):44–5.
29. Spiller HA, Ramoska EA, Krenzelok EP, et al. Bupropion overdose: a 3-year multicenter retrospective analysis. Am J Emerg Med 1994;12(1):43–5.
30. Curry SC, Kashani JS, LoVecchio F, et al. Intraventricular conduction delay after bupropion overdose. J Emerg Med 2005;29(3):299–305.
31. Hernández JL, Ramos FJ, Infante J, et al. Severe serotonin syndrome induced by mirtazapine monotherapy. Ann Pharmacother 2002;36(4):641–3.
32. Isbister GK, Whyte IM. Adverse reactions to mirtazapine are unlikely to be serotonin toxicity. Clin Neuropharmacol 2003;26(6):287–8.
33. Vieweg WV, Wood MA. Tricyclic antidepressants, QT interval prolongation, and torsade de pointes. Psychosomatics 2004;45(5):371–7.
34. Thanacoody HR, Thomas SH. Tricyclic antidepressant poisoning. Toxicol Rev 2005;24(3):205–14.

35. Brown C, Taniguchi G, Yip K. The monoamine oxidase inhibitor—tyramine interaction. J Clin Pharmacol 1989;29(6):529–32.
36. Linden CH, Rumack BH, Strehlke C. Monoamine oxidase inhibitor overdose. Ann Emerg Med 1984;13(12):1137–44.
37. McLean MM, Sherwin H, Madabhushi V, et al. A 17-year-old female patient with a lithium overdose. Air Med J 2015;34(4):162–5.
38. Okusa MD, Crystal LJ. Clinical manifestations and management of acute lithium intoxication. Am J Med 1994;97:383–9.
39. Ferron G, Debray M, Buneaux F, et al. Pharmacokinetics of lithium in plasma and red blood cells in acute and chronic intoxicated patients. Int J Clin Pharmacol Ther 1995;33:351–5.
40. Atherton JC, Doyle A, Gee A, et al. Lithium clearance: modification by the loop of Henle in man. J Physiol 1991;437(1):377–91.
41. Munshi KR, Thampy A. The syndrome of irreversible lithium-effectuated neurotoxicity. Clin Neuropharmacol 2005;28(1):38–49.
42. Stone KA. Lithium-induced nephrogenic diabetes insipidus. J Am Board Fam Pract 1999;12(1):43–7.
43. Gill J, Singh H, Nugent K. Acute lithium intoxication and neuroleptic malignant syndrome. Pharmacotherapy 2003;23(6):811–5.
44. Serinken M, Karcioglu O, Korkmaz A. Rarely seen cardiotoxicity of lithium overdose: complete heart block. Int J Cardiol 2009;132(2):276–8.
45. Gerstner T, Buesing D, Longin E, et al. Valproic acid induced encephalopathy–19 new cases in Germany from 1994 to 2003–a side effect associated to VPA-therapy not only in young children. Seizure 2006;15(6):443–8.
46. Ohtani Y, Endo F, Matsuda I. Carnitine deficiency and hyperammonemia associated with valproic acid therapy. J Pediatr 1982;101(5):782–5.
47. Spiller HA, Hays HL, Aleguas A Jr. Overdose of drugs for attention-deficit hyperactivity disorder: clinical presentation, mechanisms of toxicity, and management. CNS Drugs 2013;27(7):531–43.
48. Kashani J, Ruha AM. Isolated atomoxetine overdose resulting in seizure. J Emerg Med 2007;32(2):175–8.
49. Seger DL. Clonidine toxicity revisited. J Toxicol Clin Toxicol 2002;40(2):145–55.
50. Greenblatt DJ, Allen MD, Noel BJ, et al. Acute overdosage with benzodiazepine derivatives. Clin Pharmacol Ther 1977;21(4):497–514.
51. Greenblatt DJ, Allen MD, Harmatz JS, et al. Overdosage with pentobarbital and secobarbital: assessment of factors related to outcome. J Clin Pharmacol 1979; 19(11):758–68.
52. Botero M, Enneking FK. Reversal of prolonged unconsciousness by naloxone after an intravascular injection of a local anesthetic and clonidine. Anesth Analg 1999;88(5):1185–6.
53. Kulig K, Duffy J, Rumack BH, et al. Naloxone for treatment of clonidine overdose. JAMA 1982;247(12):1697.
54. Tsze DS, Dayan PS. Treatment of guanfacine toxicity with naloxone. Pediatr Emerg Care 2012;28(10):1060–1.
55. Roberge RJ, Francis EH. Use of naloxone in valproic acid overdose: case report and review. J Emerg Med 2002;22(1):67–70.
56. Boyer EW. Management of opioid analgesic overdose. N Engl J Med 2012; 367(2):146–55.
57. Buajordet I, Naess A, Jacobsen D, et al. Adverse events after naloxone treatment of episodes of suspected acute opioid overdose. Eur J Emerg Med 2004;11: 19–23.

58. Moore PW, Donovan JW, Burkhart KK, et al. Safety and efficacy of flumazenil for reversal of iatrogenic benzodiazepine-associated delirium toxicity during treatment of alcohol withdrawal, a retrospective review at one center. J Med Toxicol 2014;10(2):126–32.
59. Veiraiah A, Dyas J, Cooper G, et al. Flumazenil use in benzodiazepine overdose in the UK: a retrospective survey of NPIS data. Emerg Med J 2012;29(7):565–9.
60. Blackman K, Brown SG, Wilkes GJ. Plasma alkalinization for tricyclic antidepressant toxicity: a systematic review. Emerg Med 2001;13(2):204–10.
61. Seger DL, Hantsch C, Zavoral T, et al. Variability of recommendations for serum alkalinization in tricyclic antidepressant overdose: a survey of U.S. Poison Center medical directors. J Toxicol Clin Toxicol 2003;41(4):331–8.
62. Tenenbein M. Do you really need that emergency drug screen? Clin Toxicol 2009; 47(4):286–91.
63. Greene S, Harris C, Singer J. Gastrointestinal decontamination of the poisoned patient. Pediatr Emerg Care 2008;24(3):176–86.
64. Bretaudeau Deguigne M, Hamel JF, Boels D, et al. Lithium poisoning: the value of early digestive tract decontamination. Clin Toxicol 2013;51(4):243–8.
65. Burns MJ, Linden CH, Graudins A, et al. A comparison of physostigmine and benzodiazepines for the treatment of anticholinergic poisoning. Ann Emerg Med 2000;35(4):374–81.
66. Suchard JR. Assessing physostigmine's contraindication in cyclic antidepressant ingestions. J Emerg Med 2003;25(2):185–91.
67. Perrott J, Murphy NG, Zed PJ. L-carnitine for acute valproic acid overdose: a systematic review of published cases. Ann Pharmacother 2010;44(7–8):1287–93.
68. Jaeger A, Sauder P, Kopferschmitt J, et al. When should dialysis be performed in lithium poisoning? A kinetic study 14 cases lithium poisoning. J Toxicol Clin Toxicol 1993;31(3):429–47.
69. Proudfoot AT, Krenzelok EP, Vale JA. Position paper on urine alkalinization. J Toxicol Clin Toxicol 2004;42(1):1–26.
70. Mactier R, Laliberté M, Mardini J, et al, EXTRIP Workgroup. Extracorporeal treatment for barbiturate poisoning: recommendations from the EXTRIP Workgroup. Am J Kidney Dis 2014;64(3):347–58.
71. Ghannoum M, Laliberté M, Nolin TD, et al. Extracorporeal treatment for valproic acid poisoning: systematic review and recommendations from the EXTRIP workgroup. Clin Toxicol 2015;53(5):454–65.

The Changing Health Policy Environment and Behavioral Health Services Delivery

Laura N. Medford-Davis, MD, MS[a,*], Rakel C. Beall, MD, MPH[b]

KEYWORDS

- Deinstitutionalization • Insurance coverage • Health policy
- Affordable Care Act (ACA) • Mental Health Parity and Addiction Equity Act (MHPAEA)
- Psychiatric crisis • Opioid addiction • Drug abuse

KEY POINTS

- Deinstitutionalization began closing inpatient psychiatric beds in the 1950s, and the United States now has less than 25% of the number of beds needed for the population size.
- Cuts to public funding and limited insurance coverage of mental health care have also severely limited access to outpatient psychiatric care.
- The Mental Health Parity and Addiction Equity Act of 2008, the Affordable Care Act of 2010, and subsequent federal regulations improve access to mental health services, but lack of funding and poor enforcement of new rules continue to hinder progress.
- Without reliable access to outpatient care, many patients with mental illness find themselves in an acute psychiatric crisis, shifting mental health care to the criminal justice system and emergency departments.
- Substance abuse often compounds or mimics acute psychiatric crisis.

DEINSTITUTIONALIZATION: THE DECLINE OF INPATIENT PSYCHIATRIC BED AVAILABILITY

Beginning in the 1950s, deinstitutionalization called for the transfer of psychiatric care from inpatient and residential facilities to the outpatient setting. The result has been the steady closure of state inpatient facilities and a critical shortage of psychiatric treatment because inpatient closures have not been matched by a commensurate increase in outpatient treatment options. Instead total state spending on public mental health services, both inpatient and outpatient, decreased 30% from 1955 to 1997.[1]

[a] Department of Emergency Medicine, Baylor College of Medicine, 1504 Taub Loop, Houston, TX 77030, USA; [b] Meninger Department of Psychiatry, Baylor College of Medicine, One Baylor Plaza - BCM350, Houston, TX 77030, USA
* Corresponding author.
E-mail address: medford.davis@gmail.com

Psychiatr Clin N Am 40 (2017) 533–540
http://dx.doi.org/10.1016/j.psc.2017.05.013
0193-953X/17/© 2017 Elsevier Inc. All rights reserved.

Between 2005 and 2010, 13 states closed more than 25% of their beds and 4 closed more than half of their beds.[2]

The minimum standard for state inpatient psychiatric beds is 50 beds per 100,000 population census, but in 2016 the United States provided 11.7 per 100,000, just 23% of those needed.[2] The current bed count is less than in 1850 when inpatient psychiatric treatment first began, and only 3.5% of the beds available in 1955 before deinstitutionalization began.[2] Only 1 state and the District of Columbia have more than 20 beds per 100,000, whereas 16 states have less than 10 beds per 100,000, 4 states have less than 5 per 100,000, and Iowa has only 2 per 100,000.[3]

In addition, almost half of these state inpatient beds are used by patients charged with or convicted of crimes, leaving even fewer beds available for patients in psychiatric crisis living in the general population.[3] Inadequate staffing ratios can prevent existing beds from being occupied, further exacerbating the shortage.[4] Bed closures are not limited to public facilities. Nonpublic beds also shrunk 62% from 1970 to 2000, with 32% of the reduction occurring between 1990 and 2000. Adding nonstate inpatient beds to the national census brings the number available up to 25 per 100,000, still only half of those required.[3,4]

THE SIMULTANEOUS CRISIS IN OUTPATIENT PSYCHIATRIC CARE AVAILABILITY

Outpatient access to psychiatric care is also nearly nonexistent. More than half of US counties have no psychiatrist, psychologist, or social worker.[3] The number of psychiatrists declined by 10% relative to the population in the first decade of the twenty-first century.[5] Even in urban areas, after discharge from the emergency department (ED) only 22% of privately insured and 12% of Medicaid patients were able to make a follow-up appointment for depression.[6] This dearth of outpatient services contributes both to the lack of inpatient beds available, and to the number of patients in crisis needing an inpatient bed. Inpatients who have recovered enough to transfer to outpatient care continue to await outpatient service availability before discharge, worsening the inpatient bed availability crisis.[7] Meanwhile insurance ceases to cover their ongoing inpatient services because they no longer meet inpatient criteria, driving inpatient services into operating losses, which then cause more inpatient beds to close.

Patients with psychiatric illness living in the community also cannot access timely outpatient care due to the shortage, so their conditions deteriorate until they arrive to the ED in crisis requiring an inpatient admission.[2,4,7] This shortage of outpatient care creates a revolving door in which patients continually cycle through the ED and inpatient care but never link into the long-term care they need to control their illness and prevent crisis.[4] Besides time spent in the ED awaiting psychiatric care, many mentally ill patients who cannot access needed care end up homeless or incarcerated, with as many as two-thirds of the homeless population suffering from mental illness.[2]

INSURANCE ISSUES

Poor insurance coverage of psychiatric services further limits access to outpatient treatment. Among the limited number of psychiatrists who practice, the specialty is less likely to accept any type of insurance. Only 55.3% accept private insurance, 55% accept Medicare, and 43% accept Medicaid.[8] Historically, many private insurance plans have not covered mental health treatment or have provided minimal coverage with high out-of-pocket costs, strict limits on annual spending, prior authorization requirements, and frequent denials. Uninsured patients have even fewer options, and patients with mental illness are more likely to allow their insurance to lapse or to experience disorganized social situations such as homelessness that make it difficult to maintain insurance coverage. Uninsured patients are almost 4 times less likely to be admitted when presenting to the ED for psychiatric illness, perhaps due to difficulty finding placement rather than a lack of need.[9]

Medicaid is the largest payer of mental health services.[10] However, the Institutions for Mental Diseases exclusion prevents federal Medicaid funds from paying for inpatient treatment in dedicated psychiatric facilities with more than 16 beds for patients aged 21 to 64 years. This exclusion has limited the available inpatient treatment options for many Medicaid patients, increasing their boarding times. In May of 2016, the Centers for Medicare and Medicaid Services issued a new rule allowing payment to these facilities but only for Medicaid-managed care organizations.[11] The exclusion continues to limit care for fee-for-service Medicaid recipients, although a demonstration by the Innovation Center under the Affordable Care Act (ACA) is testing the feasibility and outcomes of waiving this rule in 11 states and the District of Columbia.[12]

Poor insurance coverage coupled with a limited number of inpatient beds, outpatient centers, and psychiatrists leads to a serious shortage of needed psychiatric care. Many states shift the high cost of psychiatric care to the federal government by placing dual eligible patients in nursing homes instead of state inpatient facilities, or to the criminal justice system in which the cost of treatment is less per patient than in state inpatient facilities.[2] As a result, more than a third of adults with serious mental illness receive no treatment in any given year, and the percentage has increased from 2008 to 2012.[13] Access to treatment varies by state, with 57% of adults untreated in Vermont but only 30% in Hawaii.[13]

THE ROLE OF THE CRIMINAL JUSTICE SYSTEM

During the crises caused by the lack of available psychiatric care, many mentally ill patients act out or break laws and are arrested as a result. Anywhere from 20% to 50% of incarcerated persons suffer from serious mental illness, and improved treatment of their mental illness might have prevented many from committing the crimes that led to their arrest.[3] Research shows a correlation between cuts to psychiatric inpatient funding and increases in both violent crimes and arrest-related deaths.[2]

Due to the lack of psychiatric treatment, which increases mental health crises and subsequent crimes committed by the mentally ill, prisons and jails have become the de facto replacements for inpatient psychiatric care. In 44 states, jails hold more mentally ill persons than state hospitals[3] and nationwide there are 3 times more mentally ill in jails and prisons than in hospitals.[2] The biggest inpatient psychiatric bed facilities are now found in the county jails of the 3 largest US cities.[2] New Hampshire even sends noncriminal patients to jail facilities for psychiatric treatment due to a lack of available civil options.

Unfortunately, in many states, even while incarcerated, 84% of patients with mental illness in jail and 75% of those in prison do not receive needed mental health treatment.[2] Many of these patients are placed on waiting lists for treatment in the limited number of state inpatient psychiatric beds. With an insufficient quantity of these beds, states must choose between leaving incarcerated patients in jail without treatment for long periods, increasing violence, suicide, and self-mutilation within jails, or leaving the nonincarcerated mentally ill without access to care, increasing violent crime in the public sphere.[3]

EMERGENCY DEPARTMENT BOARDING

Those patients in acute psychiatric crisis who escape being arrested are often brought to general hospital EDs for care. Limited availability of psychiatric care has increased the number of psychiatric patients presenting to EDs in such crises, while simultaneously increasing wait times for the evaluation and inpatient placement of psychiatric patients held in EDs. Boarding, the time between the decision to admit a patient and when the patient leaves the ED, is particularly burdensome for psychiatric patients who remain in the ED 3.2 times longer than nonpsychiatric patients awaiting admission.[14]

Providers cite a lack of inpatient beds as the biggest contributor to boarding.[4] One ED saw a threefold increase in ED visits requiring psychiatric evaluation, a 64% increase in wait times for psychiatric evaluation, and an overall fivefold increase in the hours ED beds were occupied by psychiatric patients when a neighboring inpatient and outpatient psychiatric treatment center closed.[15] Due to the lack of inpatient beds to transfer patients to, some patients who psychiatrists recommend for inpatient care are instead transferred to lower levels of care or discharged home when no inpatient facility can be found,[16] whereas others are admitted to medical beds from which they continue to await a psychiatric bed in which they can receive the psychiatric treatment they actually need.[4] Other factors contributing to long boarding times include lack of insurance, public insurance, restraint use, alcohol intoxication, and the need for transfer to an outside facility.[16–18]

National surveys of the extent of the problem have found that 60% of psychiatric patients in 86% of hospitals experience long boarding times: 24 to 48 hours in 50% of hospitals and 5 days or more in 21% of hospitals.[19,20] Psychiatric boarding lasts so long that each bed occupied by a psychiatric boarder could have turned over for 2 additional patients, increasing crowding and wait times for all ED patients.[14,21] This is especially concerning because longer boarding times increase subsequent in-hospital length of stay and mortality.[22] In most EDs, psychiatric patients are not receiving any psychiatric treatment to improve their acute psychiatric illness while boarding[19] and the chaotic ED environment may actually worsen their symptoms.[4,23] In addition to worsening patient outcomes, long psychiatric boarding times burden hospitals with increased costs for staff, security, and meals, even though hospitals do not receive additional reimbursement for a longer length of stay in the ED.[24]

Several solutions to boarding have been proposed.[25] Treatment protocols and dedicated psychiatric observation units within EDs can expedite the stabilization of psychiatric crises while patients board. Telemedicine can connect trained mental health providers with patients, expediting the initial evaluation and recommendation. In addition to increasing the number of available inpatient beds, statewide dashboards that match waiting patients to current bed availability, and mobile crisis units and ED case management that can find outpatient services for patients who may be well enough for discharge, can all decrease wait times for placement.

IMPACT OF THE MENTAL HEALTH PARITY AND ADDICTION EQUITY ACT (2008) AND THE AFFORDABLE CARE ACT (2010)

Several new laws and regulations in the past few years have improved access to mental health care. The Mental Health Parity Act of 1996 prohibited large group insurance plans from making lifetime or annual spending limits for mental health benefits that were more stringent than limits for medical or surgical benefits. The Mental Health Parity and Addiction Equity Act (MHPAEA) of 2008 extended parity to substance abuse benefits and to all aspects of coverage for mental health and substance use disorders, not just spending limits.[26] However, neither of these laws required coverage of mental health care; they only required parity when mental health coverage was offered. In addition the laws applied only to large private group plans with at least

50 employees but not to Medicaid or Medicare, although simultaneously the Medicare Improvements for Patients and Providers Act of 2008 eliminated higher copayments for mental health treatments within the Medicare program.[26] In 2009, the Children's Health Insurance Program (CHIP) Reauthorization Act applied similar parity requirements to CHIP coverage.[26]

The ACA of 2010 made 2 major improvements to mental health access. It was the first law to mandate coverage of mental health and substance abuse services as an essential health benefit. The ACA also extended the MHPAEA parity requirements to individual and small group plans, and to Medicaid. Most recently, a Department of Defense rule in 2016 mandated parity for Tricare recipients.[26]

However, challenges still remain and enforcement has been limited. A review of plans offered to individuals through the ACA marketplace found that 25% of plans offered were not consistent with MHPAEA requirements.[27] In addition, denials remain more commonplace, and medical necessity and prior authorization were invoked twice as often to deny mental health services despite the protections of the MHPAEA.[27] Many plans do not cover common psychiatric medications, and in-network psychiatric providers are limited and have long wait times for appointments.[27]

SUBSTANCE ABUSE AND MISUSE

Any discussion of mental health care delivery in or outside of the ED or criminal justice system must also include acknowledgment that many emergent psychiatric and behavioral health crises arise in the context of acute substance intoxication, withdrawal, or dependence. Although many patients present to the nation's EDs with

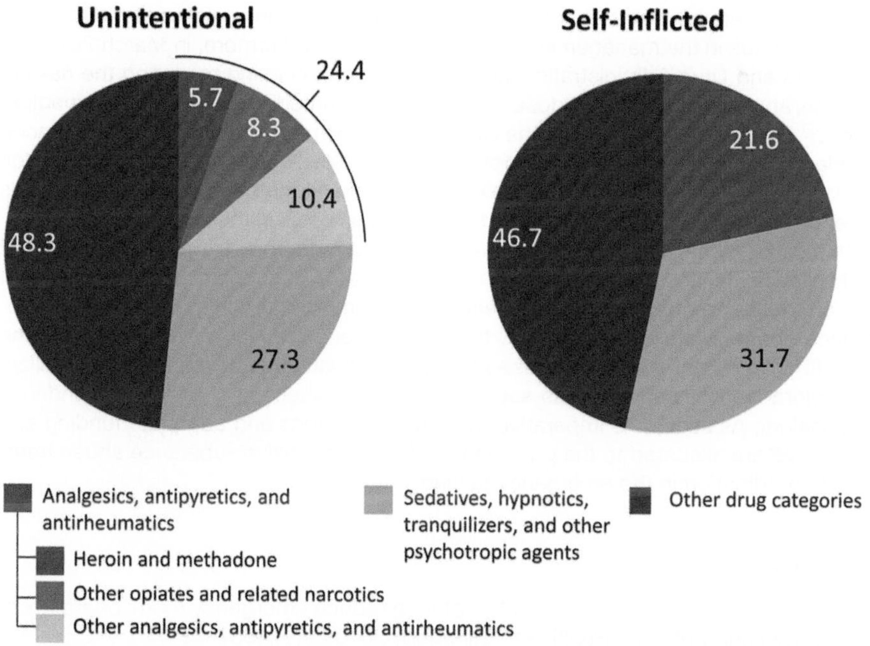

Fig. 1. Percentage of ED visits for drug poisoning, by intent and drug category: United States 2008 to 2011. (*From* Albert M, McCaig LF, Uddin S. Emergency department visits for drug poisoning: United States, 2008-2011. NCHS data brief, no 196. Hyattsville (MD): National Center for Health Statistics. 2015.)

primary nonsubstance-related changes in mental status, many others are doing so primarily due to their misuse of both medical and recreational psychotropic drugs. Between 2008 and 2011, about one-half of visits for both intentional and accidental drug poisoning (suicidal or recreational) resulted from poisoning by drugs in the categories of analgesics, antipyretics, and antirheumatics, or sedatives, hypnotics, tranquilizers, and other psychotropic agents (**Fig. 1**).[28] This means that, not only are psychiatrically ill patients misusing their prescribed medications to harm themselves intentionally, many others are presenting in crisis because they are misusing licit and illicit psychotropic substances recreationally.

Moreover, intentional misuse of prescription medications has now overtaken that of illicit drugs in the emergency setting. ED visits involving recreational use of pharmaceuticals (either alone or in combination with another drug) increased 98.4% between 2004 and 2009, from 627,291 visits to 1,244,679, respectively.[29] Likewise, the Drug Abuse Warning Network estimates that of the 2.1 million drug abuse visits in 2009, 27.1% involved recreational use of pharmaceuticals, whereas 21.2% involved illicit drugs. As such, the aforementioned heavy reliance on the criminal justice system to house and treat psychiatric patients does very little to stem the tide of ED patients made ill by legal pharmaceutical substances. In fact, the pharmaceuticals most largely involved in the staggering increase in drug-related ED visits were oxycodone products (242.2% increase), alprazolam (148.3% increase), and hydrocodone products (124.5%).[29]

Whether these medications are obtained legally from a doctor's office or via diversion methods in the community, many patients who are misusing them do not come into contact with the criminal justice system but instead with the ED. This presents a unique challenge to policymakers, in that harm-reduction efforts must also be aimed at modifying prescriber behaviors. The opioid epidemic has resulted in the recent issuance of Centers for Disease Control and Prevention guidelines aimed at reducing the use of opiates in the management of chronic pain.[30] Furthermore, in March 2016, the US Food and Drug Administration issued a black box warning regarding the risks of misuse, abuse, addiction, overdose, and death with immediate-release opioid medications.[31] Finally, in October 2016, the US Drug Enforcement Administration announced its plans to reduce the amount of almost every schedule II opiate and opioid medication produced in America by 25% or more in 2017.[32] Taken together, these policy changes offer a glimpse of hope for stemming the tide of this crisis in the coming years.

In the meantime, it will fall to emergency physicians to absorb a population that not only has very limited resources for singular psychiatric or substance abuse treatment but also a dearth of dual-diagnosis treatment of comorbid psychiatric illness and substance abuse. More often than not, these physicians are also doing so without the benefit of assistance from in-house psychiatric consultants or appropriate ancillary behavioral health staff, such as social workers and licensed chemical dependency counselors. As such, it is imperative that policy solutions and adequate funding and resources are allocated to the purveyance of comprehensive substance abuse treatment coordination in the emergency setting.

REFERENCES

1. Alakeson V, Pande N, Ludwig M. A plan to reduce emergency room 'boarding' of psychiatric patients. Health Aff (Millwood) 2010;29(9):1637–42.

2. Torrey EF, Fuller DA, Geller J, et al. No room at the Inn: trends and consequences of closing public psychiatric hospitals 2005-2010. Arlington (VA): Treatment Advocacy Center; 2012.

3. Fuller DA, Sinclair E, Geller J, et al. Going, going, gone: trends and consequences of eliminating state psychiatric beds. Arlington (VA): Treatment Advocacy Center; 2016.
4. Bender D, Pande N, Ludwig M. U.S. Department of Health and Human Services Assistant Secretary for Planning and Evaluation Office of Disability, Aging and Long-Term Care Policy. A Literature Review: Psychiatric Boarding. Washington, DC: U.S. Department of Health and Human Services; 2008.
5. Bishop TF, Seirup JK, Pincus HA, et al. Population of US Practicing psychiatrists declined, 2003-13, which may help explain poor access to mental health care. Health Aff (Millwood) 2016;35(7):1271–7.
6. Rhodes KV, Vieth TL, Kushner H, et al. Referral without access: for psychiatric services, wait for the beep. Ann Emerg Med 2009;54(2):272–8.
7. Appelbaum PS. The 'quiet' crisis in mental health services. Health Aff (Millwood) 2003;22(5):110–6.
8. Bishop TF, Press MJ, Keyhani S, et al. Acceptance of insurance by psychiatrists and the implications for access to mental health care. JAMA Psychiatry 2014; 71(2):176–81.
9. Owens PL, Mutter R, Stocks C. Mental Health and Substance Abuse-Related Emergency Department Visits among Adults, 2007. HCUP Statistical Brief #92. Rockville (MD): Agency for Healthcare Research and Quality; 2010.
10. Medicaid.gov Behavioral Health Services. Available at: https://www.medicaid.gov/medicaid/benefits/bhs/index.html. Accessed November 26, 2016.
11. Centers for Medicare & Medicaid Services (CMS), HHS. Medicaid and Children's Health Insurance Program (CHIP) Programs; Medicaid Managed Care, CHIP Delivered in Managed Care, and Revisions to Third Party Liability. Fed Regist 2016;81:27497–901.
12. Medicaid Emergency Psychiatric demonstration frequently asked questions. Available at: https://innovation.cms.gov/initiatives/medicaid-emergency-psychiatric-demo/faq.html. Accessed November 26, 2016.
13. Substance Abuse and Mental Health Services Administration. Behavioral Health Barometer: United States, 2013. Rockville (MD): U.S. Department of Health and Human Services; 2013.
14. Nicks BA, Manthey DM. The impact of psychiatric patient boarding in emergency departments. Emerg Med Int 2012;2012:360308.
15. Nesper AC, Morris BA, Scher LM, et al. Effect of decreasing county mental health services on the emergency department. Ann Emerg Med 2016;67(4):525–30.
16. Park JM, Park LT, Siefert CJ, et al. Factors associated with extended length of stay for patients presenting to an urban psychiatric emergency service: a case-control study. J Behav Health Serv Res 2009;36(3):300–8.
17. Chang G, Weiss A, Kosowsky JM, et al. Characteristics of adult psychiatric patients with stays of 24 hours or more in the emergency department. Psychiatr Serv 2012;63(3):283–6.
18. Weiss AP, Chang G, Rauch SL, et al. Patient- and practice-related determinants of emergency department length of stay for patients with psychiatric illness. Ann Emerg Med 2012;60(2):162–71.e165.
19. Psychiatric and Substance Abuse Survey. Irving (TX): American College for Emergency Physicians; 2008.
20. Emergency Department Challenges and Trends 2010 Survey of Hospital Emergency Department Administrators. Lafayette (LA): Schumacher Group; 2010.
21. Falvo T, Grove L, Stachura R, et al. The opportunity loss of boarding admitted patients in the emergency department. Acad Emerg Med 2007;14(4):332–7.

22. Singer AJ, Thode HC Jr, Viccellio P, et al. The association between length of emergency department boarding and mortality. Acad Emerg Med 2011;18(12): 1324–9.
23. Manton A. Psychiatric patients in the Emergency Department: The dilemma of extended lengths of stay. Falls Church (VA): American Psychiatric Nurses Association; 2010.
24. Bender D, Pande N, Ludwig M. Psychiatric Boarding Interview Summary. Washington, DC: U.S. Department of Health and Human Services; 2009.
25. American College of Emergency Physicians Emergency Medicine Practice Committee. Practical solutions to boarding of psychiatric patients in the Emergency Department: does your Emergency Department have a psychiatric boarding problem? Irving (TX): American College of Emergency Physicians; 2015.
26. Executive Office of the President of the United States. The mental health and substance use disorder parity task force: final report. Washington, DC: U.S. Department of Health and Human Services; 2016.
27. Health Policy Brief: Enforcing Mental Health Parity. Health Affairs, November 9, 2015.
28. Albert M, McCaig L, Uddin S. Emergency Department visits for drug poisoning: United States, 2008-2011. NCHS data brief, no 196. Hyattsville (MD): National Center for Health Statistics; 2015.
29. National Institute on Drug Abuse. Drug Facts. Drug-Related Hospital Emergency Room Visits. Rockville (MD): National Institute on Drug Abuse; National Institutes of Health; U.S. Department of Health and Human Services; 2011.
30. Dowell D, Haegerich TM, Chou R. CDC guideline for prescribing opioids for chronic pain - United States, 2016. MMWR Recomm Rep 2016;65(1):1–49.
31. FDA News Release. FDA announces enhanced warnings for immediate-release opioid pain medications related to risks of misuse, abuse, addiction, overdose and death [press release]. Silver Spring (MD): U.S. Food & Drug Administration; 2016.
32. Barrett J. DEA Reduces Opioid Manufacturing for 2017. Pharmacy Times October 4, 2016.

Legal and Ethical Challenges, Part 1

General Population

Britta Ostermeyer, MD, MBA[a,*], Anim N. Shoaib, BS[b], Swapna Deshpande, MD[c]

KEYWORDS

• Emergency medicine • Emergency psychiatry • Ethics • Law • Legal principles

KEY POINTS

- The practice of emergency clinicians is governed by specific legal and ethical principles.
- Emergency clinicians are expected to provide care to patients in the emergency department, which often establishes a patient-physician relationship without a prior formal agreement.
- Under certain circumstances, emergency clinicians must breach confidentiality.
- In emergency medicine and psychiatry, there can be an exception to the informed-consent-to-treatment process in emergency situations.
- Patients can be placed on emergency holds, can receive medication over objection, and can be transferred voluntarily or involuntarily to an inpatient psychiatric setting.

PHYSICIAN-PATIENT RELATIONSHIP

The physician-patient relationship is a special relationship that remains the cornerstone of health care. Mutual trust and confidence by patients and physicians are essential to this *fiduciary* relationship in which physicians take care of patients. This special relationship demands a higher degree of care and responsibility from trusted physicians toward patients, who depend on knowledgeable physicians for help and care.

In the physician-patient relationship, emergency psychiatrists and clinicians have duties of *beneficence, nonmaleficence, respect for patient autonomy,* and *justice.*[1] *Beneficence* means that emergency clinicians act in the best interest of their patients

---

Disclosures: The authors have nothing to disclose.

[a] Department of Psychiatry and Behavioral Sciences, University of Oklahoma, 920 Stanton L. Young Boulevard, Oklahoma City, OK 73104, USA; [b] The Honors College, University of Houston, 212 M.D. Anderson Library, Houston, TX 77204, USA; [c] Department of Psychiatry and Behavioral Sciences, University of Oklahoma, 920 Stanton L. Young Boulevard, Oklahoma City, OK 73104, USA
* Corresponding author.
E-mail address: britta-ostermeyer@ouhsc.edu

Psychiatr Clin N Am 40 (2017) 541–553
http://dx.doi.org/10.1016/j.psc.2017.05.003
0193-953X/17/© 2017 Elsevier Inc. All rights reserved.

by responding promptly to acute illness to alleviate suffering and to minimize risk of injury or loss of life. *Nonmaleficence* is ensured by the emergency clinician's priority to refrain from inflicting harm to patients. This principle is essential to clinician integrity and patient trust. Emergency clinicians must respect *patients' autonomy* as adult patients with decision-making capacity who have the right to accept or refuse treatment even in the emergency department (ED). However, in a clear emergency situation whereby the patient is unable to consent, the emergency clinician can provide treatment necessary to stabilize the patient's condition to prevent injury or loss of life (see exceptions to informed consent discussed later). The principle of *justice* is understood as acting impartial and fair. Emergency clinicians provide care to patients regardless of race, color, sex, nationality, religious faith, or other properties.

As part of the physician-patient relationship, a physician is expected to practice within the standard of care for his or her profession, which is a *reasonable person's standard*. This medical standard of care is defined as providing the type of care that would be provided by other ordinary competent and skilled medical professionals with similar backgrounds and under similar patient circumstances in the same community. Of note, the reasonable person standard requires the provision of average care, not excellent or superior care.[2]

Often the question is, when is the physician-patient relationship established? Although states vary in how they define a physician-patient relationship, the relationship is generally established when a physician affirmatively acts in a patient's case by advising, examining, diagnosing, treating, or agreeing to treat.[3] Hence, in the ED, the relationship starts when physicians, even in the absence of written consent for treatment, attend to the medical needs of patients with an acute condition.

Although a general nonemergency physician is not obligated to treat patients whom he or she does not wish to treat, even by arbitrary standards, the obligation to treat is different for emergency physicians and psychiatrists in designated urgent care or emergency care centers. When it becomes apparent that patients are in need of immediate intervention, a therapeutic relationship is assumed to exist.[4] Therefore, when patients arrive at an urgent or emergency care center, the emergency physician has a duty to provide emergency medical and/or mental health care because patients may be in imminent need of services and arrived with the expectation of urgent treatment. Before such patients can leave the ED, the emergency clinician must ensure that no further immediate interventions are required.[4]

Once physicians enters into a physician-patient relationship, a legal contract is formed under which physicians owe a duty to patients to continue to treat patients until this relationship is properly terminated.[5] Commonly, physician abandonment of patients occurs when the physician terminates the relationship either at an unreasonable time or without affording patients some reasonable time to find a new physician to ensure continuum of care.[3] In general, once a duty of care is established, the emergency clinician's obligations are to (1) evaluate, treat, and stabilize patients and (2) properly identify patients' disposition. Emergency clinicians have 3 disposition options: (1) discharge with no further treatment, (2) discharge with outpatient treatment, or (3) admission for inpatient hospitalization.[4] Hence, in order to ensure a continuum of care for patients, emergency clinicians must provide discharge follow-up care plans with provider resources to patients who are in need of outpatient care on discharge from the ED.

MALPRACTICE

Malpractice falls under the legal category of a tort, which is a civil wrong in which a person damages a second person, who is then requesting compensation for damages.[2,4] Malpractice is a negligent tort in which a physician/clinician unintentionally failed to exercise the usual standard of care (see standard of care definition discussed earlier).

Psychiatric malpractice claims are less frequent than in other specialties and most often concern wrongful treatment, suicide, or drug reactions in psychiatry.[2,5–7] On the other hand, psychiatrists are at increased risk for disciplinary actions by medical licensing boards compared with other specialties.[7] Board-certified female psychiatrists who have been in practice for a short period of time have a lower incidence of board disciplinary actions.[7]

In order for a patient plaintiff to successfully sue a physician defendant in a malpractice lawsuit, the patient plaintiff must prove the following 4 elements (known as the *4 Ds*).[2,5]

1. *Duty*: The physician must have had a duty to the patient as part of a physician-patient relationship.
2. *Dereliction:* There must be a dereliction or breach of duty in which the physician provided less than the standard of care.
3. *Direct causation:* The physician's dereliction must have directly caused the patient damage.
4. *Damage:* The patient must have damage as a result of the dereliction.

Although in the past the standard of care was measured by local practices, today's standard of care has shifted to a national standard based on national practice guidelines. In litigation, the standard of care is established through the use of authoritative professional literature, practice guidelines, medication package inserts, applicable governmental regulation, hospital and clinic policies, accreditation standards, and expert witness testimony.[2,5] Evidence-based medicine has been introduced as well to help identify appropriate care. The American Association of Emergency Psychiatry can be a good resource as well.[8]

CONFIDENTIALITY, PRIVILEGE, AND DUTY TO REPORT

As part of the physician-patient relationship, confidentiality is the physician's obligation to not reveal any information about patients to anyone unless required to do so by law.[9,10] Federal laws, and typically state laws, stipulate a higher level of privacy pertaining to patients' mental health and substance use. The circle of confidentiality includes patients, current physicians and consulting physicians, and current medical treatment team members (eg, nurses and technicians). Those outside the circle of confidentiality include adult patients' family, friends, attorneys, outside physicians and therapists, and previous physicians, therapists, and medical team members. It is important to know that the federal Health Insurance Portability and Accountability Act law is additive to whatever laws exist in the state in which the physician practices; thus, clinicians must follow whatever laws protect more confidentiality.[9]

Although confidentiality is the physician's obligation to silence, privilege is the patients' legal right to bar a physician from testifying about the patients' information.[9,10] However, this patient privilege only applies to judicial settings and there are several exceptions, such as when patients are litigants, in court-ordered evaluations, or when patients represent a danger to self or others.

Under certain duties to report, physicians must breach confidentiality.[4,9,10] Some of these situations include (1) reporting child abuse to child protective services, (2) reporting abuse of elderly and/or intellectually disabled persons (in some states), (3) reporting a gunshot wound, (4) reporting a reportable contagious illness, or (5) warning third parties of a planned crime (in some states).[9]

The obligation to warn third parties of a planned crime is often referred to as the *Tarasoff warning* related to *Tarasoff v Regents of University of California* (*Tarasoff I,* 1974; revised in *Tarasoff II,* 1976),[11] which applies to many states, such as California. It is helpful to know that the Supreme Court of California in the later 1976 *Tarasoff II* decision stated,

> *"When a therapist determines...that his patient presents a serious danger of violence to another, he incurs an obligation to use reasonable care to protect the intended victim against such danger. The discharge of his duty may require the therapist to take one or more of various steps. Thus, it may call for him to warn the intended victim, to notify the police, or to take whatever steps are reasonably necessary under the circumstances."*[11]

It is important to note that the court changed the former *duty to warn* from the 1974 *Tarasoff I* decision to a *duty to protect* in the subsequent 1976 *Tarasoff II* decision. Therefore, the *Tarasoff warning* calls for a duty to protect, not a duty to warn, which is often misunderstood.[9] In the ED, reasonable steps to protect often include transferring mentally ill patients for inpatient psychiatric treatment.

It is permissible for physicians in their fiduciary duty to their patients to disclose certain limited information in a clear emergency situation without consent. For example, if a psychotic patient in the ED refuses to grant consent to the emergency physician to contact the patient's outpatient physician for clinical information, including history and prescribed medications, the emergency situation allows the emergency physician to contact and consult with the outpatient physician in an effort to effectively treat the patient.[4,10]

INFORMED CONSENT

In the case of *Schloendorff v Society of New York Hospital* (1914) establishing the principle of informed consent,[12] Justice Benjamin Cardozo wrote in the court's opinion:

> *Every human being of adult years and sound mind has a right to determine what shall be done with his body; and a surgeon who performs an operation without his patient's consent commits an assault for which he is liable in damages. This is true except in cases of emergency where the patient is unconscious and where it is necessary to operate before consent can be obtained.*[12]

The required medical-legal informed consent process to medical treatment necessitates the presence of the following 3 elements.

1. *Knowledge:* Patients have the knowledge or information pertaining to the health care decision they are to make.
2. *Competency:* Patients are competent (see later discussion).
3. *Voluntary:* Patients make their treatment decision voluntarily and were not coerced. An involuntary consent would make the clinician liable for battery.[5,13]

When it comes to the question of how much medical information a clinician is to convey to patients in the consent process, the court formulated the *Materiality of Information Standard* in the landmark case of *Canterbury v Spence,* Washington DC (1972).[14] In this case, the United States Court of Appeals for the District of Columbia Circuit ruled that the standard is what a *reasonable* person needs to know for his or her medical decision-making, to include the following: (1) the condition being treated; (2) the proposed treatment; (3) the anticipated results; (4) recognized risks and benefits; and (5) known alternative forms of treatment, including the likely outcome if left untreated.

There are 4 stipulated exceptions to the informed consent process before a medical intervention: (1) emergency, (2) waiver, (3) therapeutic privilege, and (4) incompetence.[4,5,13] The *emergency* exception stipulates that if incompetent or nonresponsive patients are in need of emergency treatment to prevent serious injury or death and are unable to consent, a physician can provide standard-of-care medical treatment to stabilize patients. In a *waiver* situation, patients agree to give the physician some leverage over treatment decisions and release from liability, for example, a patient undergoing scheduled surgery may agree for the surgeon to extend the anticipated scope of surgery if needed. A clinician may use *therapeutic privilege* when revealing information to patients with unstable medical conditions, for example, an acute myocardial infarction, which could seriously worsen the patients' unstable condition. *Incompetence* and *capacity* in medical decision-making are discussed in detail in the later sections. It is important to understand that, although competent patients can refuse treatment, they do not have a right to demand specific treatments that clinicians think are not indicated or are harmful.[13]

MEDICAL DECISION-MAKING CAPACITY

Patients' medical decision-making capability is called *capacity* by clinicians in medical settings, and courts refer to capacity as *competency* when adjudicating a person's decision-making capabilities in the legal setting.[13] In this medical article, the authors use the term *capacity* to designate patients' medical decision-making capabilities.

The law assumes that all persons of adult age are presumed to be competent to make their own medical treatment decisions. A medical capacity evaluation is conducted when patients exhibit decision-making difficulties. Grisso and Appelbaum[15] have formulated a model that requires the following 4 abilities for medical decision-making capacity.

1. The ability to express a choice
2. The ability to understand information relevant to treatment decision-making
3. The ability to appreciate the significance of that information for one's own situation, in particular to one's illness and the probable consequences of one's treatment options
4. The ability to reason with the relevant information so as to engage in a logical process of weighing different treatment options[15]

Capacity is time specific and can change over time, that is, patients might lack the capacity while psychiatrically ill but may have regained full medical decision-making capacity on stabilization. Clinicians must, therefore, reevaluate patients' capacity when their medical situation changes.[13]

Most clinicians approach capacity as task-specific and depends on the likely anticipated decisional consequences to patients, which is referred to as the *sliding scale approach*.[13,16] In this model, high-risk decisions with a potential for negative consequences, such as the consent for brain surgery, require more patient capacity to consent in that patients are required to have a greater capability to examine and weigh the facts and potential treatment consequences. Low-risk decisions with a low risk of side effects and a high likelihood of benefits, such as the consent for much-needed dialysis in renal failure, require less capacity by patients in that patients simply have to evaluate fewer facts and the choice might be obvious, that is, dialysis for renal failure in order to survive. Hence, a person with advanced dementia might be able to consent to low-risk procedures, such as blood drawings or dialysis, but may lack the capacity to consent to elective brain surgery because of a mismatch between the task-specific demands and patients' limited/impaired ability. Conversely, demented patients may lack capacity to refuse a low-risk procedure if not undergoing such a low-risk procedure could result in probable loss of limb or life.

VICARIOUS DECISION-MAKING

When patients are no longer competent, the clinician needs to follow applicable federal and state laws pertaining to vicarious decision-making.[13,16] All states in the United States encourage competent patients to sign an *advance directive* (living will) for resolution of future medical decisions in the event patients become no longer competent. If patients have an advanced directive, the clinician must follow the patients' explicit choice as per their advance directive. Additionally, patients can appoint a health care agent (also known as proxy, surrogate, or conservator) in their advance directive to ensure that the clinician follows the patients' advance directive.

In the absence of an advanced directive, clinicians must contact patients' next of kin. Although there is some state-to-state variability, a close family member is usually asked to make medical decisions on behalf of incompetent patients. Most jurisdictions stipulate that first the patients' spouse, then the patients' adult children, and then the patients' siblings are to be consulted regarding medical treatment decisions. States typically stipulate that the vicarious decision makers replicate decisions that (formerly competent) patients would have made given the specific circumstances and situation. This is referred to as *substituted judgment*.[16] If the patients' preferences are unknown, such as in patients with intellectual disability with no prior history of competence, the vicarious decision maker should use the *best interest standard*, that is, the surrogate must decide in the best interest of the patients' well-being and health.[16]

EMERGENCY MEDICAL TREATMENT AND LABOR ACT

Enacted in 1986, the Emergency Medical Treatment and Labor Act (EMTALA) is a federal law that mandates any patient presenting to the ED with an emergent medical condition be treated and stabilized.[17] The law is famously known as the antidumping law as it prevents EDs from denying care to patients based on ability to pay, insurance status, race, sex, ethnicity, or creed.

Before the EMTALA was enacted, many private hospitals would transfer patients who were unable to pay to public hospitals. These patients, transferred without any medical examination or treatment, would often face severe complications in their conditions during the transfer process. Through the EMTALA, the US Congress sought to change this by mandating that emergency physicians perform a medical screening examination on any person who arrives at the emergency department. This examination is used to determine if patients' complaints are, in fact, an emergent medical condition. The EMTALA defines such an emergent condition as "a condition manifesting itself by acute symptoms of sufficient severity (including severe pain) such that the absence of immediate medical attention could reasonably be expected to result in placing the individual's health or the health of an unborn child in serious jeopardy, serious impairment to bodily functions, or serious dysfunction of bodily organs."[17] If an emergency physician finds such a condition or has sufficient reason to think that such a condition may be present, then they are obligated under the EMTALA to, at the minimum, provide stabilizing treatment to the best of their ability.

Patients with emergency conditions whose medical needs cannot be met by the ED's facility may be transferred to a facility that meets patients' needs in what

EMTALA defines as an appropriate transfer.[17] Such a transfer can only be performed if the following conditions are satisfied:

1. The ED provides stabilizing treatment to the best of their capacity to patients.
2. The risks of transferring patients are outweighed by the benefits of treatment at the receiving hospital.
3. The receiving hospital is confirmed to have the required services available and accepts the incoming patient transfer.

The EMTALA's guidelines carry significant penalties if violated and, thus, operate as an emergency physician's standard of care. Many uninsured and impoverished individuals gain access to health care through the EMTALA; therefore, EDs receive many types of medical cases, including psychiatric cases. Because the EMTALA's guidelines equally apply to psychiatric patients, emergency physicians must stabilize these patients on presentation to the ED.

RIGHT TO TREATMENT AND HOSPITAL ADMISSION

The right to mental health treatment dates back to the eighteenth century and the British Parliament's Vagrancy Act in which it was first recognized that persons with mental illness require treatment.[18] In 1960, Dr Morton Birnbaum first requested that courts grant a constitutionally protected right to treatment when persons with mental illness are deprived of their freedom and are institutionalized. This request refers to the underlying principle of quid pro quo (this for that) in which the mentally ill person gives away his or her liberty in exchange for treatment, which is one of the principles of involuntary hospital admission.[18]

In the case of *Rouse v Cameron,* Washington DC (1966), Judge Bazelon of the United States Court of Appeals for the District of Columbia recognized for the first time the right to treatment and wrote "the purpose of involuntary hospitalization is treatment, not punishment."[19] In that case, the court also stipulated that the hospital does not need to show that treatment will cure or improve the person but that there is a "bona fide effort to do so." In addition, the court articulated the concept of individual treatment plans and that "failure to provide suitable and adequate treatment cannot be justified by lack of staff or facility."[18,19]

All states allow adult patients to voluntarily enter a psychiatric hospital with statutory requirements that patients are in need of mental health care and the facility is equipped to provide the needed care. There is state variability at which age adolescents can consent to inpatient psychiatric treatment, with a range of 12 to 18 years.[4] Some states require that patients are competent to sign in for a voluntary psychiatric admission, whereas other states do not specify this requirement, likely because of concerns of depriving persons of needed inpatient care.[4] In the Florida case of *Zinermon v Burch* (1990), the US Supreme Court held in a narrow focus that patient Burch could raise a claim under a specific section of the federal civil rights. Burch alleged that he was deprived of his liberty without due process when he was admitted voluntarily as he was incompetent to give informed consent.[20]

The American Psychiatric Association (APA) task force on consent to voluntary hospitalization recognizes the many advantages of a voluntary admission over an involuntary admission because it maintains the patients' autonomy, maximizes patients' rights, reduces stigma, broadens access to inpatient care as many patients do not meet the criteria for involuntary admission, may allow for earlier treatment initiation before patients are more deteriorated, enhances the collaborative treatment relationship, may lead to more favorable outcome, and avoids increased costs for the mental health system and the courts that are incurred by involuntary admission processes.[21] Although the APA task force recommended screening each patient for capacity to sign for voluntary psychiatric admission, only a minimum level of capacity is required. Gutheil and Appelbaum[4] state that patients who understand that they are entering a hospital and recognize that they may not be able to leave at will if they are deemed to be a danger to self or others meet sufficient criteria for capacity to sign for voluntary psychiatric admission.[4]

Most states allow for a *conditional* voluntary status admission, which allows the facility to hold patients for a certain period of time, usually hours to a few days, even on voluntarily admitted patients' request to leave. This time interval is designed to allow clinicians to evaluate if patients meet the criteria for conversion to involuntary status and for the preparation of discharge planning in case the patients must be released.[4]

INVOLUNTARY COMMITMENT

The historical principles for involuntary hospitalization of the mentally ill are parens patriae and the state's *police power. Parens patriae* means "parent of the country" and goes back to Anglo-American law and the power of English kings, who were viewed as the fathers of their people.[4] This principle is one of the underlying principles for commitment laws that grant the government/state the public policy power to intervene, protect, and make decisions for persons who are unable to care for themselves. *Police power* gives the government the right to protect its citizens from harm and to maintain safety in society.

Most states allow for short-term hospitalizations (emergency holds) of patients in psychiatric emergency situations for a limited amount until a court hearing can take place.[4] The time interval for such holds varies from state to state and is usually between 2 days to 3 weeks. A physician, psychiatrist, or psychologist (or, in some states, other licensed mental health professionals) must sign a mental health emergency certificate attesting that patients are mentally ill and because of mental illness are a danger to self or others. Patients can then be held in the ED for that state's legislatively specified amount of time. At the end of this strict time period, the facility must decide whether to release patients or petition for court-ordered involuntary hospitalization.

Although involuntary commitment standards vary from state to state, all have standards that are based on the presence of mental illness and danger to self or others.[4] In addition, some states have commitment standards that also allow for an involuntary admission for persons with mental illness who are unable to care for themselves, in need of treatment, or at risk of deterioration.

The American College of Emergency Physicians urges all emergency physicians participating in commitment procedures to consider all relevant laws, regulations, institutional policies, documentation, and patients' rights.[22] Furthermore, the college supports the use of ED guidelines pertaining to the commitment of emergency patients and strongly supports access for these patients to appropriate consultations by mental health professionals in the emergency care setting.

It is of the utmost importance for every clinician to review his or her state's commitment statue and other relevant legislative information. In case of an involuntary admission, the clinician and facility must ensure that the proper due process is followed, that is, the state's commitment statues are properly applied and patients meet the specified commitment criteria, all necessary papers and certificates are filled out and are filed with the court, and all specified time periods are properly followed. This obligation is critically important as patients might otherwise allege *false imprisonment*, which occurs when a clinician deprives a person of his or her freedom in an unjustified manner.[5]

Although malpractice is classified as an unintentional tort, *false imprisonment* is classified as an intentional tort, meaning the clinician willfully deprived patients of their freedom while being aware that the patients did not meet the legally mandated commitment criteria.

FORCED MEDICATIONS

Justifications to force medications on patients against their will also date back to the principles of parens patriae and police power.[18] The latter principle justifies forced medication administration to persons in psychiatric emergency situations when there is an imminent risk of harm to self or others, that is, ED medical staff.[23] In these emergency situations, the clinician is allowed to administer medication to treat patients and move them away from danger. In the ED, clinicians typically use the so-called cocktail of intramuscular haloperidol, lorazepam, and diphenhydramine. It is important to clearly document in the patients' chart the observations and events that necessitated such psychiatric emergency medication order.[18]

Aside from such clear psychiatric emergencies, the clinician is not permitted to force patients to take medication against objection unless the clinician was granted a court order to administer medications. Some states (eg, Utah) allow a clinician to treat patients against objection when patients are involuntarily admitted to the hospital. With such involuntary admission, patients are also declared incompetent to make medical decisions as a condition for the commitment,[18] which emphasizes the parens patriae concept.

CHILD ABUSE AND NEGLECT

In 1962 Kemp and colleagues[24] originally described the battered child syndrome, a clinical condition in young children with serious physical abuse. According to the National Child Abuse and Neglect Data System, which collects child maltreatment data from all states, most states recognize 4 types of abuse, including neglect, emotional abuse, physical abuse, and sexual abuse.[25] Neglect is the most commonly reported child maltreatment (75% of cases) and can be in the form of physical, educational, and emotional neglect or child endangerment. Physical abuse is reported in 17% of the maltreatment cases followed by sexual abuse (8.3%). Parents or parents with other persons are described as perpetrators in 80% of reported child maltreatment cases.

In 2014, child protective agencies received an estimated 3.6 million reports of child maltreatment involving approximately 6.6 million children, out of which 2.2 million referrals were screened in (60.7%).[25] It was estimated that 1580 children died as a result of abuse and neglect, with 70.7% of these fatalities occurring in children less than 3 years of age. At least one parent was identified as the perpetrator in 79.3% of these cases.

Child abuse and neglect is associated with significant morbidity and mortality and can have considerable impact on the short- and long-term physical and emotional health of a child. There have been tremendous advances in this field in last 30 years, with increasing evidence of how child abuse leads to persistent biological alterations in the body and the brain.[26] For example, child abuse and neglect not only increase the risk of major psychiatric disorders but also worsen the course of such disorders in abused persons.[26] Additionally, the abused population is at higher risk for other medical disorders, including cardiovascular disorders, diabetes, asthma, irritable bowel syndrome, and other conditions.

Identification of child abuse is crucial; physicians should have a high index of suspicion for abuse or neglect in patients with unexplained injuries, subdural hematomas, skin and soft tissue bruises, multiple fractures at different stages of healing, and/or failure to thrive. Suspected child abuse can elicit strong and uncomfortable reactions in physicians; at times, a physician's reluctance to think that parents could be aggressive to the child might serve as a barrier to proper identification of abuse.[24]

Since1966 all states have had mandatory statutory requirements for physicians and others, such as nurses and teachers, to report child maltreatment. Some states require that *all* persons with knowledge of child abuse must report the maltreatment. Typically, states require that a report must be made if the reporter has a *reasonable* cause to know, suspect, or think that a child has been abused or neglected.[27] This requirement represents a low threshold intended to ensure that cases are not missed. Additionally, immunity from liability is provided for the reporting entity.

Failure to report child maltreatment can have serious legal consequences.[28] Although in most states failure to report suspected abuse is classified as a misdemeanor or a similar legal charge, the state of Florida can impose a felony. In Arizona and Minnesota misdemeanors are upgraded to felonies for failure to report more serious abuse situations, and several states upgrade second or subsequent violations to felonies. In the California case of *Landeros v Flood* (1976), the California Supreme Court held that doctors are expected to diagnose child abuse,[29] that failure to diagnose and report child abuse is a valid malpractice cause of action, and the mother's intervening abuse does not preclude liability for the physician.

In addition to the identification and reporting of suspected abuse, the role of the emergency physician may include supporting affected families and coordinating care with community agencies and other professionals. At times, physicians may have to provide written reports to child protective services or appear in court for testimony.[30]

ELDER ABUSE

Elder abuse refers to a knowing, intentional, or negligent act by a caregiver or another person that inflicts harm or a risk of serious harm to a vulnerable adult.[31] Victims are typically older, frail, vulnerable, and depend on others; they often suffer in silence from the abuse and/or neglect. A change in an elder's personality or behavior should be questioned in order to investigate and understand what is occurring. Elder abuse may manifest in the form of physical, sexual, or emotional abuse, neglect, exploitation, abandonment, or self-neglect. The self-neglected elderly are often depressed and withdrawn. Telltale signs of elder abuse are bruises, broken bones, unexplained withdrawal from normal daily activities, or a sudden change in alertness. Bruises around the breasts and genitalia may occur secondary to sexual abuse, whereas bedsores, unattended medical needs, poor hygiene, and weight loss can be signs of neglect. Family member behaviors, such as threats, belittling, or control, are often indicators of emotional abuse. Of particular importance is that elders can also be abused and/or neglected by nursing home staff. Tense relationships and frequent arguments between an elderly person and a caregiver are also often telltale signs of abuse.

The most recent incident data available report that approximately 450,000 elderly persons in domestic settings were abuse and/or neglected in 1996.[32] When self-neglect is added, the number increases to approximately 551,000. It is thought that this number only represents the tip of the iceberg. In almost 90% of the reported cases, the perpetrator is a family member, with two-thirds of these perpetrators being adult children and spouses. Female elderly are abused at a higher rate than male elderly.

Although all 50 states have passed some form of elder abuse prevention law, states frequently have no formal organized and mandatory reporting system similar to the child abuse system. Suspected elder abuse cases are commonly reported to adult protective services. In some states, elderly abuse is a crime and suspected abuse may have to be reported to law enforcement. In cases of suspected elder abuse in nursing homes, clinicians can contact their state's *Long Term Care Ombudsman Program* to investigate and resolve such complaints. The Web page of the National Center on Elder Abuse provides helpful information.[33]

PHYSICIAN REPORTING OF IMPAIRED DRIVERS

The American College of Emergency Physicians opposes the reporting of entire classes of patients or diagnoses, for example, epilepsy, unless compelling evidence exists for public benefit of such reporting.[34] For instance, the college advises physicians to individualize reporting to a patient's given clinical condition and the clear risk posed by driving to the individual patient and to the public. Additionally, the college advocates that physicians who report patients in good faith to the state's motor vehicle department should have protection from liability for such action.

SUMMARY

Emergency medical and psychiatric operations must have a good awareness and understanding of the numerous ethical and legal concepts inherent in treating patients in emergency situations. The importance of checking federal and state laws pertaining to these significant medical-legal issues cannot be overstated.

REFERENCES

1. American College of Emergency Physicians. Code of ethics for emergency physicians. Available at: http://www.acep.org/Clinical--Practice-Management/Code-of-Ethics-for-Emergency-Physicians/. Accessed November 25, 2016.
2. Resnick PJ. Psychiatric malpractice. In: Resnick PJ, editor. Syllabus. Forensic psychiatry review course. Bloomfield (CT): American Academy of Psychiatry and the Law; 2014. p. 1001–54.
3. Blake V. When is a patient-physician relationship established? Virtual Mentor 2012;14(5):403–6.
4. Gutheil TG, Appelbaum PS. Legal issues in emergency psychiatry. In: Gutheil TG, Appelbaum PS, editors. Clinical handbook of psychiatry and the law. 4th edition. Philadelphia: Lippincott Williams & Wilkins; 2007. p. 33–68.
5. Gutheil TG, Appelbaum PS. Malpractice and other forms of liability. In: Gutheil TG, Appelbaum PS, editors. Clinical handbook of psychiatry and the law. 4th edition. Philadelphia: Lippincott Williams & Wilkins; 2007. p. 111–76.
6. Wettstein RM. Specific issues in psychiatric malpractice. In: Rosner R, editor. Principles & practice of forensic psychiatry. 2nd edition. New York: Oxford Press; 2003. p. 249–59.
7. Reich JH, Moldonado J. Empirical findings on legal difficulties among practicing psychiatrists. Ann Clin Psychiatry 2011;23:297–307.
8. The American Association of Emergency Psychiatry. Available at: http://www.emergencypsychiatry.org/. Accessed November 26, 2016.
9. Resnick PJ. Confidentiality and Tarasoff. In: Resnick PJ, editor. Syllabus. Forensic psychiatry review course. Bloomfield (CT): American Academy of Psychiatry and the Law; 2014. p. 1099–126.

10. Gutheil TG, Appelbaum PS. Confidentiality and privilege. In: Gutheil TG, Appelbaum PS, editors. Clinical handbook of psychiatry and the law. 4th edition. Philadelphia: Lippincott Williams & Wilkins; 2007. p. 1–32.
11. Tarasoff V. Regents of the University of California, 551 P.2d 334 (1976) 872–3.
12. Schloendorff v. Society of New York Hospital, 105 N.E. 92 N.Y. (1914).
13. Ostermeyer B, Flores A, Dukes C, et al. Medical decision-making capacity in depression. Psychiatr Ann 2016;46(4):247–52.
14. Canterbury v. Spence, 464 F.2d 722 (1972) 863.
15. Grisso T, Appelbaum PS. Assessing competence to consent to treatment: a guide for physicians and other health professionals. New York: Oxford University Press; 1998.
16. Gutheil TG, Appelbaum PS. Competence and substitute decision-making. In: Gutheil TG, Appelbaum PS, editors. Clinical handbook of psychiatry and the law. 4th edition. Philadelphia: Lippincott Williams & Wilkins; 2007. p. 177–214.
17. Emergency Medical Treatment and Labor Act (EMTALA). Available at: http://emtala.com. Accessed November 26, 2016.
18. Scott CL. Right to treatment. In: Resnick PJ, editor. Syllabus. Forensic psychiatry review course. Bloomfield (CT): American Academy of Psychiatry and the Law; 2014. p. 327–76.
19. Rouse v. Cameron, 373 F.2d 451 (1966) 855.
20. Zinermon v. Burch, 494 U.S. 113 (1990) 854–855.
21. Cournos F, Faulkner L, Fitzgerald L, et al. Report of the task force on consent to voluntary hospitalization. Bull Am Acad Psychiatry Law 1993;21(3):293–307.
22. American College of Emergency Physicians. Available at: https://www.acep.org/. Accessed November 25, 2016.
23. Gutheil TG, Appelbaum PS. Legal issues in inpatient psychiatry. In: Gutheil TG, Appelbaum PS, editors. Clinical handbook of psychiatry and the law. 4th edition. Philadelphia: Lippincott Williams & Wilkins; 2007. p. 69–110.
24. Kempe CH, Silverman FN, Steele BF, et al. The battered-child syndrome. In: Kempe CH, editor. A 50 year legacy to the field of child abuse and neglect. New York: Springer; 2013. p. 23–38.
25. US Department of Health & Human Services, Administration for Children and Families Administration on Children, Youth, and Families. Child maltreatment. 2014. Available at: http://www.acf.hhs.gov/programs/cb/research-data-technology/statistics-research/child-maltreatment. Accessed November 22, 2016.
26. Nemeroff CB. Paradise lost: the neurobiological and clinical consequences of child abuse and neglect. Neuron 2016;89(5):892–909.
27. Scott CL. Child abuse child witness testimony. In: Syllabus. Forensic psychiatry review course. Bloomfield (CT): American Academy of Psychiatry and the Law; 2014. p. 377–430.
28. US Department of Health and Human Services, Administration for Children and Families, Administration on Children, Youth, and Families, Children's Bureau. Penalties for failure to report and false reporting of child abuse and neglect. Available at: https://childwelfare.gov/pubPDFs/report.pdf. Accessed November 23, 2016.
29. Landeros v Flood, 551 P.2d 389 (1976) 826–827.
30. Christian CW. The evaluation of suspected child physical abuse. Pediatrics 2015;135(5):1337–54.
31. US Department of Health and Human Services Administration for Community Living. Available at: http://www.aoa.acl.gov_Programs/Elder_Rights/Elder_Abuse/Index.aspx. Accessed November 25, 2016.

32. National Center on Elderly Abuse, The American Public Human Services Association in collaboration with Westat, Inc. The National Elderly Abuse Incidence Study. Final report. 1998. Available at: http://www.aoa.acl.gov_Programs/Elder_Rights/Elder_Abuse/docs/AbuseReport_Full.pdf. Accessed November 25, 2016.
33. National Center on Elder Abuse. Available at: https://ncea.acl.gov/suspectabuse/index.html. Accessed November 26, 2016.
34. American College of Emergency Physicians. Available at: https://www.acep.org/clinical--practice-management/physician-reporting-of-potentially-impaired-drivers/. Accessed November 26, 2016.

Legal and Ethical Challenges in Emergency Psychiatry, Part 2

Management of Inmates

Andrew Foote, MD[a], Britta Ostermeyer, MD, MBA[b,*]

KEYWORDS

• Emergency psychiatry • Inmates • Ethics • Legal

KEY POINTS

- Physicians and clinicians need to provide care and treatment of jail and prison inmates with the same medical professional and ethical standards.
- Inmates have a right to treatment/right to refuse treatment. Although their treatment choices may be limited, they have to undergo the informed consent process.
- Inmates have limited confidentiality: clinicians have to balance an inmate's needs/right to confidentiality with a facility's responsibilities for safety of other inmates and correctional staff.
- Inmates have unique situational and correctional facility challenges that have to be carefully factored into the disposition and treatment planning processes.
- Inmates have a high suicide risk. Clinicians need to ascertain additional inmate-specific risk factors into their suicide risk assessment and intervention.

INTRODUCTION

In 2014, the number of incarcerated individuals in the United States totaled 744,660 for jails and 1,561,550 for prisons.[1] Approximately 16% of inmates in jails and prisons have serious mental illness[2] and suicide is the leading cause of death in jails.[3] More than two-thirds of individuals meet criteria for a substance use disorder at the time of entry to jail.[4] Correctional facilities often use community medical resources, especially for emergency medical and psychiatric services.[5]

Disclosures: The authors have nothing to disclose.
[a] Variety Care, 1025 Straka Terrace, Oklahoma City, OK 73139, USA; [b] Department of Psychiatry and Behavioral Sciences, University of Oklahoma, 920 Stanton L. Young Boulevard, Oklahoma City, OK 73104, USA
* Corresponding author.
E-mail address: britta-ostermeyer@ouhsc.edu

Psychiatr Clin N Am 40 (2017) 555–564
http://dx.doi.org/10.1016/j.psc.2017.05.004
0193-953X/17/© 2017 Elsevier Inc. All rights reserved.

Psychiatrists may be asked to evaluate inmates in an emergency department, which presents unique ethical and legal issues. For psychiatrists who seldom encounter an inmate patient, this may be an unfamiliar situation. A basic outline of correctional facilities and systems is given to assist psychiatrists in these situations. The ethical and legal issues examined include the constitutional right to treatment and to refuse treatment, the physician-patient relationship, confidentiality, and the importance of suicide prevention. Lastly, practical general guidelines provided by the American College of Emergency Physicians may also be helpful for psychiatrists working with inmates in emergency departments.

CORRECTIONAL SYSTEMS

A typical inmate patient scenario presenting to an emergency department is the case of a 55-year-old man who is brought in from the local county jail after being found in his cell hanging from the ventilation grate by bed sheets around his neck.

When treating inmates from a correctional facility, it is important to have an understanding of correctional systems and their settings. In general, individuals held in a correctional facility are referred to as *detainees* before trial and as *offenders* after sentencing.[6] For simplicity, this article uses inmates to refer to both despite clear legal differences. Correctional facilities generally include lockups, jails, and prisons that are maintained by local, state, and federal agencies, respectively. Lockups are temporary holding facilities (usually <48 hours) typically located in police departments. They hold individuals who have been arrested or charged and have completed the initial administrative booking process and are waiting for court arraignment. Additionally, police may bring individuals requiring a mental health evaluation to an emergency department prior to arrest or booking.

Jails are locally operated facilities that generally hold both detainees awaiting trial and offenders convicted of misdemeanors and other minor crimes with a sentence of up to 1 year. Prisons are operated by state or federal governments and typically confine offenders convicted of a felony with a minimum of a 1-year sentence.[6]

Individuals recently arrested and waiting in jail for a court date must adjust to acutely high stress levels with tremendous uncertainty about their legal and personal future.[7] Individuals who have been sentenced have a more certain legal future (unless they acquire additional charges) but must continue to adjust to separation from family and established social support systems and contend with potential relational institutional conflicts.

RIGHT TO TREATMENT AND RIGHT TO REFUSE TREATMENT

Over the past 40 years, many legal cases have brought reform for inmates with mental illness, which have addressed both the right to treatment and the right to refuse treatment. The US Supreme Court in *Estelle v Gamble* (1976) held that officials must provide adequate medical care to convicted prisoners.[8] Failure to provide care violates the prohibition of cruel and unusual punishment in the Eighth Amendment. The Fourth Circuit Court of Appeals in *Bowing v Godwin* (1977) clarified this requirement to include mental health treatment.[9] The right to treatment was extended to pretrial detainees by the US Supreme Court decision *Bell v Wolfish* (1979) based on the Due Process Clause of the Fourteenth Amendment.[10] In *Ruiz v Estelle* (1980), the Southern District of Texas Court set minimum standards for mental health treatment of prisoners.[11] The US Supreme Court annotated procedural protections in *Vitek v Jones* (1980) for prisoners who may be involuntarily transferred to psychiatric hospitals.[12] This included the right to an adversarial hearing and legal assistance and the opportunity to present evidence and to challenge the state's evidence. In *Washington v Harper* (1990), the US Supreme Court held that a judicial hearing was not required for involuntarily medicating prisoners over their objection for mental health treatment.[13] They indicated that an internal administrative hearing at the correctional facility provided for sufficient due process. Many state laws, however, have higher standards than the *Harper* process for treatment over objection.[2,14] Lastly, the US Supreme Court in *Sell v United States* (2003) established the criteria for involuntary medication for a mentally ill pretrial detainee for competency to stand trial restoration, even in the absence of being dangerous or gravely disabled.[15]

PHYSICIAN-PATIENT RELATIONSHIP

An inmate becomes a patient when the clinician (physician) treatment relationship is established. *The Principles of Medical Ethics with Annotations Especially Applicable to Psychiatry* by the American Psychiatric Association (APA) applies to inmates.[16] The standards of compassion, respect for human rights, dignity, autonomy (including informed consent), professionalism, and access to care are equally applicable to inmates. Inmates must depend on correctional staff and administrators to get access to, attention to, and treatment of their medical and mental health needs (*Estelle v Gamble* [1976]).[8] The APA guidelines in *Psychiatric Services in Correctional Facilities*[2] note that although the situation of the correctional facility may limit the available treatment choices, an inmate retains the ability to make medical decisions within the given scope.

The APA's *Principles* prohibit "the psychiatric evaluation of any person charged with criminal acts prior to access to, or availability of, legal counsel." The permissible exception is for "rendering of care to the person for the sole purpose of medical treatment." Thus, an emphasis is placed on protecting the rights of the accused. Additionally, the *Ethics Guidelines for the Practice of Forensic Psychiatry* adopted by the American Academy of Psychiatry and the Law warn against dual roles, stating that a treating psychiatrist should "generally avoid...performing evaluations of their patients for legal purposes."[17] Therefore, a treating psychiatrist is not to address and opine as an expert witness on forensic medical-legal questions, such as competency to stand trial or criminal responsibility, for patients to whom the psychiatrist is providing or has provided psychiatric or medical care. As with any physician-patient relationship, the primary duty and responsibility is to the patient.[13] The treating physician clearly is to serve the patient's interests (beneficence), whereas an expert witness in a forensic medical-legal scenario serves the court's interests in a quest for truth. The truth may harm the interests of the evaluee (inmate in criminal proceedings), which would represent a conflict to the core medical principle of "Do no harm" (nonmaleficience). Patients may have disclosed information confidentially in treatment under the protection of the physician-patient relationship. Disclosure of such confidential treatment information later on as an expert witness poses great ethical concerns and may harm the patient. Thus, there is a clear distinction between a treating responsibility and a medical-legal evaluation obligation.[2]

COUNTERTRANSFERENCE

Interactions with inmates may evoke a spectrum of countertransference feelings. Particularly heinous offenses, objectionable personality traits, or suspicion of malingering may stimulate negative responses, whereas positive feelings may lead to over-identification and risk boundary violations.[18] An awareness of these feelings helps maintain a nonjudgmental approach, facilitate therapeutic rapport, and reduce the risk of bias and diagnostic inaccuracy.

MALINGERING

Malingering is the intentional production of false or grossly exaggerated physical or psychological symptoms motivated by conscious external incentives and rewards, such as avoiding work or jail, avoiding criminal prosecution, obtaining drugs, or obtaining financial compensation or disability.[19] Although malingering was removed from the index of the *Diagnostic and Statistical Manual of Mental Disorders* (5th edition), it remains a V code.[20]

While maintaining an empathic stance, psychiatrists and clinicians are encouraged to be aware of malingering, in particular in patients in jail and in prison inmates or in persons brought in from the street under police arrest. Such patients may try to malinger to seek admission to a hospital, avoiding the less desired correctional setting, escape more easily in the less secured hospital setting, receive drugs, and/or avoid criminal proceedings.

To detect malingering, clinicians should use multiple sources of data, including the clinical interview of the inmate as well as interviews of collateral informants, such as the guards on duty with the inmate, staff at the facility, or family members. In addition, psychometric tests usually performed by psychologists can shed light on the situation. Reliance alone on the clinical interview of the inmate only allows for detection of malingering in obvious cases.[19]

When malingering is suspected, a clinician should focus on asking open-ended questions to avoid giving clues about symptoms, allow the inmate to explain, and listen to the inmate. The clinician should look for inconsistencies in the presenting history and symptoms, such inconsistencies in an inmate's self-report, discrepancies between the history and symptoms, inconsistencies in symptom observation, or discrepancies between reported symptoms and how genuine symptoms are manifested.[19]

Malingerers often thrust their symptoms forward in an effort to gain a clinician's attention, whereas patients with genuine psychosis are often more guarded, are not forthcoming, and may exhibit negative symptoms of psychosis. In addition, it is more difficult for malingerers to portray negative psychotic symptoms and the more subtle cognitive impairments that are seen in patients with genuine psychosis. In general, malingering patients who falsify psychotic symptoms often overact their part. They may attempt to look as bizarre as possible to be perceived as more psychotic, and they often overact in feigning intellectual defects as well.[19]

A clinician may pose obvious improbable symptoms to ascertain if a malingering inmate will endorse them.[19] Resnick[19] suggests mentioning some easily imitated symptoms within earshot of the malingerer. The sudden report or appearance of such symptoms is suggestive of malingering as well. Resnick also states that clinicians require detailed knowledge of genuine psychiatric symptoms, such as auditory and visual hallucinations, delusions, and other psychiatric symptom manifestations, to better detect malingering.

It is important for clinicians to maintain a positive and caring rapport with inmate patients because any irritation over being deceived by a clinician usually forces a patient into a more defensive position, which may not be conducive to the evaluation process.[19] When a clinician confronts a patient with a concern over malingering, it is important to make efforts to enable the patient to be able to save face. For example, if a clinician suspects that a patient is not forthcoming, the clinician may inquire about additional information and encourage the patient to share, or the clinician may emphatically endorse that symptoms are different to see if the patient agrees.

CONFIDENTIALITY AND PRIVACY

When treating inmates, limited disclosure of protected health information beyond conventional exceptions to nonclinical correctional staff (officers or administrators) may be necessary to maintain the safety and security of the correctional environment and staff. The APA guidelines on *Psychiatric Services in Correctional Facilities*[2] advise that the limits of confidentiality in the community also apply to the correctional setting: suicide risk, assault/homicide risk, and grave disability or inability to care for oneself. Furthermore, the guidelines note possible additional limitations on confidentiality applicable to the correctional population: (1) significant escape risk, (2) security threat to institution (eg, riot), (3) active illicit substance use, and (4) a patient's care requires movement to a special unit or off-site facility for assessment and management of an acute psychiatric episode.[2] The guidelines reinforce the ethical principle of confidentiality and note that for inmates with mental illness, "the importance of private space for confidential doctor-patient interactions cannot be overstated."[2] If safety concerns require the presence of a police/correctional officer to the extent of compromising auditory confidentiality, the psychiatrist should appreciate the potential limitations to the inmate's response transparency. Legally, the Health Information Portability and Accountability Act Privacy Rule (45 CFR. Subtitle A, §164.512[5] [i]) permits the disclosure of protected health information to correctional institutions and law enforcement when necessary for the health and safety of an individual, other inmates, staff, and other employees and for the "administration and maintenance of the safety, security, and good order of the correctional institution."[21] Thus, a psychiatrist treating inmates is tasked with the complex ethical issue of balancing the importance of confidentiality in the therapeutic relationship with the institutional needs for security and stability.

SUICIDE RISK FACTORS

Suicide has continued to be the most frequent cause of death in jails since 2000.[3] In 2013, suicide was the sixth most frequent cause of death in prisons, and drug or alcohol intoxication was the fourth most frequent cause of death in jails.[3]

Several suicide risk factors in correctional facilities have been identified. A recent national jail study on suicide revealed many important findings: 20% of the inmates who committed suicide were intoxicated at the time of their deaths; 93% committed suicide by hanging; and approximately one-third of the suicides occurred close to the date of a court hearing.[7] This study also found that 22% of inmate suicides occurred close to the date of a telephone call or visit, which suggests that receiving bad news may increase suicide risk. Studies of the nation's 2 largest state prison populations demonstrated an increase suicide risk in inmates with a significant change in legal status (eg, denial of parole and additional charges),[22] inmates who expressed safety concerns with associated anxiety and agitation,[22] and inmates with a diagnosis of major depressive disorder, bipolar disorder, schizophrenia, or nonschizophrenic psychotic disorder.[21,23]

Several factors have been identified that correlate with increased suicide risk in both jail and prison inmates: white race, male gender, arrest/conviction of violent offense, history of mental health problems, history of substance use disorder, and history of suicide behavior or attempts.[7,22] Additionally, housing arrangements that facilitate isolation, such as single cell, administrative segregation, and multioccupancy cells with absent cellmates, increase the risk of suicide in both jails and prisons.[7,24]

Some notable contrasts have also been identified. In jails, the suicide rate has tended to increase with age, with higher rates occurring in inmates older than age 55, whereas suicide rates in prisons tend to be evenly distributed across the adult age range.[3] In jails, approximately 50% of suicides occurred within 2 weeks of incarceration, whereas prison suicides were less concentrated at the time of admission, with only a 7% suicide rate within the first month.[25]

SUICIDE SCREEN/ASSESSMENT

Every inmate should be screened for suicide risk as part of the initial booking process into a correctional facility.[26] This is often accomplished by a trained correctional officer or nursing staff member. In addition to traditional suicide risk factors (eg, past suicide attempts and prior psychiatric hospitalization), inmate screening may include recent significant loss (eg, death of family member, loss of job, or loss of status in community due to legal concerns), suicide risk during prior confinement, and arresting/transporting officer's beliefs that inmate is currently at risk.[27] A positive suicide screen should initiate a further assessment by a qualified mental health professional (QMHP).

As discussed previously, situational events that warrant a more extensive suicide risk assessment include recent court proceedings, contact with family members/significant others that may lead to change in behavior, transfer to different prison facility (proximity to family/social support), and placement in segregated or restrictive housing.[27] Therefore, a psychiatrist who evaluates an inmate for suicide risk and safety should inquire carefully about situations pertaining to the inmate's legal process or sentence (eg, court dates or problems with probation) and the inmate's situation at the correctional facility (eg, safety concerns by other inmates or single-cell segregation). An appreciation of these principles assist psychiatrists in performing a comprehensive suicidal risk assessment when evaluating inmates in an emergency department.

SUICIDE PREVENTION PLAN

After the evaluation and conceptualization of a treatment plan for an inmate, it is critically important for a clinician to determine how the correctional facility can realistically implement the treatment recommendations when the inmate is stable enough to be discharged from the emergency department back to the correctional facility.[28] This requires understanding of the correctional facility's physical plant structure and resources at the facility, including potential housing and observation options, such as a psychiatric unit. In addition, it requires knowledge about the available medical and mental health staff and other QMHPs.

In a national survey of jails and lockups, 87% of the respondents indicated that inmates on suicide precaution were observed at 15-minute intervals (close observation), with only 2% reporting constant observation as an available option.[7] Lockups were less likely to maintain a suicide precaution protocol and often do not have QMHPs.[7] Additionally, communication breakdown between correctional, medical, and mental health staff is a common factor in the reviews of many inmate suicides.[29]

The psychiatrist should call the correctional facility and inquire about the facility-specific treatment and observation options as well as the mental health/medical staff composition. Facility-specific factors and limitations must be included in the treatment and disposition planning processes. Facilities with crisis stabilization units that provide 24/7 coverage by nursing and custodial staff should be able to appropriately manage inmates requiring suicide precautions.[30] Additionally, the psychiatrist should inform the facility's staff, preferably the mental health staff, if available, about the inmate's assessment and recommended treatment plan to ensure proper follow-up and safety.

If an inmate's safety and follow-up care needs cannot be ensured after a psychiatrist's discussion with the facility staff, the psychiatrist or emergency physician may consider hospital admission for the inmate. Much like other patients, inmates can be admitted to inpatient psychiatric units. As discussed previously, inmates involuntarily transferred from a correctional facility to an inpatient psychiatric facility must have the minimum due process, including an adversarial hearing, established by the Supreme Court in *Vitek v Jones* (1980).[12] Additionally, some jurisdictions have statutory or case law that requires additional procedures for a *Vitek* hearing beyond the Supreme Court minimum.[14] Some states may incorporate elements of involuntary commitment procedures to satisfy *Vitek* requirements.[31] *Vitek* hearings, however, are not required for short-term crisis stabilization in psychiatric emergencies.[32] Nonetheless, clinicians should be familiar with law in their jurisdiction pertaining to the transfer of inmates to psychiatric hospitals for long-term treatment.

In the event of a hospital inpatient admission, the psychiatrist should contact the correctional facility regarding hospital admission preferences because correctional facilities typically have contractual arrangements with certain hospitals for their inmates' inpatient treatment needs. Such hospitals are also accustomed to the additional requirements that are required to admit an inmate to an inpatient psychiatric unit, such as a single room with an arrangement for the presence of a correctional officer without disturbing the inpatient treatment milieu for other patients.

Once the correctional authorities are notified about the recommendation for hospitalization and the need for further economic expenditures, they may decide to drop the charges or release the inmate on their own recognizance. In such cases, the alleged offense is usually a minor or nonviolent charge. When the inmate is no longer in custody, the physician may proceed with standard hospitalization procedures. Alternatively, the authorities may determine that an inmate is too dangerous to be transferred to an inpatient psychiatric hospital and chooses to return the inmate back to the correctional facility.

Unfortunately, many jails do not have direct access to psychiatric inpatient care often due to unresolved differences with the community hospital about the requirements for admission and safety concerns.[30] Thus, access to inpatient psychiatric care for some jail inmates may be limited to the state hospital as part of a competency to stand trial evaluation or restoration.

ADDITIONAL PRACTICAL GUIDELINES

The American College of Emergency Physicians has developed general guidelines for the medical care of inmates that may provide additional practical principles for psychiatrists.[28] Examination and treatment should be thorough and unbiased by officers. Restraints may need to be removed but should not jeopardize the safety of the health care worker. The assessment and treatment plan should be reviewed with the inmate in the same manner as for a noninmate patient. The attending officer should be informed regarding physical or medical limitations that may have an impact on restraints or transport. Similarly, in addition to contacting medical staff at the receiving facility, the psychiatrist may advise the officer when recommendations include transfer to a specialized unit for management of an acute psychiatric episode.

SUMMARY

Psychiatrists treating inmates in emergency departments need to be equipped with an appreciation of relevant ethical and legal issues pertaining to the management of jail and prison inmates. As physicians, they must not abandon the ethical standards of professionalism and should strive to establish the parameters of the therapeutic relationship while acknowledging the limitations and the additional needs for security in the correctional system. The courts have established both the right to mental health treatment and the right to refuse mental health treatment of inmates in prisons and jails. Because the suicide risk for inmates continues to be a significant concern, the importance of screening, assessment, and ensuring follow-up remains paramount. When equipped with an awareness of inmate suicide risk factors and a realistic understanding of a correctional facility's plant layout and resources as well as the facility's medical staffing situation, psychiatrists can make a meaningful impact on suicide prevention and in the amelioration of painful psychiatric symptoms for patients who happen to be inmates.

ACKNOWLEDGMENTS

The authors would like to thank Dr Jeff Metzner for his helpful guidance with this article.

REFERENCES

1. Kaeble D, Glaze L, Tsoutis A, et al. Correctional populations in the United States, 2014. Washington DC: US Department of Justice, Office of Justice Programs, Bureau of Justice Statistics; 2016. Available at: http://www.bjs.gov/content/pub/pdf/cpus14.pdf. Accessed September 23, 2016.
2. American Psychiatric Association, Work Group to Revise the APA Guidelines on Psychiatric Services in Correctional Facilities. Psychiatric services in correctional facilities/The American Psychiatric Association Work Group to revise the APA guidelines on psychiatric services in correctional facilities. 3rd edition. Arlington (VA): American Psychiatric Publishing; 2016.
3. Noonan M. Mortality in local jails and state prisons, 2000-2013-statistical tables. Washington, DC: US Department of Justice, Office of Justice Programs, Bureau of Justice Statistics; 2015. Available at: http://www.bjs.gov/content/pub/pdf/mljsp0013st.pdf. Accessed September 23, 2016.
4. Karberg JC, James DJ. Substance dependence, abuse, and treatment of jail inmates, 2002. Washington, DC: US Department of Justice, Office of Justice Programs, Bureau of Justice Statistics Special Report; 2005. Available at: http://www.bjs.gov/content/pub/pdf/sdatji02.pdf. Accessed September 23, 2016.
5. Eiting E, Lopez S, Harrison D, et al. Reduction in jail emergency department visits and closure after implementation of a new jail urgent care staffing model. Ann Emer Med 2014;64(4):S11.
6. Scott CL. Overview of the criminal justice system. In: Scott CL, editor. Textbook of correctional mental health. 2nd edition. Washington, DC: American Psychiatric Publishing; 2010. p. 3–23.
7. Hayes HM. National study of jail suicide: 20 years later. J Correct Health Care 2012;18(3):233–45.
8. Estelle v. Gamble, 429 U.S. 97 (1976).
9. Bowring v. Godwin, 551 F2d 44 (4th Cir 1977).
10. Bell v. Wolfish, 441 U.S. 520 (1979).
11. Ruiz v. Estelle, 503 F. Supp. 1265 (S.D. Tex. 1980).
12. Vitek v. Jones, 445 U.S. 480 (1980).
13. Washington v. Harper, 494 U.S. 210 (1990).

14. Norco MA, Burns CG, Dike C. Hospitalization. In: Trestman RL, Appelbaum KL, Metzner JL, editors. Oxford textbook of correctional psychiatry. New York: Oxford University Press; 2015. p. 141–5.
15. Sell v. U.S. 539 U.S. 166 (2003).
16. American Psychiatric Association. The principles of medical ethics with annotations especially applicable to psychiatry, 2013 edition. Arlington (VA): American Psychiatric Association; 2013. Available at: https://www.psychiatry.org/File%20Library/Psychiatrists/Practice/Ethics/principles-medical-ethics.pdf. Accessed October 4, 2106.
17. American Academy of Psychiatry and the Law. Ethics guidelines for the practice of forensic psychiatry, adopted May 2005. Bloomfield (CT). Available at: http://www.aapl.org/ethics.htm. Accessed October 4, 2016.
18. Lee L. Interviewing in correctional settings. In: Trestman RL, Applebaum KL, Metzner JL, editors. Oxford textbook of correctional psychiatry. New York: Oxford University Press; 2015. p. 62–70.
19. Resnick PJ. Malingering. In: Rosner R, editor. Principles & practice of forensic psychiatry. 2nd edition. New York: Oxford University Press; 2003. p. 543–54.
20. Scott CL. DSM-5 and malingering. Available at: http://oxfordmedicine.com/oso/search:downloadsearchresultaspdf;jsessionid=6403D2C76F7C1D7B40EEE3EFFF4FD3D6?isQuickSearch=true&pageSize=10&q=DSM&sort=relevance. Accessed November 29, 2016.
21. Health Information Portability and Accountability Act (HIPPA) Privacy Rule (45 C.F.R. Subtitle A, §164.512(5)(i)). Available at: https://www.law.cornell.edu/cfr/text/45/164.512. Accessed November 29, 2016.
22. Patterson R, Hughes K. Review of completed suicides in the California department of corrections and rehabilitation, 1999 to 2004. Psychiatr Serv 2008;59:676–82.
23. Baillargeon J, Penn JV, Thomas CR, et al. Psychiatric disorders and suicide in the nation's largest state prison system. J Am Acad Psychiatry Law 2009;37:188–93.
24. Reeves R, Tamburello A. Single cells, segregated housing, and suicide in the New Jersey department of corrections. J Am Acad Psychiatry Law 2014;42:484–8.
25. Mumola CJ. Suicide and homicide in state prison and local jails. Washington, DC: US Department of Justice, Office of Justice Programs, Bureau of Justice Statistics Special Report; 2005. Available at: https://www.bjs.gov/content/pub/pdf/shsplj.pdf. Accessed September 23, 2016.
26. Malony MP, Dvoskin J, Metzner JL. Mental health screening and brief assessments. In: Trestman RL, Applebaum KL, Metzner JL, editors. Oxford textbook of correctional psychiatry. New York: Oxford University Press; 2015. p. 57–61.
27. Hughes KC, Metzner JL. Suicide risk management. In: Trestman RL, Appelbaum KL, Metzner JL, editors. Oxford textbook of correctional psychiatry. New York: Oxford University Press; 2015. p. 237–44.
28. American College of Emergency Physicians Public Health Committee. Recognizing the needs of incarcerated patients in the Emergency Department. American College of Emergency Physicians. 2006. Available at: https://www.acep.org/content.aspx?id=30164. Accessed September 16, 2016.
29. Hayes LM. Toward a better understanding of suicide prevention in correctional facilities. In: Scott CL, editor. Handbook of correctional mental health. 2nd edition. Washington, DC: American Psychiatric Publishing; 2010. p. 231–54.

30. Metzner JL, Appelbaum KL. Levels of care. In: Trestman RL, Appelbaum KL, Metzner JL, editors. Oxford textbook of correctional psychiatry. New York: Oxford University Press; 2015. p. 112–6.
31. State of Oklahoma Department of Mental Health and Substance Abuse Services. 43A O.S. § 3–702. Available at: https://www.ok.gov/odmhsas/documents/2010%20-%2043A.pdf. Accessed November 29, 2016.
32. Scott CL. Legal issues regarding the provision of care in a correctional setting. In: Scott CL, editor. Textbook of correctional mental health. 2nd edition. Washington, DC: American Psychiatric Publishing; 2010. p. 63–88.

International Emergency Psychiatry Challenges

Disaster Medicine, War, Human Trafficking, Displaced Persons

Michael Jaung, MD[a], Suni Jani, MD, MPH[b], Sophia Banu, MD[c],
Joy M. Mackey, MD[a,*]

KEYWORDS

• International psychiatry • Disaster • Conflict • Trafficking • Displaced persons

KEY POINTS

- Mental health disorders are a major cause of morbidity measured by disability-adjusted life years and a growing burden in low- and middle-income countries; but there is little existing literature on the detailed epidemiology, diagnosis, and treatment in low-resource settings.
- Differences in culture, language, and symptoms that may not fit into Western paradigms are significant barriers to identifying and treating mental health disorders in the international population.
- Preflight stressors, trauma, and prolonged displacement contribute to posttraumatic stress disorder, depression, and other mental health disorders among refugees and internally displaced persons.
- Assessment and treatment of human trafficking victims should take into account the continuum of experience of patients and cultural sensitivity to the trauma and use a community-based approach that allows individuals to feel connected and validated in their experience.

INTRODUCTION

One could hardly open a newspaper in the current day and age without encountering a story about refugees. Sad and heart-wrenching, these often remind the reader of the fragility of the human condition, but also its tenacity and strong will to live. However,

---

Disclosure statement: The authors have no disclosures to make.
[a] Department of Emergency Medicine, Baylor College of Medicine, 1504 Taub Loop, Houston, TX 77030, USA; [b] Massachusetts General Hospital, McLean Department of Child and Adolescent Psychiatry, Yawkey Center for Outpatient Care, 6A, 55 Fruit Street, Boston, MA 02114, USA; [c] Department of Psychiatry, Baylor College of Medicine, One Baylor Plaza, BCM350, Houston, TX 77030, USA
* Corresponding author.
E-mail address: jmmackey@bcm.edu

Psychiatr Clin N Am 40 (2017) 565–574
http://dx.doi.org/10.1016/j.psc.2017.05.015
psych.theclinics.com
0193-953X/17/© 2017 Elsevier Inc. All rights reserved.

we also need to go no further than our emergency departments to see these stories unfold every day, as refugees tend to need emergency care quite often and with specific parameters that may go above and beyond the routine care paradigms providers are used to. By the United Nations High Commissioner for Refugees' (UNHCR) definition, a refugee is "someone who has been forced to flee his or her country because of persecution, war, or violence."[1] At the end of 2015, UNHCR estimated there was a total of 24.5 million refugees and asylum seekers and an additional 40.8 million internally displaced people (IDP).[1] Each of these terms denote a different legal status, and asylum seekers with pending applications may not be afforded similar protections or resources as refugees (**Box 1**). Each population has unique characteristics due to being exposed to both acute and chronic stressors that contribute to mental health disorders.

With affected populations spanning the globe, the number of refugees has been increasing since 2011 with affected populations spanning the globe. The distribution of refugees in the UNHCR-Bureau region is shown in **Fig. 1**. An estimated 86% of refugees were hosted in developing countries. Unfortunately, these countries are often the least able to provide the resources for these vulnerable populations. **Table 1** highlights this inequity by showing the countries at the end of 2015 from where the most refugees originated to where most sought asylum and the number of refugees hosted per 1 US dollar gross domestic product based on purchasing-power-parity. Programs serving refugee populations must address these gaps by evaluating the distribution of resources and effectiveness of interventions, including mental health programs, in developing country settings.

Box 1
Definitions

- *Humanitarian emergency:* an event that overwhelms local capacity to manage and provide basic services, such as shelter, health care, and security to the affected population.
- *Refugee* (UNHCR): "someone who has been forced to flee his or her country because of persecution, war, or violence."
- *IDP* (UNHCR): "while they may have fled for similar reasons [to a refugee], IDPs stay within their own country and remain under the protection of its government, even if that government is the reason for their displacement."
- *Human trafficking* (UNODC): "the recruitment, transportation, transfer, harboring or receipt of persons, by means of the threat or use of force or other forms of coercion, of abduction, of fraud, of deception, of the abuse of power or of a position of vulnerability or of the giving or receiving of payments or benefits to achieve the consent of a person having control over another person, for the purpose of exploitation."
- *Sexual and gender-based violence* (UNHCR): "violence that is directed at a person on the basis of gender or sex. It includes acts that inflict physical, mental, or sexual harm or suffering, threat of such acts, coercion and other deprivations of liberty."
- *Torture* (UN Convention): "any act by which severe pain or suffering, whether physical or mental, is intentionally inflicted on a person for such purposes as obtaining from him or her or a third person information or a confession, punishing him for an act he or a third person has committed, or intimidating or coercing him or a third person, or for any reason based on dis-crimination of any kind, when such suffering is inflicted by or at the instigation of or with the consent or acquiescence of a public official or other person acting in an official capacity. It does not include pain or suffering arising from, inherent in or incidental to lawful sanctions."

Abbreviations: UN, United Nations; UNODC, United Nations Office on Drugs and Crime.
Data from Refs.[1,25,26]

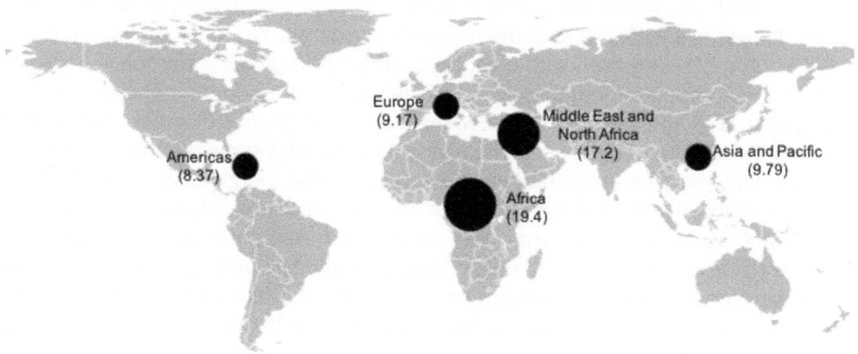

Fig. 1. Refugees, asylum seekers, IDP, and other populations of concern to UNHCR by UNHCR-Bureau region (millions). *Data from* UNHCR. UNHCR global trends 2015. Geneva (Switzerland); 2016.

Table 1
Distribution of refugee populations

Rank	Country	Number
Major source countries of refugees		
1	Syrian Arab Republic	4,872,585
2	Afghanistan	2,666,254
3	Somalia	1,123,052
4	South Sudan	778,697
5	Sudan	628,770
Refugees by country of asylum		
1	Turkey	2,541,352
2	Pakistan	1,561,162
3	Lebanon	1,070,854
4	Iran (Islamic Republic of)	979,437
5	Ethiopia	736,086
—	United States	58,624
—	Canada	46,925
Number of refugees hosted per 1 USD GDP (PPP) per capita		
1	Democratic Republic of the Congo	471
2	Ethiopia	453
3	Pakistan	317
4	Uganda	233
5	Kenya	180
—	United States	4.7
—	Canada	2.9

Abbreviations: GDP (PPP), gross domestic product based on purchasing-power-parity; USD, US dollar.

Data from UNHCR. UNHCR Global Trends 2015. Geneva (Switzerland); 2016.

Mental health disorders are a major cause of morbidity measured by disability-adjusted life years (DALYs) and, combined with neurologic disorders, are the most significant source of years lived with disability.[2] They are a growing burden in low- and middle-income countries; but there is little existing literature on the detailed epidemiology, diagnosis, and treatment in low-resource settings. Part of the challenge in assessing the burden of disease is identifying and classifying mental health disorders that may not fit into Western paradigms. Language is also a significant barrier to accurately describing signs and symptoms of mental disorders. Variation in spiritual, religious, and family structures may also contribute to the perception and approach to mental disorders in these settings. Although stigma toward people with mental health disorders remains a significant issue in high- and low-resource settings, the lack of a biopsychosocial approach to mental health and inadequate access to treatment further inhibits the acceptance of treatment.

There is limited research on the implementation and outcomes of various treatment modalities for mental health disorders in low- and middle-income countries. In many low-resource settings, lack of access to primary caregivers and specialists limits the evaluation, monitoring, diagnosis, and management. Most research has examined chronic management for these disorders; however, and integrated health care approach should include management of severe, refractory, or emergency presentations in these populations as well that require emergency and specialist care.[2] This review article examines the existing knowledge of mental health disorders with a specific focus in psychiatric emergencies in the setting of disasters and conflict and among people who are refugees, internally displaced, and victims of human trafficking.

MENTAL HEALTH IN THE SETTING OF HUMANITARIAN EMERGENCIES

Epidemiology

Humanitarian emergencies caused by conflict or natural disasters pose added disruptions to displaced populations. These crises commonly lead to prolonged exposure to potentially traumatic events as well as collapse of psychosocial support networks.[3] Trauma in these settings can be both physical trauma, including traumatic brain injury, and psychological trauma through witnessing the loss of family, property, and communities. In various conflicts, specific methods of physical trauma have been observed. Studies of resettled refugees have found as many as 55% of refugees from a specific conflict experienced torture.[4] In other studies, there have been high rates of sex and gender-based violence affecting women, children, and, less frequently, men.[4,5]

The burden of mental health disorders in humanitarian emergencies have been studied in many different crises. Most studies use Western tools to identify cases of posttraumatic stress disorder (PTSD), depression, and other disorders. A meta-analysis of PTSD and depression prevalence in postconflict populations found that the cumulative prevalence of PTSD and depression were 30.6% and 30.8%, respectively.[6] In this analysis, exposure to torture was the strongest predictor for PTSD. Children and adolescents are a significant proportion of the population affected by humanitarian crises. Specific problems arise from disruption from families and education, female genital mutilation, child marriage, and early pregnancy, warranting specific interventions for mental health services in these populations.[7]

Few of the studies examining the burden of mental health disorders characterized in detail the incidence of psychiatric emergencies, such as suicidality, among those identified with PTSD or depression. One study in Kashmir, an area with chronic conflict, many suicide attempts were reported over an 8-year period; the researchers found a high comorbidity of adjustment disorder, depression, and PTSD.[8] Another study among mothers with sexual violence–related pregnancies in the setting of chronic conflict in the Democratic Republic of Congo found that 34.2% of respondents reported prior suicide ideation or suicide attempt.[5] Women in this study who reported current stigma due to being a victim of sexual violence and other social stressors were significantly more likely to report suicidality as well as meet criteria for depression, PTSD, and anxiety.

Psychiatric emergencies may occur in the context of PTSD and depression in humanitarian crises, but patients with other mental health disorders are also at risk of exacerbation from disruption of their psychosocial environment and previous support. These conditions include schizophrenia, other forms of psychosis, substance abuse, adjustment disorder, and other unclassified severe neuropsychiatric disorders. A limited number of studies have quantified the burden of these mental health disorders; but a systematic review found a significant prevalence of severe mental disorders, especially psychosis.[9] Of the specific studies included in this analysis, it was found that in cases whereby treatment programs for psychosis and severe mental health disorders were established, researchers found a steadily increasing incidence as more patients were referred or presented to care.

In the setting of a humanitarian emergency, some mental health programs have included the diagnosis and treatment of epilepsy and other neurologic disorders. Like mental health disorders, epilepsy and many neurologic disorders are chronically disabling; diagnosis and treatment in humanitarian settings are limited by stigma, poor understanding of disease processes, and lack of trained providers and other resources.[2,9] Although these conditions can often present as emergencies to a health facility, diagnosis and treatment of neurologic disorders are outside the scope of this review.

Diagnosis and Treatment

By definition, humanitarian emergencies overwhelm local capacity to manage and provide basic services, such as shelter, health care, and security to affected populations. Regardless of development status of the affected community, mental health services are often under-resourced before emergencies. When working with preexisting health systems during humanitarian crises, it has been recommended that organizations and health facilities should work to develop durable programs that can deliver care to patients with mental health disorders but also lead to lasting improvement and change in these systems.[2]

In a review of specific mental health treatment programs during humanitarian crises, the most often-implemented activities were provided by peers and general practitioners.[10] These activities included basic counseling for individuals, groups, and families; facilitation of community awareness and support; child-friendly spaces and structured recreational activities; and nonpharmacologic management of mental health disorders. Relatively few randomized controlled trials (RCTs) have been done for these interventions. There is evidence for modest improvements in PTSD symptoms seen with narrative exposure therapy among adults but differing efficacy for other interventions.[10] This review also found differing efficacies for treatment programs for children and adolescents.

No clinical studies on specific interventions for psychiatric emergencies, such as suicidality or acute psychosis, in humanitarian crises were found for this review. The approach to identification and stabilization of psychiatric emergencies should be evidence based, and the efficacy of specific treatments may not differ from other clinical settings. Instead, experts have recommended that interventions in humanitarian crises focus on training providers and strengthening health systems.[9] Examples include long-term training for general practitioners working in humanitarian settings, deployment and training of mental health specialists, and developing clinical protocols and guidelines to channel procurement of medications and supplies.

PSYCHIATRIC EMERGENCIES FACING FORCED MIGRANTS, REFUGEES, AND INTERNALLY DISPLACED PEOPLE

The burden of mental health disorders during humanitarian crises and disasters is part of the spectrum of the challenges facing forced migrants. Prolonged displacement, return to the community of origin, or screening and resettlement to a new country pose difficulties in the care for patients with mental health disorders.

Epidemiology

There is a high prevalence of PTSD and depression among refugees, but there has been significant variance in prevalence among different studies. The prevalence ranged from 20% to 74% for PTSD and 39% to 64% for depression.[11] An earlier review of studies to refugees already resettled in Western countries found aggregate prevalence of 9% for PTSD and 5% for depression.[12] Another systematic review found that the high prevalence of mental disorders persisted even 5 years after displacement.[13]

In all 3 of these reviews, there were few studies examining other severe mental disorders and psychiatric emergencies. A meta-analysis of studies in general immigrant populations in Europe and Australia found an increased rate of schizophrenia, and a higher risk of the disease was found in populations immigrating from countries with a lower level of economic development.[14] This higher rate of psychotic disorders was also observed in refugees resettled in Western countries.[12]

Although the diagnosis and management of mental health disorders of refugees resettled in high-income countries often takes place in primary care or psychiatry outpatient settings, there can be gaps in care; they may first present to an emergency department with decompensation of a mental health disorder or seeking enrollment in care.[4]

It has been seen that refuges with severe cases of mental illness present to the emergency department; there are many others with mild to moderate mental illness who do not receive any treatment for many reasons. One is that the case managers who take care of them are overwhelmed with the number of cases they have, so unless they are clearly hallucinating or express suicidal ideation or homicidal ideation (in which case they are taken to the emergency department), they do not come on the radar of the overworked case manager, who is busy taking care of the basic needs of the refugees.

The other reason is the background and the culture of the refugee; there are refugees who do not want to complain and report everything is fine even when it is not.

In a 3-year case series of refugees presenting to an emergency department in Switzerland, researchers found that psychiatric complaints were the third most common type of complaint following trauma and infectious disease.[3]

As far as compliance with medications and psychotherapy follow-up appointments in mental health clinics, despite an increasing evidence base demonstrating the success of mental health care in the developed countries, patient participation remains the key factor in its success. Individuals who have engaged in mental health services are aware of the time commitment, monitoring, lifestyle modifications, and frequent follow-up appointments necessary for recovery from mental illness to be a possibility. Arriving to weekly or sometimes daily appointments, group therapy, meetings, and medical follow-up can be difficult for individuals who work full-time and lack consistent transportation. As a result, mental health providers must obtain a strong social history before initiating what may seem to be the ideal treatment of their patients. Although biweekly therapy with psychopharmacology may be indicated for patients initially, it may not be what is best for patients who cannot afford medication or take time off from social or occupational commitments. This concept is crucial to understand before initiating treatment of refugee patients who may not adhere to treatment as it occurs in the context of relearning a new way of life. In the case of refugees, the presence of a well-matched case worker to assist them in activities of daily living, such as use of or procuring transportation, bill paying, educational support for children, and job seeking, is imperative for adaptive functioning in a new community. However, even with assistance in social functioning, even well-educated refugee patients may struggle to comprehend the mechanics of individual therapy, as they do not understand it because of it being a foreign concept, stigma, or language barriers. Although the presence of an interpreter may assist with this, finding an interpreter with the same dialect as patients who understands the nuances of explanation and comprehension of mental health care is difficult. The intervention with the best risk profile and outcome for patients who are at risk of poor follow-up is using the treatment time when they do present to engage in motivational interviewing, empathy, and the growth of the therapeutic alliance, which may eventually empower patients to discover their own feasible path to treatment.

Among forced migrants, there are 2 populations that warrant special attention. Asylum seekers, people who apply for asylum after arrival in another country, face specific challenges in treatment because of the instability of care and possible reliance of mental health status for success in application for asylum status.[11] IDP is a second group distinct from refugees. Like refugees, they often experience the same preflight phase stressors, trauma during flight, and prolonged displacement; studies have shown they also suffer from high rates of PTSD, depression, and other mental health disorders.[15] However, IDP do not cross recognized national boundaries and they are not protected by international refugee laws leading in most situations to less attention, aid, or direct services. This circumstance is exacerbated by the fact that many IDP already live in low- or middle-income countries that may have few existing mental health services.

PSYCHIATRIC EMERGENCIES FACING VICTIMS OF HUMAN TRAFFICKING

Epidemiology

Several meta-analyses have established evidence that human trafficking is associated with a large prevalence and increased relative risk of health problems and violence associated with premigration, migration, and postmigration dangers, stresses, and traumas.[16] The most commonly reported mental health sequelae of these experiences are anxiety, depression, and posttraumatic stress disorder, which affect functioning in a myriad of ways but can result in psychiatric emergencies of harm to self and others through suicide and neglect of self and families.[17] Although a psychiatric emergency is apparent to the eyes of a community in a suicide attempt or bizarre, maladaptive behavior in a cultural context, the pathway to worsening mental health following human trafficking is indolent and often overlooked because of the differences in resilience, pretrafficking and post-trafficking traumas, education, stigma, willingness to seek care, and presentation of premorbid symptoms.[18]

Diagnosis and Treatment

Although symptoms of trauma, depression, and anxiety may decline over time for human trafficking victims without psychiatric intervention, they remain higher than the general population and are at risk of worsening to an emergent state without proper intervention.[18] One of the major symptoms of trauma is dissociation, an experience of being separate from the body when encountering traumatic stimuli, which can result in memory loss and have significant legal and psychiatric implications during any interview process.[18] Some victims of sex trafficking have reported delays in cognitive, social, and emotional development beyond their expected trajectory that result in poor rehabilitation even after rescue.[19] Other associated symptoms of trauma include hypervigilance, reexperiencing traumas, behavioral regression, shame, psychosomatic symptoms, and mistrust in new and preexisting relationships with loved ones.[20] The inability to trust may manifest as internal stigma that prevents victims of human trafficking and other traumas from meaningfully engaging in treatment or in the community, a major risk factor for suicide and self-harm.[21] Furthermore, some victims of trafficking have been forced into drug addiction as part of their situation and continue afterward to use drugs to manage their psychiatric symptoms, further exacerbating their risk of suicide and revictimization.[22]

Despite the near-universal exploitation of the victims of human trafficking, the psychological effects are varied by individual. Individuals demonstrate a variety of symptoms based on their personalities, existing resources, immigration statuses, familial connections, severity of substance use, and extent of hope as well as any associated legal issues when addressing their psychiatric emergency. In addition to psychiatric management, the differences in psychosocial barriers require case management that can identify social barriers to recovery, such as food, shelter, clothing, emergency medical treatment, legal representation for repatriation or relocation, crisis intervention, and safety planning regarding revictimization risks.[23]

The comprehensive psychiatric assessment of an emergency facing human trafficking victims should focus on understanding patients before trafficking and the idiosyncratic experience of being trafficked. Therapy should focus on trauma-related aspects of symptoms while concurrently treating other disorders as they arise, including personality traits, substance use disorders, and comorbid medical conditions that exist.[24] Survivors of human trafficking require cultural sensitivity to the trauma that led them to experience isolation from their culture of choice and identity, whether in an emergency situation or long-term care. A community-based approach that allows individuals to feel connected and validated in their experience by the provider is necessary in alliance building at every step.[19]

SUMMARY

In conclusion, mental health disorders are a major cause of morbidity measured by DALYs and a growing burden in low- and middle-income countries; but there is little existing literature on the detailed epidemiology, diagnosis, and treatment in low-resource settings. Barriers, such as access to care, language and cultural differences, stigma, and lack of social support, limit effective diagnosis and treatment. Special situations with vulnerable populations, such as those created by international humanitarian emergencies, refugees or IDPs, and victims of human trafficking, are increasing in prevalence. PTSD is common among this population who are often victims of extreme hardship, conflict, torture, or sexual violence. These victims are often resettled in developed countries and come to the emergency department seeking care. To better care for these populations, knowledge of specialized psychosocial and cultural considerations should inform the comprehensive psychiatric assessment and treatment plan.

REFERENCES

1. United Nations High Commission on Refugees. UNHCR global trends 2015. Geneva (Switzerland): The United Nations High Commission for Refugees; 2016. Available at: http://www.unhcr.org/statistics. Accessed June 21, 2017.
2. Patel V, Chisholm D, Parikh R, et al. Addressing the burden of mental, neurological, and substance use disorders: key messages from disease control priorities, 3rd edition. Lancet 2016;387(10028):1672–85.
3. Miller KE, Rasmussen A. War exposure, daily stressors, and mental health in conflict and post-conflict settings: bridging the divide between trauma-focused and psychosocial frameworks. Soc Sci Med 2010;70(1):7–16.
4. Crosby SS. Primary care management of non–English-speaking refugees who have experienced trauma. JAMA 2013;310(5):519–28.
5. Scott J, Rouhani S, Greiner A, et al. Respondent-driven sampling to assess mental health outcomes, stigma and acceptance among women raising children born from sexual violence-related pregnancies in eastern Democratic Republic of Congo. BMJ Open 2015;5(4):e007057.
6. Steel Z, Chey T, Marnane C, et al. Association of torture and other potentially traumatic events with mental health outcomes among populations exposed to mass conflict and displacement. JAMA 2009;302(5):537–49.
7. Hirani K, Payne D, Mutch R, et al. Health of adolescent refugees resettling in high-income countries. Arch Dis Child 2016;101(7):670–6.
8. Wani ZA, Hussain A, Khan AW, et al. Are health care systems insensitive to needs of suicidal patients in times of conflict? The Kashmir experience. Ment Illn 2011;3: 11–3.
9. Jones L, Asare JB, El Masri M, et al. Severe mental disorders in complex emergencies. Lancet 2009;374(9690):654–61.
10. Tol WA, Barbui C, Galappatti A, et al. Mental health and psychosocial support in humanitarian settings: linking practice and research. Lancet 2011;378(9802): 1581–91.
11. Slobodin O, De Jong JT. Mental health interventions for traumatized asylum seekers and refugees: what do we know about their efficacy? Int J Soc Psychiatry 2015;61(1):17–26.
12. Fazel M, Wheeler M, Danesh J. Prevalence of serious mental disorder in 7000 refugees resettled in western countries: a systematic review. Lancet 2005; 366(9497):1605.
13. Bogic M, Njoku A, Priebe S. Long-term mental health of war-refugees: a systematic literature review. BMC Int Health Hum Rights 2015;15(1):29.
14. Cantor-Graae E, Selten JP. Schizophrenia and migration: a meta-analysis and review. Am J Psychiatry 2005;162(1):12–24.
15. Siriwardhana C, Stewart R. Forced migration and mental health: prolonged internal displacement, return migration and resilience. Int Health 2013;5(1):19–23.
16. Ottisova L, Hemmings S, Howard LM, et al. Prevalence and risk of violence and the mental, physical and sexual health problems associated with human trafficking: an updated systematic review. Epidemiol Psychiatr Sci 2016;25(4): 317–41.

17. Oram S, Khondoker M, Abas M, et al. Characteristics of trafficked adults and children with severe mental illness: a historical cohort study. Lancet Psychiatry 2015; 2(12):1084–91.
18. Abas M, Ostrovschi NV, Prince M, et al. Risk factors for mental disorders in women survivors of human trafficking: a historical cohort study. BMC Psychiatry 2013;13:204.
19. Patel RA, Ahn R, Burke TF. Human trafficking in the emergency department. West J Emerg Med 2010;11(5):402–4.
20. Brunovskis A, Surtees R. Coming home: challenges in family reintegration for trafficked women. Qual Social Work 2012;454–72.
21. Zimmerman C, Hossain M, Watts C. Human trafficking and health: a conceptual model to inform policy, intervention and research. Soc Sci Med 2011;73(2): 327–35.
22. Deshpande NA, Nour NM. Sex trafficking of women and girls. Rev Obstet Gynecol 2013;6(1):e22–7.
23. Hemmings S, Jakobowitz S, Abas M, et al. Responding to the health needs of survivors of human trafficking: a systematic review. BMC Health Serv Res 2016;16:320.
24. Pascual-Leone AK, Kim J, Morrison OP. Working with victims of human trafficking. J Contemp Psychotherapy 2016;1–9.
25. United Nations Office on Drugs and Crime. Available at: https://www.unodc.org/unodc/en/human-trafficking/what-is-human-trafficking.html. Accessed June 21, 2017.
26. United Nation Convention Against Torture. Available at: http://www.ohchr.org/EN/ProfessionalInterest/Pages/CAT.aspx. Accessed June 21, 2017.

Violence in the Emergency Department

A Global Problem

Allison Tadros, MD*, Christopher Kiefer, MD

KEYWORDS

• Patient violence • Emergency department • Health care workers

KEY POINTS

- In one survey, emergency department (ED) nurses reported both verbal (100%) and physical (82%) assaults by patients.
- A combination of the ED environment and the population they care for puts emergency workers at particular risk for violence.
- All heath care providers should be trained to manage workplace violence, and all acts of violence should be reported to hospital administration.
- Physicians and nurses should be familiar with medications available to sedate agitated patients. Protocols for physical restraints should be adhered to, and patients must be closely monitored to prevent morbidity or death.
- Laws to protect health care workers from violence should be both enacted and enforced.

INTRODUCTION

A cardiothoracic surgeon was fatally wounded in 2015 after being shot by a patient's family member inside Brigham and Women's Hospital in Boston.[1] Similarly, in 2010 an orthopedic surgeon was nonfatally shot by a patient's family member while he was discussing with him the patient's treatment.[2] Young adults deciding on a profession choose medicine to treat and prevent disease and improve public health. However, unlike those choosing such careers as law enforcement or the military, doctors and nurses likely do not realize that they are entering a job that has one of the highest rates of nonfatal assaults against workers in the United States. The emergency department (ED) is a particularly vulnerable setting.[3,4] This article explores possible reasons for the high rates of violent incidents, reviews laws regarding workplace violence in health care settings, discusses controversies on the subject, and suggests steps that can

---

Disclosure: The authors have nothing to disclose.
Department of Emergency Medicine, Health Science Center, West Virginia University, PO Box 9149, Morgantown, WV 26506, USA
* Corresponding author.
E-mail address: atadros@hsc.wvu.edu

Psychiatr Clin N Am 40 (2017) 575–584
http://dx.doi.org/10.1016/j.psc.2017.05.016
0193-953X/17/© 2017 Elsevier Inc. All rights reserved.

be taken to manage agitated patients and, therefore, mitigate violence toward health care providers.

SCOPE OF THE PROBLEM

Health care workers are 4 times more likely to have serious workplace injuries related to violence than workers in private industry.[5] In 1999, the National Institute for Occupational Health and Safety reported a rate of 8.3 nonfatal violent assaults for every 10,000 health care workers compared with a rate of 2 for every 10,000 workers in private non–health care sectors.[6] More recent data from the Bureau of Labor Statistics revealed that 15.7% of all workplace assaults between 2003 and 2007 occurred in the health care industry.[5] Psychiatric hospitals and EDs are the 2 areas where violence is most likely to be encountered.[7] Among health care workers, nurses are at higher risk than doctors, possibly because of the increased contact time with patients.[8,9]

EPIDEMIOLOGY OF VIOLENCE IN UNITED STATES EMERGENCY DEPARTMENTS

Although the statistics provided by governmental agencies do not specifically provide the prevalence of violent behavior and assaults in the ED, it does make clear that violence in the general health care setting is a serious problem. A survey of residents and attending physicians working in academic EDs has revealed that up to 78% of them had experienced an episode of workplace violence in the prior year; although verbal assaults were more common, up to 21% had experienced an episode of physical violence.[4] Similarly, a study of attending physicians working in EDs in the state of Michigan revealed that 74.9% of physicians had received a verbal threat or assault, with 28.1% reporting a physical assault. The most common perpetrators in this study were the patients themselves, who initiated 71.9% of the reported verbal threats and 89.1% of the reported assaults. Although this certainly represents most assaults and verbal threats, it is important to keep in mind that the remainder of assaults and threats were initiated by patients' family members or friends; ED safety efforts should focus on these individuals as well.[10]

The available data suggest that nurses seem to fare even worse than physicians. In a survey of hospital nurses, ED nurses reported a 100% incidence of verbal assaults and 82% had experienced physical assault.[11] The most common type of verbal assault was being yelled or sworn at, whereas the most common kind of physical assault was being grabbed or pulled.[12]

Although the previously described studies were performed in the mid to late 2000s, a more recent prospective survey of nurses, physicians, and allied health staff working in level 1 trauma centers, urban nontrauma hospitals, as well as suburban nontrauma hospitals over a 9-month period reveals that health care workers in the ED setting experienced 4.15 violent events during the 9 months, with the most common event again being verbal in nature. Additionally, health care workers in this study experienced physical assault at a rate of 1.13 events per person during the 9-month period, with the most common assault being hitting or kicking.[8] These more recent findings suggest that violence in the workplace is a tangible, ongoing threat to those individuals working on a daily basis in US EDs.

EPIDEMIOLOGY OF VIOLENCE IN EMERGENCY DEPARTMENTS OUTSIDE THE UNITED STATES

Unfortunately, violence in the ED is not isolated to the United States. A survey of ED providers in Turkey found statistics similar to those found in the surveys based in the United States, with 74% of ED workers reporting that they had been subject to verbal or physical assault during the course of their jobs in the past.[13] Additionally, surveys of all providers working in the National Health System in the United Kingdom revealed that 28% of providers had experienced an act of workplace violence. Half of those respondents did not report the incident to a superior, with the most common reason being that they thought violence was part of their job.[14] Both in the United States and abroad, it is clear that health care providers in the ED face the threat of violence on a regular basis; it is essential to better understand not only the scope of this problem but also the downstream effect on workers. As part of the societal safety net, providers in the ED who cannot choose their patients or refuse to serve those who are aggressive or violent must have strategies ready to safely care for these patients.

FACTORS LEADING TO VIOLENCE IN EMERGENCY DEPARTMENTS

There are factors inherent to EDs that may lead to stress and violence in patients and their family members. Gang violence and domestic disputes can, at times, overflow from the streets into the ED. Opposing gang members with injuries could be treated in close proximity in the same ED, where hostilities may continue. Long wait times before patients are brought back from the waiting room or seen by a provider frequently leads to anger and frustration in patients before the patient-provider encounter even starts. EDs are often noisy and crowded. There may be little privacy for patients, as the only thing separating patients at times is a curtain and patient care sometimes takes place in the hallway. Patients also may have unrealistic expectations for what will occur during their ED visit. For example, they may desire to have testing or procedures that are not feasibly done through the ED or may not be indicated. In addition, they may expect to be admitted to the hospital when this is not deemed to be clinically appropriate by the provider.

There are patient factors that inevitably lead to increased violence in the ED. A large portion of the violence in the ED is perpetrated by patients who are under the influence of drugs and/or alcohol.[15] There is no other health care setting where such a large volume of patients are acutely intoxicated at the time of their visit.[11] Both intoxicated and psychiatric patients may be brought in by law enforcement against their will or be given the choice between transport to the ED or transport to jail.[16] Patient violence related to drugs may result from either patient intoxication or anger over not being prescribed a controlled substance the patients were hoping to procure.

There are other potential factors at play that may expose EDs to violence. The last several decades have seen a sharp decline in the number of psychiatric beds available in the United States. This decline has led to the deinstitutionalization of patients who are chronically mentally ill.[17,18] Patients who need acute psychiatric care, therefore, have no choice but to come to the ED. Once there, they often wait for hours or days until a psychiatric bed becomes available.[19] A patient already in crisis may become violent when they are not given proper psychiatric treatment in a crowded and chaotic ED.

CLUES TO IMPENDING VIOLENCE

When faced with agitated violent patients in the ED, the clinician must ensure the safety of the patients, the safety of ED team members, and evaluate patients for possible medical causes of agitated delirium that may be the underlying cause of the aggressive behavior. An important first step toward ensuring the safety of patients and ED staff is for the clinician to be aware of cues in the patients' presentation that may alert the clinician to the threat of impending violence.

It is incumbent on the emergency physician to be aware of risk factors for potential violence as well as clinical clues that a clinical situation may escalate to one that is violent or abusive. Potentially violent patients may at first become agitated, with increasingly higher volumes of speech and use of hand gestures.[20] Interventions to help de-escalate patients at this stage of aggression should focus on caring for patients and may include comforting gestures in the forms of food or blankets as well as verbal reassurance that the ED is a safe place and the staff will do all they can to care for patients.[20,21]

If the situation further escalates, agitated and restless patients may become defensive, as they think they are losing control over the situation and may begin to use aggressive or abusive language toward staff or other patients. Once this stage of aggression has been reached with patients behaving inappropriately, ED physicians and staff need to set firm boundaries for their behavior. In a calm, nonjudgmental tone, the physician should relay those boundaries to patients along with the consequences should patients fail to comply with expectations.[20,21]

Despite the best intentions of the treatment team, it is entirely possible that the behavior previously outlined will continue to escalate and result in physical violence against the providers. In order to ensure the safety of patients and the safety of the staff, the usage of medications to help calm patients or physical restraints, both in a nonpunitive manner, should be considered by the treating physician; their appropriate and safe usage is detailed next.

MEDICATION OPTIONS

Once the physician has decided that patients must be restrained or sedated in order to maintain the physical safety of the patients and providers, he or she must do so in a manner that is efficacious and provides the least potential for complications and lowest level of sedation for the patients. Typically, physicians have chosen a benzodiazepine or antipsychotic medication, with the agents either given as monotherapy or used together simultaneously.

Benzodiazepines

Lorazepam is the most common benzodiazepine administered for control of aggressive and violent behavior in the ED. It is most often given via the intramuscular (IM) route in doses ranging from 0.5 mg to 2.0 mg as frequently as every 15 minutes.[20] This agent has a relatively quick time of onset of 15 to 30 minutes following IM administration and can have sedative effects for greater than 3 hours.[20]

IM lorazepam has been shown to be as effective as a 5-mg dose of the antipsychotic medication haloperidol in treating agitation and aggressive behavior.[22] With regard to side effects, benzodiazepines, including lorazepam and midazolam, do not have the risk of extrapyramidal side effects, such as akathisia, dystonia, or tardive dyskinesia, that are associated with the neuroleptic antipsychotic agents. However, when deciding on whether or not to give an additional dose of lorazepam, clinicians must be aware that this medication can lead to oversedation and respiratory depression and must balance the need for safe control of the patients and environment with the risk of respiratory depression and resultant hypoxia.

Midazolam is an additional benzodiazepine option that can be used for sedation and control of acutely agitated patients. A 5-mg dose of midazolam IM has been shown to be superior to a 10-mg dose of haloperidol.[22] One potential advantage for using midazolam is the rapidity of clinical effect, with a reported mean time of onset of

18 minutes. However, this is coupled with a relatively short half-life of 1.5 to 2.5 hours, which may lead to a repeat episode of agitation or the need for redosing.[22]

Typical Antipsychotics

Haloperidol is a typical neuroleptic medication that uses dopamine blockade at the D2 receptor in the central nervous system as its main mechanism of action. It may be given in acutely agitated patients in doses between 2.5 mg and 10.0 mg every 30 to 60 minutes with an onset of action of 15 to 30 minutes and a duration of action of 4 hours.[20] Given its reliance on dopaminergic blockade, administration can result in extrapyramidal symptoms, such as akathisia or dystonia. If this should occur, patients may be given an anticholinergic agent, such as diphenhydramine or benztropine.

Droperidol is an additional typical antipsychotic agent that has a relatively fast onset of action and is reported to produce greater sedation than haloperidol. Its duration of action is approximately 2 hours and may be given in 2.5- to 5.0-mg doses every 15 minutes.[20] Although all antipsychotic agents are known to prolong the QTc interval, droperidol was previously removed from the market following a Food and Drug Administration black box warning related to prolonged QTc leading to cardiac dysrhythmia and death. A retrospective study evaluating an alternative usage of droperidol as any postoperative antiemetic failed to reveal a patient who developed torsades de pointes following administration of low-dose droperidol.[23] The black box warning was ultimately dropped, and droperidol returned to the market; however, usage of this medication for control of agitation is currently off label, and the drug is experiencing shortages in the United States at the time of this publication.[20]

Atypical Antipsychotics

There are 3 atypical antipsychotics available for control of agitated patients currently: olanzapine, ziprasidone, and risperidone. These medications exert their mechanism of action through dopamine blockade at the D2 receptor and additionally have antiserotonergic properties. Given this mechanism of action, these medications are able to effectively sedate acutely agitated patients but are associated with a decreased incidence of extrapyramidal side effects. Despite this positive difference in side effect profile, all of these agents are still associated with QTc prolongation, although generally to a lesser degree than the typical antipsychotics.[22]

Two of these medications, olanzapine and risperidone, are available in oral formulations, in the form of both standard tablets and orally dissolving tablets. The orally dissolving forms do not reach the time to peak effect faster than other orally available forms but are a potential option in more compliant patients.[22]

Combination Therapy

Many providers empirically treat acutely agitated violent patients with combination therapy in the form of 5 mg of IM haloperidol coupled with 2 mg of IM lorazepam in an attempt to rapidly gain control over acutely agitated patients. A prospective, double-blind study performed in the ED setting revealed that patients achieved tranquilization with combination therapy more than with haloperidol or lorazepam administered in isolation.[24] This study also revealed a lower incidence of extrapyramidal symptoms with combination therapy when compared with monotherapy with haloperidol; however, clinicians must be cognizant of the possibility of prolonged sedation with combination therapy.[24]

PHYSICAL RESTRAINTS

As with medications used to control agitation and violent behavior, the decision to use physical restraints can only be made to keep patients and providers safe, with the primary goal of preventing patients from harming themselves or others while being cautious to avoid complications that may arise from prolonged or unsafe restraint practices. The exact policy and type of restraint used varies between institutions; therefore, this review focuses on general principles surrounding their usage.

The most common types of restraints used in the emergent setting are soft cloth and leather restraints safely affixed to patients' extremities (either 2 or all 4) to the frame of the bed, not the side rails. Leather restraints have a lock and key mechanism, are relatively fixed, and do not tighten as patients struggle against them.[20,21] Soft restraints are easier for the health care providers to place on the patient. However, they can tighten around the distal extremity as patients move and, therefore, may lead to compromised circulation.[20,21]

When restraining patients, if all 4 extremities are to be restrained, the clinician leading the team should ensure that one arm be fixed to the gurney in the up position with the other arm in the down position, which will reduce the risk of patients generating significant enough force to overturn the gurney. Care should also be taken to ensure that patients are not placed in the prone position to avoid the risk of suffocation from the bedding.[21] Providers should also comply with their individual hospital policies regarding frequent reassessment of restrained patients to ensure that complications of restraint are not occurring.

COMPLICATIONS OF RESTRAINT USAGE

Following a decision to physically restrain a patient that is centered on the need to keep the patient and health care providers protected, the physician must be vigilant to ensure that the patient remains safe during the period of physical restraint. As previously mentioned, patients should never be restrained in a prone position as asphyxia can develop. Patients should be placed on their side or in the supine position, with the supine position avoided in patients who are at risk for vomiting and subsequent aspiration.[21]

Although data are somewhat limited regarding the rate of complications in physically restrained patients, Zun[25] performed a prospective, observational study evaluating the rate of complications in restrained patients over a 1-year period in a community-based, urban ED. In the group of 298 restrained patients, only 7% experienced complications, with the most common complication being that the patient removed the restraint device. Three patients in this study population vomited, with no patients suffering hypoxic events or fatal complications.[25] These data suggest that when appropriate patients are selected, restrained appropriately, and monitored closely, the complication rate for physical restraint is low.

ORGANIC CAUSES OF AGITATION

Although this review article focuses largely on maintaining the safety of acutely violent patients, clinicians must include the possibility of medical causes for acutely agitated patients. Factors that should cause clinicians to expand the differential diagnosis include new-onset agitation or psychosis in adult patients; the presence of visual hallucinations; and the presence of associated systemic symptoms or fever that may suggest the presence of an infectious process, such as urinary tract infection, meningitis, or encephalitis, leading to an acute encephalopathy and agitation.

Although all agitated patients do not require dedicated laboratory testing or imaging studies to evaluate for a potential organic cause, the clinician may consider obtaining a urinalysis, computed tomography of the head, electrolyte studies, or a lumbar puncture, depending on the clinical presentation of patients.

LAWS REGARDING PATIENT VIOLENCE AND BARRIERS TO REPORTING

Currently in the United States, 39 states have laws criminalizing violent behavior against health care providers, with states varying on whether the action is classified as a felony or a misdemeanor.[7] An additional 8 states have laws criminalizing assault against emergency medical service or first responder personnel only.[7,12] Despite the very real risk of harm to the health care provider, most assaults likely go unreported to superiors or to law enforcement officials and prosecution does not frequently occur.

Barriers that providers have reported in the past to reporting assaults that have occurred in the workplace include feelings that patients may not be responsible for their behavior because of their psychosis.[7,26] Once a verbal or physical assault has occurred, health care workers are not likely to report the incident to hospital authorities. In one survey, 65% of health care workers who had experienced violence in the ED had not reported the incident.[27] Some people consider it to be part of the job or fear that they will be seen as incompetent by supervisors. Others may think that there will be no consequences to the perpetrator resulting from the complaint. Almost half of nurses surveyed responded that no action was taken when they reported a verbal or physical assault.[12] And as there is a push toward improved customer service and satisfaction in medicine currently, health care workers may think that the hospital administration will not be supportive or take action. Because of underreporting, hospital administrators may not be aware of the extent of the problem, making them less likely to dedicate resources or policies to minimize it.

Furthermore, when considering reporting an assault to authorities, it is possible that clinicians may simply want to avoid the hassle of participating in the legal system; they may also be met with legal authorities who do not wish to pursue the case further given the mental illness of the individual who perpetrated the assault.[26]

In addition to the physical injuries that may be incurred, health care workers who are victims of workplace violence may have an even bigger psychological impact. This impact may include fear of returning to work, feeling guilty, feeling powerless, and fear of reaction by supervisors.[28] Physicians and nurses who experience workplace violence may have lower job satisfaction and early burnout.[11] Immediately following an assault, workers reported they were less able to handle their workload and provide patient care. One survey found that more than 80% of providers felt fearful of violence in their workplace.[8,10]

CONTROVERSIES

There are many controversies surrounding preventative measures. Whether one thinks that the availability of guns leads to more violence or not, there has been a marked increase in the number of guns purchased by US citizens over the past decade, and keeping guns out of the ED seems to be a reasonable measure.[29] Metal detectors are estimated to be present in one-third of US hospitals.[30] One study found that the presence of a metal detector increased the number of weapons confiscated but did not lead to a decrease in violent episodes reported.[31] Metal detectors may lead to a false sense of security by staff. In addition, patients arriving by ambulance are not usually screened and there is commonly more than one way to gain access to an ED, both of which limit the utility of metal detectors located at the front door of the ED.[32]

Handheld metal detecting devices are an option for patients who arrive via ambulance or enter through an alternate door and are not screened in the ED entrance. Studies have not been able to demonstrate the effectiveness of metal detectors at decreasing violence in the ED. Other physical safety measures include panic buttons, video surveillance, adequate lighting, and having more than one exit route.

Many hospitals use security officers who can assist in various roles in violence prevention. They may assist in taking down aggressive patients or they may carry handcuffs. About half of surveyed security personnel reported that they carry hand guns (52%) or Tasers (47%).[30] There is the possibility though that the officer's weapon could be taken by agitated patients. In addition, there is also concern that officers inadequately trained in health care settings may add an extra layer of danger to an already tense situation.

SUMMARY

Violent behavior in the ED is a multifactorial problem potentially affecting the safety and well-being of all providers who work in this health care setting. In order to maintain their safety, physicians and other professionals in the ED must be aware of the inherent risk factors that can incite agitation and violent behavior, be ready to safely and appropriately restrain patients and evaluate them for potential psychiatric and organic conditions, and work with law enforcement and hospital administration to ensure that violent behavior is reported and appropriate steps are taken to reduce the risk of potential future violence.

REFERENCES

1. CBS News. Cardiac surgeon dies after shooting at Boston hospital; suspect dead. Available at: http://www.cbsnews.com/news/cardiac-surgeon-shot-at-boston-hospital-suspect-dead/. Accessed June 26, 2017.
2. ABC News. Johns Hopkins hospital Gunman shoots doctor, then kills self and mother. Available at: http://abcnews.go.com/US/shooting-inside-baltimores-johns-hopkins-hospital/story?id=11654462. Accessed June 26, 2017.
3. Janoch JA , Smith TS. Workplace safety and health in the health care and social assistance industry, 2003-2007. In: U.S. Bureau of Labor and Statistics. Available at: http://www.bls.gov/opub/mlr/cwc/workplace-safety-and-health-in-the-health-care-and-social-assistance-industry-2003-07.pdf. Accessed June 26, 2017.
4. Behnam M, Tillotson RD, Davis SM, et al. Violence in the emergency department: a national survey of emergency medicine residents and attending physicians. J Emerg Med 2011;40:565–79.
5. Worker safety in hospitals: Caring for our caregivers. In: U.S. Department of Labor. Available at: https://www.osha.gov/dsg/hospitals/workplace_violence.html. Accessed June 26, 2017.
6. CDC, National Institute for Occupational Safety and Health. Violence and occupational hazards in hospitals. Available at: http://www.cdc.gov/niosh/docs/2002-101/. Accessed November 12, 2016.
7. Phillips JP. Workplace violence against health care workers in the United States. N Engl J Med 2016;374:1661–9.
8. Kowalenko T, Gates D, Gillespie GL, et al. Prospective study of violence against ED workers. Am J Emerg Med 2013;31(1):197–205.
9. Lehmann LS, McCormick RA, Kizer KW. A survey of assaultive behavior in Veterans Health Administration facilities. Psychiatr Serv 1999;50(3):384–9.

10. Kowalenko T, Walters BL, Khare RK, et al. Workplace violence: a survey of emergency physicians in the state of Michigan. Ann Emerg Med 2005;46:142–7.
11. May DD, Grubbs LM. The extent, nature, and precipitating factors of nurse assault among three groups of registered nurses in a regional medical center. J Emerg Nurs 2002;28(1):11–7.
12. Emergency Nurses Association. Emergency department violence surveillance study: November 2011. Available at: https://www.ena.org/practice-research/research/Documents/ENAEDVSReportNovember2011.pdf. Accessed June 26, 2017.
13. Cikriklar H, Yurumez Y, Gungor B, et al. Violence against emergency department employees and the attitude of employees towards violence. Hong Kong Med J 2016;22:464–71.
14. Dubb SS. It doesn't "come with the job": violence against doctors at work must stop. BMJ 2015;350:h2870.
15. Crilly J, Chaboyer W, Creedy D. Violence towards emergency department nurses by patients. Accid Emerg Nurs 2004;12(2):67–73.
16. Kowalenko T, Cunningham R, Sachs CJ, et al. Workplace violence in emergency medicine: current knowledge and future directions. J Emerg Med 2012;43(3):523–31.
17. Sharfstein SS, Dickerson FB. Hospital psychiatry for the twenty-first century. Health Aff (Millwood) 2009;28(3):685–8.
18. Fuller Torry E, Entsminger K, Geller J, et al. The shortage of public hospital beds for mentally ill persons: a report of the treatment advocacy center. Available at: http://www.treatmentadvocacycenter.org/storage/documents/the_shortage_of_publichospital_beds.pdf. Accessed June 26, 2017.
19. Brauser D. Psychiatric patients often warehoused in emergency departments for a week or more. In: Medscape. Available at: http://www.medscape.com/viewarticle/736187#vp_1. Accessed June 26, 2017.
20. Isaacs E. The violent patient. In: Adams JG, Barton ED, Collins JL, et al, editors. Emergency medicine: clinical essentials. 2nd edition. Philadelphia: Elsevier Saunders; 2013. p. 1630–8.
21. Coburn MA, Mycyk MB. Physical and chemical restrains. Emerg Med Clin North Am 2009;27:655–67.
22. Rund DA, Ewing JD, Mitzel K, et al. The use of intramuscular benzodiazepines and antipsychotic agents in the treatment of acute agitation or violence in the emergency department. J Emerg Med 2006;31:317–24.
23. Nuttall GA, Eckerman KM, Jacob KA, et al. Does low-dose droperidol administration increase the risk of drug-induced QT prolongation and torsade de pointes in the general surgical population? Anesthesiology 2007;107:531–6.
24. Battaglia J, Moss S, Rush J, et al. Haloperidol, lorazepam, or both for psychotic agitation? A multicenter, prospective, double-blind, emergency department study. Am J Emerg Med 1997;15:335–40.
25. Zun LS. A prospective study of the complication rate of use of patient restraint in the emergency department. J Emerg Med 2003;24(2):119–24.
26. Miller RD, Maier GJ. Factors affecting the decision to prosecute mental patients for criminal behavior. Hosp Community Psychiatry 1987;38:50–5.
27. Gates DM, Ross CS, McQueen L. Violence against emergency department workers. J Emerg Med 2006;31:331–7.
28. Guidelines for preventing work place violence for healthcare and social service workers. In: U.S. Department of Labor, Occupational Safety and Health

Administration. Available at: https://www.osha.gov/Publications/osha3148.pdf. Accessed June 26, 2017.

29. Horsley S. Guns in America, by the numbers. Available at: http://www.npr.org/2016/01/05/462017461/guns-in-america-by-the-numbers. Accessed June 26, 2017.
30. Schoenfisch A , Pompeii L. Weapon use among hospital security personnel. In: IHSS Foundation. Available at: https://www.canadiansecuritymag.com/news/health-care/ihssf-releases-study-on-weapons-use-among-hospital-security-personnel-2502. Accessed June 26, 2017.
31. Rankins RC, Hendey GW. Effect of a security system on violent incidents and hidden weapons in the emergency department. Ann Emerg Med 1999;33(6):676–9.
32. Violence against ED workers a growing problem. In: Emergency physicians monthly. Available at: http://epmonthly.com/article/violence-against-ed-workers-a-growing-problem/. Accessed June 26, 2017.

Highlight in Telepsychiatry and Behavioral Health Emergencies

James Rachal, MD[a], Wayne Sparks, MD[a],
Christine Zazzaro, MEd[b,*], Terri Blackwell, MD[a]

KEYWORDS

• Telepsychiatry • Psychiatric emergency services • Carolinas HealthCare System

KEY POINTS

- The development of emergency psychiatric care through dedicated psychiatric emergency services programs in this country has been evolving for many years because of the limitations in care delivery as outlined.
- Carolinas HealthCare System has one of the largest freestanding psychiatric emergency departments in the country.
- Carolinas HealthCare System (CHS) has developed from a small mental health center started by Charlotte Mental Hygiene Society in the 1930s serving a circumscribed population into one of the largest emergency mental health providers in the country.

INTRODUCTION

The delivery of emergency services for individuals with mental illness began as far back as the 1920s in some metropolitan areas of the United States, using psychiatric residents working in medical emergency rooms who helped evaluate and make disposition plans for challenging psychiatric cases.[1] There were many fledgling attempts to handle emergency crises over subsequent decades. However, it was not until the passage of the Community Mental Health Services Act of 1963 that dedicated services to the mentally ill began to develop more systematically throughout the country. This federal act allowed for a basic shift from containment in the hospital to less restrictive community-based alternatives.[2]

The legislation necessitated psychiatric hospitals, local health departments, and outpatient (OP) facilities work together. Clinics would offer walk-in services during the day, hospital emergency rooms would offer the service at night, and community crisis lines would offer emergency services over the telephone.[1] This was the same

[a] Department of Psychiatry, Carolinas HealthCare System, 501 Billingsley Road, Charlotte, NC 28211, USA; [b] Department of Psychiatry, Carolinas HealthCare System, 1601 Abbey Place, Charlotte, NC 28209, USA
* Corresponding author.
E-mail address: Christine.zazzaro@carolinashealthcare.org

Psychiatr Clin N Am 40 (2017) 585–596
http://dx.doi.org/10.1016/j.psc.2017.05.014

0193-953X/17/© 2017 Elsevier Inc. All rights reserved.

time that the Mecklenburg County Mental Health Clinic began offering emergency crisis services. They offered a 9 AM TO 5 PM emergency walk-in clinic and a 24-hour hotline. The emergency department (ED) continued to assess patients overnight.

A second significant wave of growth began in the 1970s after the enactment of two significant pieces of legislation. The Emergency Medical Services Systems Act of 1973 led to the development of an emergency services system, to provide "personnel, facilities and equipment for the effective and coordinated delivery" of emergency services[3]; and in 1974, the legal decision of Kovach v Schubert held that to be involuntarily committed, a patient had to be a danger to themselves or others. Previously, the law only required that two psychiatrists concur that a patient needed treatment. Patients could no longer be easily directly admitted to a hospital by their treating psychiatrists[4]; they needed to be evaluated first to determine if they were a danger to themselves. Thus there was a need to create a space to evaluate these patients safely, and the concept of a psychiatric emergency service (PES) was born. Following this movement some psychiatric hospitals began offering 24-hour walk-in centers, where a patient could receive a full evaluation and diagnosis. Carolinas HealthCare System (CHS) began offering 24-hour services in the early 1980s.

Between 1971 and 1984, there was a near doubling of hospitals that offered PES, to a total of 2178. There was also an increase by 150% of psychiatric emergency room visits during that time. As time progressed, the primary arena for emergency psychiatric care became emergency units in general hospitals,[1,5] in large part because of the impact of deinstitutionalization and other social forces on the mentally ill community. Lack of beds on inpatient (IP) units led to a higher level of acuity in OP seen in the community, and a backup of psychiatric patients seen in the general hospital emergency room, which also prevented other medical patients from being able to obtain care.[5,6]

Other contributors to the backup included diminishing access to mental health care in the community, increased rates of mental illness, shrinking mental health resources, and increasing fragmentation of resources.[7] This has led to the development of different strategies across the country to deal with the problem of treating the emergency mental health patient, including using community crisis centers to provide a space between OP and EDs, development of separate units within medical EDs for psychiatric patients,[8–10] and our own model of a free-standing dedicated psychiatric-only ED.[11–13] These increasing pressures necessitated the dramatic changes we see at CHS.

PROGRESSION OF EMERGENCY PSYCHIATRIC CARE WITHIN CAROLINAS HEALTHCARE SYSTEM

Behavioral Health–Charlotte, which was referred to as "Carolinas Medical Center-Randolph," was the Mecklenburg County Mental Health Center, although its physicians were employed by CHS. In 2013, CHS incorporated the mental health system into its network and it became a department within the larger hospital. The facility consists of 66 IP beds, OP, and partial hospitalization programs for child and adult patients. There is also a robust case management system for chronically and persistently mentally ill patients, and an OP therapy program for adults and children. Until 1988, the ED was staffed by psychiatrists who worked in these areas with coverage primarily being an on-call system where the ED nurse would contact the on-call psychiatrist from 5 PM to 8 AM to staff patients for treatment options. Those patients who were not safe or stable to be discharged were placed in observation status, with the psychiatrist giving telephone orders to the nurse, until the following morning, when a psychiatrist would be assigned to round on these patients and determine further treatment, with a recommendation either for IP or OP care.

In 1997, the current PES was started to efficiently manage psychiatric patients who presented in crisis at several local medical EDs. This was also started to consolidate call structure and have an on-site psychiatrist available in the ED to manage patients as they presented, rather than holding patients until the morning to be seen. This allowed for the on-call system to be greatly diminished, because the on-site psychiatrist managed any emergencies or on-call needs directly from in-house. This service was started with four full-time board-certified psychiatrists who worked rotating shifts, with some weekend coverage of the ED provided by other psychiatrists who worked in IP or OP areas routinely. The initial group of psychiatrists covering the ED service worked 13 weeks of each shift: morning shift of 40 hours, evening shift of 40 hours, and overnight shift of 56 hours, and 13 weeks off. The volume of patients during those beginning years was approximately 20 to 30 patients in a 24-hour period. This arrangement allowed a better system for continuity of care, and physician satisfaction was high.

Initially there was no systematic process for seeing patients, which allowed for more autonomy but also created uneven treatment plans. As we began to see more patients in the community, and became aware of the changing landscape of available resources, we became more systematic in the way we evaluated patients. We continued to improve our system to meet the changing community needs and improve overall care.

Face-to-Face Assessment

Our model for capturing as much critical current and historical information on every patient entering the emergency room includes the following components:

- Nursing triage (assigning acuity a code between 1 and 5; the lower the number the higher the acuity)
- Columbia-Suicide Severity Rating Scale (a nationally recognized rating scale for capturing past/current suicidal thoughts/behaviors[14]
- Detailed nursing assessment (assessing past psychiatric history, family history, social history, drug/alcohol use history, legal history, trauma/abuse history, and medical histories)
- Physician assessment (reviewing all of the previously mentioned information with the patient, performing a detailed mental status examination, documenting findings, and developing a preliminary diagnosis and treatment plan)

Coordination of Care

Coordination of care consists of the following:

- Admission for safety/stabilization
  - Notifying our behavioral health patient placement team that a patient requires IP stabilization (behavioral health patient placement is a centrally located remote team responsible for facilitating movement of patients from one facility to the next in a specific geographic area; discussed later)
  - Admission to observation status unit, if no beds currently available
- Discharge
  - Referral to community resources (eg, substance abuse treatment, shelter programs)
  - Linkage to follow-up appointments (therapy and psychiatrist)
  - Medication management
  - Family/collateral history and inclusion in safety planning

- Peer support
  - Peer support was added to have a specialist who can support patients and their families when presenting to the ED
  - Peer support staff use their own lived mental health and substance abuse experience to offer an empathic and supportive approach to individuals and families in crisis and guidance and education on the ED process
  - Peer support in the ED gives hope to individuals who are in a critical moment in their lives and also acts as a strong advocate within the system for patient-focused care
    - Some specific gains include adding peer support–led groups focused on coping and relaxation
    - Individual support to patients and their families
    - Advocating for the children in observation to have outside group time
    - Acting as a liaison/support person when walking patients to other programs for evaluations
    - Working with patients to reduce anxiety with the goal of reducing restraint episodes

PSYCHIATRIC BOARDING

As programs changed in OP areas across North Carolina with mental health reform and with the closure of more IP beds at the local and state level, we found that patients who had previously been managed in OP systems of care were no longer able to have consistent care. This change increased the volume of psychiatric patients coming to the stand-alone psychiatric ED, and presenting to our system medical EDs (**Fig. 1**).

Patients seeking psychiatric care make up 6% to 9% of all medical ER visits[15–17] in the United States. From 2008 to 2010, psychiatric-related ED visits in North Carolina increased by 17.7%, from 347,806 to 409,276. By 2010, ED visits for patients with mental health diagnoses accounted for 9.3% of all ED visits in North Carolina.[18] This has led to overcrowding in emergency medical centers, with extended waiting

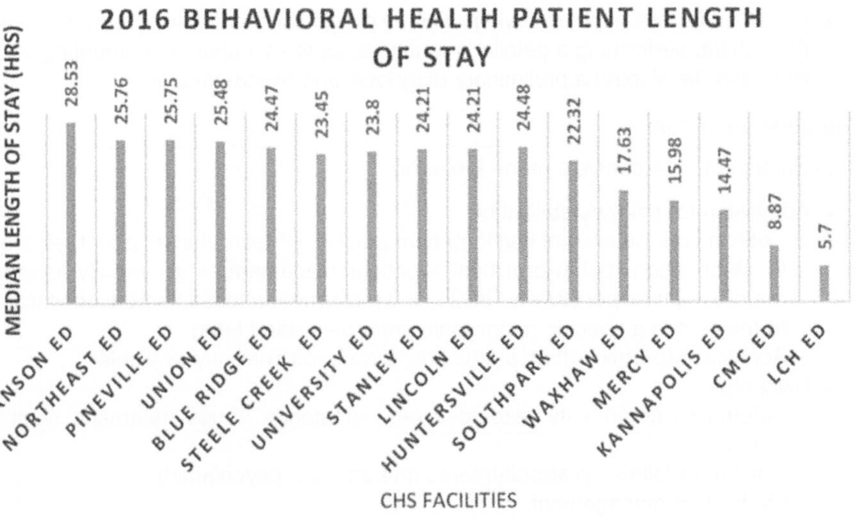

Fig. 1. Total median length of stay in psychiatric boarding.

times between initial evaluation and treatment of these patients. This practice, known as psychiatric boarding,[19] leads to several problems for psychiatric patients and medical emergency room services, including the following[20]:

- Increased psychological stress on patients who may already be in depressed or psychotic states
- Delayed mental health treatment that could mitigate the need for a mental health IP stay
- Consumption of scarce ED resources
- Worsens ED crowding
- Delays treatment of other ED patients
- Some of whom may have life-threatening conditions
- Has a significant financial impact on ED reimbursement

CHS volume and acuity of the patients have continued to increase over the years (**Table 1**). We had considerable capacity concerns in our own ED, and had limited ability to receive transfers from the medical EDs in our system. These patients now stay in medical EDs, and if we can accept a transfer to evaluate the patient psychiatrically, we send the patient back to their originating ED should they require IP treatment. This process has become cumbersome and inefficient, and not the best treatment of the patient.

Table 1
ED psychiatry volume annual comparison

Summary Table			
Reporting Period: January 1, 2016–September 30, 2016			
Report Run Date: October 31, 2016			
	2014	*2016*	*% Change*
ED Anson	94	145	54.26
ED Cleveland	343	311	−9.33
ED CMC	1446	2043	41.29
ED Harrisburg	—	40	—
ED Huntersville	54	72	33.33
ED Kannapolis	3	43	1333.33
ED Kings Mountain	555	516	−7.03
ED Lincoln	187	340	81.82
ED Mercy	102	180	76.47
ED NorthEast	869	1395	60.53
ED Pineville	459	599	30.50
ED SouthPark	8	50	525.00
ED Stanly	—	393	—
ED Steele Creek	83	94	13.25
ED Union	621	838	34.94
ED University	447	598	33.78
ED Waxhaw	12	43	258.33
LCH	59	265	349.15
Total	5342	7965	49.10
Total (minus Stanly)	5342	7572	41.74

MOVE TO VIRTUAL CARE: TELEPSYCHIATRY

The increase in the volume of psychiatric patients in the medical EDs within our system required a reimagining of how to provide service to these patients safely and more efficiently. Our ED psychiatrists had concurrently been providing occasional virtual psychiatric consultations and admissions for one system facility, and would use this process to evaluate patients who could not be transferred to our ED for other reasons, usually a medical instability. With the inability to continue accepting all psychiatric patients presenting to medical EDs in our area, we increased the use of virtual evaluations: telepsychiatry.[21,22] This started with just the medical EDs in our county of Mecklenburg, and as demand for this service grew, we have expanded to 21 EDs within the CHS system; we currently see around 1000 patients monthly in these 21 EDs (**Table 2**).

The process for telepsychiatry involves an initial interview by licensed clinical staff (licensed professional counselor, licensed clinical social worker, or a registered Nurse [RN]). This initial evaluation is like the initial evaluation completed by RNs in the PES, and includes a brief history, past psychiatric history, medical history, family and social history, and a risk assessment for suicide with the Columbia-Suicide Severity Rating Scale. The psychiatrist then reviews this information and contacts the medical ED to set up the virtual evaluation, where the patient is interviewed over secure, HIPAA-compliant video and audio lines. The assessment is documented, and recommendations for further treatment are provided to the medical ED physician, who is the primary physician managing the patient. There is an automatic alert notifying the medical ED when the consultation is complete and the assessment and recommendations are in the chart for their review.

When patients who require IP treatment cannot immediately be admitted to an IP bed, which unfortunately occurs in most the medical EDs, these patients board until a psychiatric bed becomes available.

If patients are held in the ED, they are started on medications right away for their psychiatric treatment. The consulting psychiatrist places these medication orders after evaluating the patient. Patients are rounded on by a member of the licensed clinical team daily, and the psychiatrist or psychiatric nurse practitioner rounds on patients at least every 48 hours. This allows for potential discharge to OP and avoids unnecessary IP treatment. Before using telepsychiatry, nearly all these patients would wait in a medical ED and be destined for an IP hospitalization. The current discharge rate is about 35% and with rounding on patients as they wait in the ED and receive treatment the discharge rate overall is closer to 40%.

CENTRALIZED PATIENT PLACEMENT

Telepsychiatry seemed to solve the issue of access to a psychiatric evaluation while in the medical emergency room, but there were many problems that remained in our system regarding getting those who needed further psychiatric care where they needed to be.

The previous system had each individual hospital in our system competing for the same beds with no regard to acuity or length of stay. This was a system of inefficiencies and redundancies. Hospitals we were referring to were getting hundreds of pages of patient medical records that were auto faxed with a software program regardless of bed availability. We realized it was in the best interest of the patient and the hospital teammates if a department was created with professionals who had the skills required to find and secure the appropriate placement for the patient in a timely way. If this was the sole job of this team, they could do that with little interruption and no distraction from having to also care for medically acute patients. In addition, knowing we were serving multiple facilities across a large geographic area,

Table 2
Volume of telepsychiatry patients

Year Totals	ED Volume	ED Volume Adult	ED Volume Child	% ED Volume Child	Total OBS Volume	% of ED Volume Admit to OBS	ED + OBS Volume	Telepsych Volume	Telepsych Volume Adult	Telepsych Volume Child	% Telepsych Volume Child	Combined Volume	ED Volume	OBS Volume	Telepsych Volume
2014	15,893	12,072	3821	24.00	7863	33.10	23,756	4688	4088	600	12.80	28,444	15,893	7863	4688
Average daily	44	33.1	10.5	—	21.5	—	65	12.8	11.2	1.6	12.80	77.9	43.5	21.5	12.8
2015	11,863	8329	3534	29.80	8210	40.90	20,073	7453	—	—	0.00	27,526	11,863	8210	7453
Average daily	33	23	10	—	22	—	55	20.4	0	0	15.70	75	33	22	20
2016	11,101	8066.40	3034.80	27.30	9694.80	55.90	20,796	11,517	—	—	—	32,313	11,101	9695	11,517
Average daily	30	22.1	8.3	—	27	—	57	31.6	—	—	—	89	30	27	32

Abbreviation: OBS, observation status.

we needed a virtual option, because it would not be sustainable to have staff 24/7 in all the EDs doing this work.

Carolinas HealthCare System pulled together a small team, consisting of an RN and several admission transfer coordinators who were bachelor level teammates with previous experience managing patients in psychiatric emergencies. Using professionals with this skill mix enabled us to keep our cost low while maintaining quality care. The team monitors the acuity and capacity at all our medical EDs daily to ensure we are attentive to their individual needs and the needs of the patients.

Once an IP bed is located, transport of the patient occurs with law enforcement or our contracted transport company.

TRANSPORTATION OF PSYCHIATRIC PATIENTS

In most states, the legal statute requires that the transportation of psychiatric patients in crisis happens via law enforcement.[23] In almost all of these situations these patients pose little to no safety risk, but they still have to endure transport in a police vehicle, often in handcuffs. The experience can be traumatizing. Arrival of a police vehicle to a home is embarrassing and certainly does not respect their right to privacy. This is a huge impact to the patient's experience related to getting care.

There is also a huge impact on law enforcement agencies. Law enforcement spends thousands of hours each year transporting patients to and from psychiatric facilities.[24] Often, they have to spend all day transporting one patient to a bed across the state at the expense of taxpayers. It also impacts public safety. It puts local police out of service for hours at a time and unable to respond to more urgent emergencies. We learned recently first hand that the opposite is also true. In the recent civil unrest that we experienced in Charlotte, law enforcement agencies were not able to transport any patients for many days. If we had not already had the option of an alternate transport service, our patients would have had to wait unnecessarily just for a ride to their IP facility.

The system of transport in North Carolina is much like other states. At Carolinas Healthcare System, we were pushed to explore options other than law enforcement because of the ever-growing number of patients presenting in crisis and the desire to decrease the number of patients who are involuntarily committed. It was taking sometimes 2 days or more to get transport by law enforcement. The company we chose to contract with uses unmarked vehicles, and a non-police-type uniform. They also allow the patient to choose what music they listen to and they do not use any type of restraints.

Advocacy groups who support the rights of mentally ill are advocating for lawmakers to include transport as a reimbursable expense.[25] Some states have succeeded. Minnesota Legislature took a major step to address the problem by creating a special class of nonemergency transports under state law.[26] Regardless of government or private insurance funding, the hospital can justify the expense based on the cost savings of getting patients to a psychiatric facility in a timelier manner.

FUTURE STATE: EXPANDING VIRTUAL CARE

Primary Care Integration

Our system has always been an early adopter to innovation. The move toward virtual behavioral health care was no exception to this. In addition to integrating emergency Behavioral Health care through telepsychiatry consultation and virtual rounding on patients boarding in acute care EDs, we have also invested in the integration of behavioral health support into primary care and pediatric practices.

The model for our program is based on the Impact Model created by The University of Washington, Psychiatry & Behavioral Sciences Division of Population Health.[27]

Our integration model is virtual. Although there is no clinician embedded in the practice, there is collaboration with the psychiatrist, therapist, health coach, and pharmacist, and the primary care provider or pediatrician, rather than the psychiatrist, as the primary manager of the patient's medical and psychiatric care. This more holistic approach provides the patient with support from specialists, but allows them to continue to get their care from their primary care provider, with whom they have an existing relationship.

Virtual Care Coordination

Care coordination is a part of many health care redesign efforts recently. It involves bringing together various providers, resources, and information systems to coordinate health services, patient needs, and information to help better achieve the goals of treatment and care. Research shows that care coordination increases efficiency and improves clinical outcomes and patient satisfaction with care.[28]

As the care of our patients presenting to medical EDs in crisis has moved to a virtual platform, a much-needed piece of coordinating a patient's care has been missing. The teams located in medical EDs do not have the clinical skills to evaluate behavioral health patients nor are they able to coordinate OP care or assist in meeting other needs the patient might have that contribute to the reasons they present to EDs in crisis. A psychiatrist evaluating the patient virtually might make a decision to admit a patient just to ensure they receive the necessary care coordination.

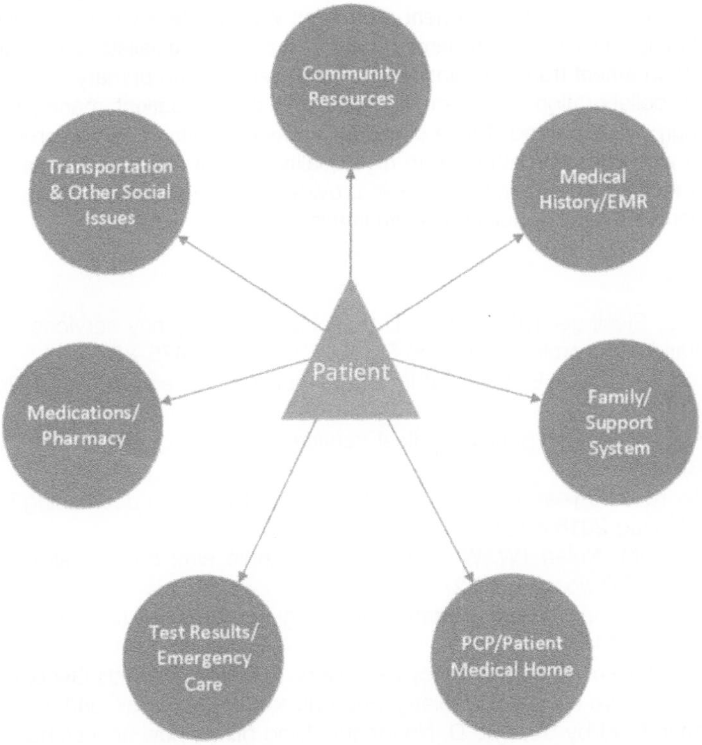

Fig. 2. Virtual care coordination model. EMR, electronic medical record; PCP, primary care provider.

Beginning in 2017, CHS will be leveraging a virtual care coordination model to assist patients in medical ED over a large geographic area get the care they need in an OP setting.

These virtual care coordinators will do what an on-site coordinator would be tasked to do, such as setting up follow-up appointments and ensuring they are able to get medications to last until the next appointment to prevent another emergent visit just for refills. They will also be able to assist with issues related to social determinants that pose barriers to the patient staying well (**Fig. 2**).

SUMMARY

The development of emergency psychiatric care through dedicated PES programs in this country has been evolving for many years because of limitations in care-delivery. CHS has one of the largest freestanding psychiatric EDs in the country. We have grown from a small mental health center started by Charlotte Mental Hygiene Society in the 1930s serving a circumscribed population to one of the largest emergency mental health providers in the country. We offer services in person and via telepsychiatry to other EDs and to primary care clinics. We dramatically decreased emergency room wait times and revolutionized where and how patients get their care. This has been the work of several different groups from many different disciplines. In some ways, Carolinas Healthcare's transition from a community mental health center to a large-scale mental health ED has been a model for the rest of the country. The evolution has continued to be rapid to meet patient needs and to address some of the limited psychiatric access across the geographic footprint of Carolinas Healthcare, by expanding with innovative assessment and treatment modalities via an extensive virtual assessment team, including clinicians, physicians, patient placement specialists, and a dedicated non–law enforcement transportation team. Our expansion into primary care OP clinics with virtual collaboration has been successful in overall patient management with continued growth expected. These changes in how care has been delivered (virtually) have been with the same attention to high quality, patient safety and satisfaction, as with the traditional care delivery, but this provides a more efficient professional team able to improve overall population health in this region.

REFERENCES

1. Wellin E, Slesinger DP, Hollister D. Psychiatric emergency services: evolution, adaptation and proliferation. Soc Sci Med 1987;24(6):475–82.
2. Gerson S, Bassuk E. Psychiatric emergencies: an overview. Am J Pscyhiatry 1980;137(1):1–11.
3. Harvey J. The emergency medical service systems act of 1973. JAMA 1974; 230(8):1139–40.
4. Zander K. A 30-year retrospective: degrees of difficulty in decreasing LOS. Prof Case Manag 2016;21(5):233–42.
5. Berwick DM, Nolan TW, Whittington J. The triple aim: care, health, and cost. Health Aff (Millwood) 2008;27:759–69.
6. Swartz MS. Emergency department boarding: nowhere else to go. Psychiatr Serv 2016;67(11):1163.
7. Pager LM, Ivkovic A. Emergency psychiatry. In: Massachusetts General Hospital comprehensive clinical psychiatry, 2nd edition 2016; 88, 937–949.e2.
8. Saurman E, Kirby SE, Lyle D. No longer 'flying blind': how access has changed emergency mental health care in rural and remote emergency departments, a qualitative study. BMC Health Serv Res 2015;15:156.

9. Wang H, Johnson C, Robinson RD, et al. Roles of disease severity and post-discharge outpatient visits as predictors of hospital readmissions. BMC Health Serv Res 2016;16(1):564.
10. Zhu JM, Singhal A, Hsia RY. Emergency department length-of-stay for psychiatric visits was significantly longer than for nonpsychiatric visits, 2002-11. Health Aff (Millwood) 2016;35(9):1698–706.
11. Wright K, McGlen I, Dykes S. Mental health emergencies: using a structured assessment framework. Emerg Nurse 2012;19:28–35.
12. Hamilton JE, Desai PV, Hoot NR, et al. Factors associated with the likelihood of hospitalization following emergency department visits for behavioral health conditions. Acad Emerg Med 2016;23(11):1257–66.
13. Kuszmar TJ, Bell L, Scholz DM. Detox in the ED: taking urgent action. JAAPA 2000;13(6):43–4, 47-8, 52-4.
14. Posner K, Brown GK, Stanley B, et al. The Columbia-Suicide Severity Rating Scale: initial validity and internal consistency findings from three multisite studies with adolescents and adults. Am J Psychiatry 2011;168(12):1266–77.
15. Hazlett SB, McCarthy ML, Londner MS, et al. Epidemiology of adult psychiatric visits to US emergency departments. Acad Emerg Med 2008;11(2):193–5.
16. Larkin GL, Claassen CA, Emond JA, et al. Trends in US emergency department visits for mental health conditions, 1992-2001. Psychiatr Serv 2005;56(6):671–7.
17. Owens P, Mutter R, Stocks C. Statistical Brief #92: mental health and substance abuse-related emergency department visits among adults. Agency for Healthcare Research and Quality; 2007.
18. Hakenewerth AM, Tintinalli JE, Waller AE, et al. Emergency department visits by patients with mental health disorders—North Carolina, 2008-2010. MMWR Morb Mortal Wkly Rep 2013;62(23):469–72.
19. Mathur H. Behavioral health patient boarding in the ED. International Association for Healthcare Security and Safety Foundation Website. 2015. Available at: https://c.ymcdn.com/sites/www.iahss.org/resource/collection/48907176-3B11-4B24-A7C0-FF756143C7DE/2015_Behavioral_Health_Patient_Boarding.pdf. Accessed November 18, 2016.
20. Alleviating ED boarding of psychiatric patients. Quick Safety, Joint Commission Website; 2015. Available at: http://www.jointcommission.org/assets/1/23/Quick_Safety_Issue_19_Dec_20151.PDF. Accessed November 18, 2016.
21. Hilty DM, Ferrer DC, Parish MB, et al. The effectiveness of telemental health: a 2013 review. Telemed J E Health 2013;19:444–54.
22. O'Neil A. The need for national data on "boarding" psychiatric patients in emergency departments. Psychiatr Serv 2016;67(3):359–60.
23. NAMI State Mental Health Legislation 2014: trends, themes & effective practices. 2014. p. 13. Available at: http://www.nami.org/legreport2014. Accessed March 2016.
24. University of Washington Psychiatry & Behavioral Sciences Division of Population Health. AIMS Center Resource Library. Advancing integrated mental health solutions web site. Available at: http://aims.uw.edu/resource-library. Accessed July 20, 2016.
25. Substance Abuse and Mental Health Services Administration. Care coordination. SAMHSA-HRSA Center for Integrated Health Solutions Web site. Available at: http://www.integration.samhsa.gov/workforce/care-coordination. Accessed November 2, 2016.
26. Barrow MW. Henderson Police Department Annual Report 2016. Henderson Police Department.

27. National Alliance on Mental Illness. Best mental health investments for 2015: NAMI Minnesota's Legislative Goals. NAMI, Minnesota. Available at: http://www.namihelps.org/blogs/best-mental-health-investments-for-2015.html. Accessed November 17, 2016.
28. National Alliance on Mental Illness Minnesota Legislature. 2015 Minnesota legislative session: summary of new laws affecting children and adults with mental illnesses and their families. NAMI Minnesota. Available at: _http://www.namihelps.org/2015-NAMI-Minnesota-Legislative-Summary.pdf. Accessed November 17, 2016.

Printed and bound by CPI Group (UK) Ltd, Croydon, CR0 4YY
03/10/2024
01040388-0003